Seizures: Diagnosis, Treatment and Related Conditions

Seizures: Diagnosis, Treatment and Related Conditions

Editor: Ezra Dixon

MURPHY & MOORE
www.murphy-moorepublishing.com

www.murphy-moorepublishing.com

MURPHY & MOORE

Cataloging-in-Publication Data

Seizures : diagnosis, treatment and related conditions / edited by Ezra Dixon.
p. cm.
Includes bibliographical references and index.
ISBN 978-1-63987-497-2
1. Spasms. 2. Spasms--Diagnosis. 3. Spasms--Treatment. 4. Epilepsy. 5. Convulsions. I. Dixon, Ezra.
RC429 .S45 2022
616.855--dc23

Murphy & Moore Publishing,
1 Rockefeller Plaza,
New York City, NY 10020, USA

ISBN 978-1-63987-497-2 (Hardback)

Contents

Preface

The medical condition which is caused by abrupt and uncontrolled electrical disturbances in the brain is called seizure. It can affect a person's movements, behavior, levels of consciousness and feelings. A few common causes of seizures are closed head injury, meningitis and stroke. Seizures are classified as either focal seizures or generalized seizures. Focal seizures are caused when there is unusual electrical activity in a particular part of the brain, while generalized seizures involve all the areas of the brain. Generalized seizures are further classified into clonic seizures, tonic seizures, atonic seizures, myoclonic seizures, etc. There are various complications and accidents which can be caused due to seizures such as falling, car accidents, drowning and emotional health issues. The book aims to shed light on some of the unexplored aspects of seizures and the recent researches in this field. It elucidates the concepts and innovative models with respect to their diagnosis and treatment. This book includes contributions of experts and scientists which will provide innovative insights into this field.

This book has been the outcome of endless efforts put in by authors and researchers on various issues and topics within the field. The book is a comprehensive collection of significant researches that are addressed in a variety of chapters. It will surely enhance the knowledge of the field among readers across the globe.

It gives us an immense pleasure to thank our researchers and authors for their efforts to submit their piece of writing before the deadlines. Finally in the end, I would like to thank my family and colleagues who have been a great source of inspiration and support.

Editor

1

Psychogenic Nonepileptic Seizures in Patients Living with Neurocysticercosis

Lourdes de Fátima Ibañez-Valdés and

Humberto Foyaca-Sibat

Abstract

Very little is known about psychogenic nonepileptic seizures (PNES) in patients with cysticercosis in the brain. We review the available medical literature on PNES in patients with neurocysticercosis and found no reports on this matter apart from our publications. Based on our previous experiences with patients presenting neurocysticercosis and associated epileptic seizures and/or PNES, we compared our results with the current advances published up to date. We also discuss the available information about epidemiology including frequency and prevalence, the role of sexual abuse on the ethiopathogenesis of PNES, clinical diagnosis and its differential diagnosis, laboratory investigations and video electroencephalogram, methods to induce PNES, medical treatment, and psychological intervention.

Keywords: psychogenic nonepileptic seizures, epileptic seizures, epilepsy, neurocysticercosis, epidemiology, diagnosis, video electroencephalogram, treatment and ethical aspects

1. Introduction

Neurocysticercosis (NCC) is a parasitic disease of central nervous system (CNS) caused by the larval stage (cysticercus cellulosae) of the pig tapeworm *Taenia solium*. This parasite is the most common helminthes to produce CNS infection in humans. The presence of acquired epilepsy in a person from an endemic region for cysticercosis or even in one living in close contact with patient who have taeniasis should suggest a diagnosis of cysticercosis of the CNS; the NCC may remain asymptomatic for months to years, and sometimes its diagnosis is made incidentally when CT/MRI scan is done. Symptoms and signs are related both to the parasite and to the inflammatory-immunological response of the host but in almost all symptomatic patients, headache and epileptic seizure (ES) are the most frequent problem. NCC is the most common cause of acquired epilepsy worldwide and most of the patients taking first line antiepileptic drugs (AED) respond very well [1]. For interested people, other aspects concerning to NCC are available online [2].

NCC is a common parasitic disease of the brain in developing countries. The clinical and pathologic features of NCC vary depending on the inflammatory/immune response around cysticerci, their number, size, and localization. Inflammation around degenerating cysticerci may have severe consequences, including focal encephalitis, edema, and vasculitis. NCC can cause a wide variety of clinical syndromes from chronic meningitis and cranial nerve palsy to spinal infarction and symptoms due to either as mass effect or, particularly in racemose disease, raised intracranial pressure.

Almost all patients living neurocysticercosis (PLNCC) have epileptic seizures (ES) due to this zoonotic parasitic infection [2]. However, an important number of those epileptic patients also present psychogenic nonepileptic seizures (PNES) because epileptic and nonepileptic seizures are not mutually exclusive phenomena and may coexist in the same patient. PNESs are defined as change in behavior or consciousness resembling epileptic seizures but which have a psychological origin. PNESs are categorized as a manifestation of dissociative or somatoform (conversion) disorders. Predisposing, precipitating, and perpetuating factors should be carefully assessed individually. The complex process of communicating the diagnosis to patients and their relatives using a multidisciplinary approach is an important and effective therapeutic step than should be performed by good skilled physician. Video-EEG (vEEG) recording of an event is the gold standard for diagnosis [3], but in many developing countries where NCC is endemic, this technology is not available.

To distinguish ES from PNES, an accurate clinical assessment is mandatory apart from other technologies. Frontal lobe seizures can be mistaken for PNES, though these tend to have shorter duration, stereotyped patterns of movements, and occurrence during sleep in spite of vEEG technology. Sometimes, elevated blood levels of serum prolactin following most tonic–clonic or complex partial ES can support a diagnosis, but because the frequency is false positive, it is not a gold standard test. The psychological mechanisms underlying PNES are poorly understood, and there is a lack of well-established, evidence-based treatments [4].

To differentiate PNES from ES in PLNCC is an important challenge for neurologists, epileptologists, internists, and pediatricians but even more for general practitioners and family doctors. PNESs, also known as nonepileptic attack disorders, are events resembling an epileptic seizure but without the characteristic electroencephalophic anomalies associated with epileptic seizures. They are common in neurological settings and often associated with considerable distress and disability.

Brown and Markus described PNES (nineteenth century), as *seizure-like attacks not related to an identified central nervous system lesion*, and are currently classified as a conversion disorder, according to the Diagnostic and Statistical Manual of Mental Disorders, fifth edition (DSM-5) [4]. While a universally accepted and unifying etiological model does not yet exist, several risk factors have been identified. Management of PNES should be based on multidisciplinary collaboration, focusing on modifiable risk factors. The first priority in the management of PNES is patient engagement that is challenging given the demonstrated low rates of treatment retention [4]. The differential diagnosis of PNES firstly involves ruling out epilepsy as the cause of the seizure episodes, along with other organic causes of nonepileptic seizures, such as syncope, migraine, vertigo, stroke, faking ES, and malingering.

Are psychogenic nonepileptic seizures just another symptom of conversion disorder?

Some authors argue that the etiological and mechanistic distinctions they support, particularly when bolstered by additional data, give reason to sustain a separation between these conditions [5].

In 2003, an international consensus group of clinician-researchers in epilepsy, neurology, neuropsychology, and neuropsychiatry from the International League Against Epilepsy Nonepileptic Seizure Task Group collaborated with the aim of developing clear guidance on standards for the diagnosis of PNES. Because the gold standard of vEEG is not available in many countries, and for every patient, the group delineated a staged approach to PNES diagnosis. Using a consensus review of the literature, this group evaluated key diagnostic approaches. These included history, EEG, ambulatory EEG, vEEG/monitoring, neurophysiologic, neurohumoral, neuroimaging, neuropsychological testing, hypnosis, and conversation analysis. Levels of diagnostic certainty are developed including possible, probable, clinically established, and documented diagnosis, based on the availability of history, witnessed event, and investigations, including vEEG. The aim and hope of this report are to provide greater clarity about the process and certainty of the diagnosis of PNES, with the intent to improve the care for people with epilepsy and PNES [6].

There is no general scientific consensus as to what causes PNES. However, some physicians [7] *believe* that *the condition may be triggered by psychological problems (irrespective of whether the patient shows any obvious psychological distress or pathology). It is estimated that 20% of seizure patients seen at specialist epilepsy clinics have PNES.*

Other author [8] believes that *PNES can significantly affect an individual's quality of life, the health care system, and even society. The first decade of the new millennium has seen renewed interest in this condition, but etiological understanding and evidence-based treatment availability remain limited. After the diagnosis of PNES is established, the first therapeutic step includes a presentation of the diagnosis that facilitates engagement in treatment.*

To date, only very narrow aspects of ethical dilemmas in PNES have been explored, but without doubt, the most important ethical values at stake include trust, transparency, confidentiality, professionalism, autonomy of all stakeholders, and justice.

> *Recently, Gul and Ahmad [9] "demonstrated cognitive impairment in terms of the interrupted ability to switch between emotion and non-emotion face categorizations in patients with PNES. In contrast, healthy individuals exhibited efficient switching between these face categorizations. They also found in patients with PNES, an asymmetric relationship between*

> *emotion and age tasks, while this asymmetry was absent in the healthy group. Their results demonstrated that patients with PNES used expressive suppression to regulate their emotions more frequently than the control group and on the other hand, patients with PNES less frequently reappraised their cognitions than healthy individuals. This is the first study demonstrating the presence of switching deficits in terms of inferior cognitive control of emotion in patients with PNES as compared to healthy individuals".*

PNESs are relatively common, accounting for 5–40% of visits to tertiary epilepsy centers. Inpatient vEEG monitoring is the gold standard for diagnosis as mentioned before, but additional positive predictive tools are necessary given vEEG's relatively scarce availability. Robbins et al. [10] investigated *if the number of patient-reported allergies distinguishes between PNES and epilepsy, using electronic medical records, ICD-9 codes, and text-identification algorithms to search EEG reports, and they identified 905 cases of confirmed PNES and 5187 controls with epilepsy but no PNES. Patients with PNES averaged more self-reported allergies than patients with epilepsy alone (1.93 vs. 1.00, $p < 0.001$).* They concluded that *"long allergy lists may help identify patients with PNES and hypothesize that a tendency to inaccurately self-report allergies reflects a maladaptive externalization of psychologic distress and that a similar mechanism may be responsible for PNES in some patients with somatic symptom disorder".*

Many patients with PNES dismiss the idea that their seizures are psychogenic, especially if the correct diagnosis comes after many years of treatment for epilepsy [11].

Outcomes in PNES are generally poor: 71% of PNES patients continue to have seizures 4 years after diagnosis and 56% are dependent on Social Security assistance. Neurologic and psychiatric factors associated with poor outcome include:

- history of epilepsy
- abnormal MRI
- presence of a psychiatric diagnosis
- age > 30
- duration of illness (the longer the patient has been treated for epilepsy, the worse the prognosis) [11].

> *In Diagnostic and Statistical Manual of Mental Disorders, fifth edition, "PNES do not have a unique classification as they can be found within different categories: conversion, dissociative, and somatization disorders. The ICD-10, instead, considers PNES within dissociative disorders, merging the dissociative disorders and conversion disorders, although the underlying defense mechanisms are different"* [12].

Last year, some authors conducted 140 empirical studies on the following aspects of PNES: life adversity, dissociation, anxiety, suggestibility, attention dysfunction, family/relationship problems, insecure attachment, defense mechanisms, somatization/conversion, coping, emotion regulation, alexithymia, emotional processing, symptom modeling, learning, and expectancy, and they concluded that:

"physical symptom reporting is elevated in patients with PNES; trait dissociation and exposure to traumatic events are common but not inevitable correlates of PNES; also, concluded that there is a mismatch between subjective reports of anxiety and physical arousal during PNES; and inconsistent findings in this area are likely to be attributable to the heterogeneity of patients with PNES" [4].

The main goal of this chapter is to compare our finding from 2003 with recent investigation on PNES to identify new knowledge and challenges.

1.1. Our study

In 2003, we studied 32 rural patients from the poorest regions in Mthatha (South Africa), diagnosed as epilepsy due to NCC presenting PNES. We found that the common clinical characteristics of this series and its psychological profile were duration of events, history of sexual abuse in females, absent of focal neurological signs, vocalization in the middle of the seizures, and lack of postictal symptoms were very useful for its differential diagnosis and the possible difference between the clinical features and psychological profile of those patients and others without PNES. Finally, some advices for the management of this condition by family doctors were delivered [13].

As mentioned [14–16], PNES *are sudden changes in behavior that resemble epileptic attack but lack organic cause and are also known by conversion seizures, dissociative seizures, hysterical seizures, psychogenic seizures, and nonepileptic seizures.* They are quite often misdiagnosed and represent the opposite end of the spectrum from seizures that mimic psychiatric disorders without organic cause and an expected EEG changes. Accurately distinguishing PNES from EP and other illnesses is difficult because of the breadth and overlap of symptoms seen in each condition and the frequent co-occurrence of PNES and epilepsy [14].

There is a general consensus about subjects with PNES that exhibited trauma-related profiles which differed significantly from those of epileptic comparison subjects and closely resembled those of individuals with a past medical history of traumatic experiences [15–17]. As we published, PNES patients frequently report a history of physical and sexual abuse, and traumatic experience is considered part of the mechanism for producing dissociation and may be a manifestation of dissociative disorders, especially when a history of sexual or physical abuse is documented [18]. In our region, sexual abuse is more frequently seen among members of the same family.

At the present moment, there exists a controversy regarding the significance of dissociation and conversion in the pathogenesis of PNES. Soon after the elimination of the term "hysterical neurosis" from the current diagnostic systems, these kinds of seizures were diagnosed as either Dissociative Disorders (ICD-10) or in the DSM IV as Somatoform disorder, most often conversion type.

"The significantly higher incidence of dissociation in the patients with PNES suggests dissociation in the pathogenesis of these seizures" [13].

Significant advances have been made in the diagnosis and treatment of epilepsy before 2003. With the introduction of vEEG monitoring, physicians are now able to reliably differentiate epilepsy from other conditions that can mimic it, including PNES. Many new AEDs have become available in recent years. The ketogenic diet is another treatment option in certain types of epilepsy and the vagus nerve stimulator, approved in 1997, represents another treatment modality for refractory epilepsy, and finally epilepsy surgery is an effective treatment for those patients with uncontrolled epilepsy.

Our study was performed at the former Transkei which was one of the three administrative authorities of the so-called independent South African homelands (Ciskei, Transkei, and the Cape Provincial Administration under different apartheid governments). It is currently named as region D and E of Eastern Cape Province, and it is also one of the poorest region of the country. That region serves as a labor reservoir for other wealthier provinces, with men leaving behind women and children, while they seek and find employment elsewhere. Our region has the most elevate indices of poverty and underdevelopment and shows a remarkable limited access to employment, cash income, primary education, safe and clean water, proper toilet facilities, proper refuse disposal, electricity, and telecommunication. Some communities still do not have easy access to any health care facility.

The aim of this study was to identify a psychological profile of a group of patients with epilepsy NCC-related presenting PNES and to detect the possible difference between the clinical features and psychological profile of patients affected by PNES and ES NCC-related and those patients in whom EPs are associated with NCC only and have been reported earlier [19–25].

We included female and male patients [13]. In this region, people beyond age of 13 are considered as adults. Therefore, people aged 13 years and older who had all developed EP fulfilling the International League Against Epilepsy criteria for epilepsy and the radiological criteria for calcified NCC (considering multiples intraparenchymal calcifications measuring between 2 and 10 mm in patients from endemic regions as pathognomonic) were selected, and others experienced more than one attack of PNES per month. Patients were excluded due to the following reasons: seizures caused by clear precipitants such as alcohol or hypoglycemia; we also excluded patients with previous medical history of head injury, syncope, stroke, brain tumor, cortical dysplasia, hyponatremia, hypomagnesaemia, hyperparathyroidism, cardiac arrhythmias, heart failure, and history of medication taken on the past 6 months such as theophylline, meperidine hydrochloride, isoniazid, antipsychotic drugs, alkylating agent, beta-lactam antibiotics, tricycle antidepressants, acyclovir, beta-blockers, and decongestants; also pregnant or breastfeeding women and patients with any medical condition that might interfere with the interpretation of the results of this study. At screening, all patients had a physical examination, including a detailed neurological examination done by one of us (FSH), routine laboratory test including hematology, urinalysis, urea, and electrolytes, glucose, plain skull X-rays, CT scan of the head, and a 32-channel digital EEG (Nihon Khoden) for 30 minutes recording using opening and closing the eyes and 3 minutes hyperventilation as activating maneuver.

Seven patients presented PNES that we could not distinguish clinically from EP; therefore, their anticonvulsant medication was rapidly tapered to provoke seizure; if the seizure did not develop, other serial maneuvers including 24 hours' sleep deprivation followed by hyperventilation and suggestion with intravenous saline injection were done. Diagnosis of PNES was considered when their seizures did not change the background EEG activity under observation plus others clinical features of PNES. All patients granted written informed consent before entering the study [13].

All patients presented radiographic signs of active and/or calcified NCC on CT scan (**Figure 1**), and signs of other stage of the parasite were also observed but the predominant finding was no less than five calcified lesions fulfilling the radiographic criteria for calcified NCC at the brain parenchyma. In this series, 37% of patients (all women) were on disability grant program for epilepsy, and that cash income was the only way for alleviating their requirements and poverty; however, evidence of malingering on this group was not be identified [13].

About 85% of the studied female patients were single mothers or married women living alone with their children, while their husband was working in gold mines very far away from home and only contact between them happened on December every year.

A total of 17 female patients from our series complained of a previous history of sexual abuse, and 14 of them physical abuse as well. Members of their own family raped 10 women, and 11 mentioned other members of their families that have had been raped during their early youth. According to information obtained from this group, some families suffered deeply when one of their members was raped and six people (not included in this series) were also murdered. Usually their father or the mother became chronically depressed, alcoholic, and their socioeconomic situation became remarkably deteriorated; for five patients to talk about this topic was rejected, and each refused to accept psychiatry or psychological referral because of financial or

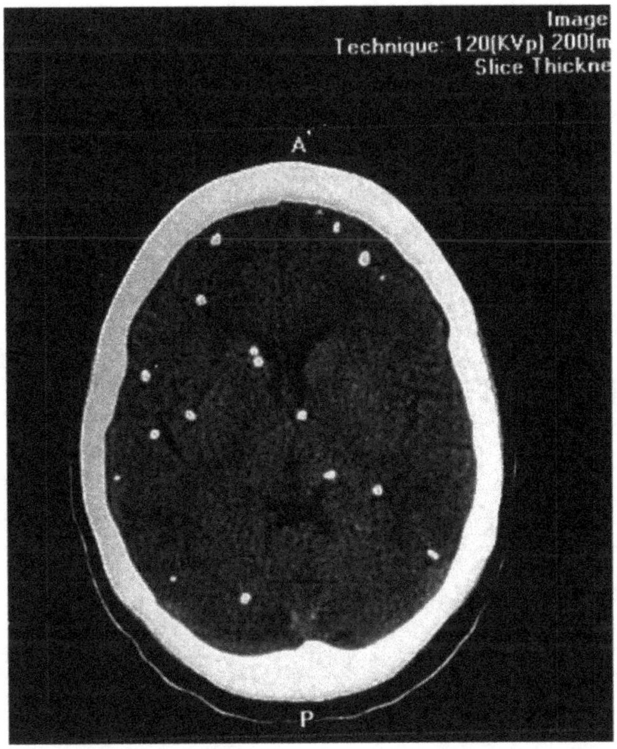

Figure 1. Bilateral calcified NCC lesions on CT scan of the brain.

transportation's problems (25%) because they did not consider it necessary (18%) or for other reasons. About 38% got injuries on both group including tongue biting [13].

Maximal duration of tonic-clonic ES was 95 seconds and for PNES was 904 seconds, and minimal duration was 45 seconds for EP and 18 seconds for PNES. See **Table 1**.

Psychic manifestations were present in different group: frontal lobe epilepsy (FLE), tonic-clonic generalized (TCG), partial complex motor seizure (PCS), and PNES: Rocking: PNES = 47, FLE = 63; PCS = 18, TCG = 5; Kicking: PNES = 60, FLE = 75, PCS = 21, TCG = 0; Cursing PNES = 54, FLE = 35, PCS = 47, TCG = 0; Babinski: PNES = 0, FLE = 65, PCS = 76, TCG = 83; Pelvic thrusting: PNES = 57, FLE = 0, PCS = 63, and TCG = 5; and other dissociative symptoms of depersonalization and deserialization were present only in patients with PCS/PNES (see **Tables 2** and **3**).

No changes of the background activity on the EEG during provocative saline infusion and the occurrence of PNES were seen.

In general, patients complained of PNES revealed higher percentage of Somatoform Disorders and Cluster B Personality Disorders. The occurrence of PNES mimicking generalized tonic-clonic ES was documented only on illiterate peoples.

Three patients complained of auditory hallucinations, two had focal complex motor seizures as well, and the third one presented TCG seizures and paranoid schizophrenia; all presented calcified NCC on the basal ganglia without active or calcified lesion of NCC on the temporal lobe. EEG under provocative saline solution done in two patients did not show changes on the background activity during the test (**Figure 2**).

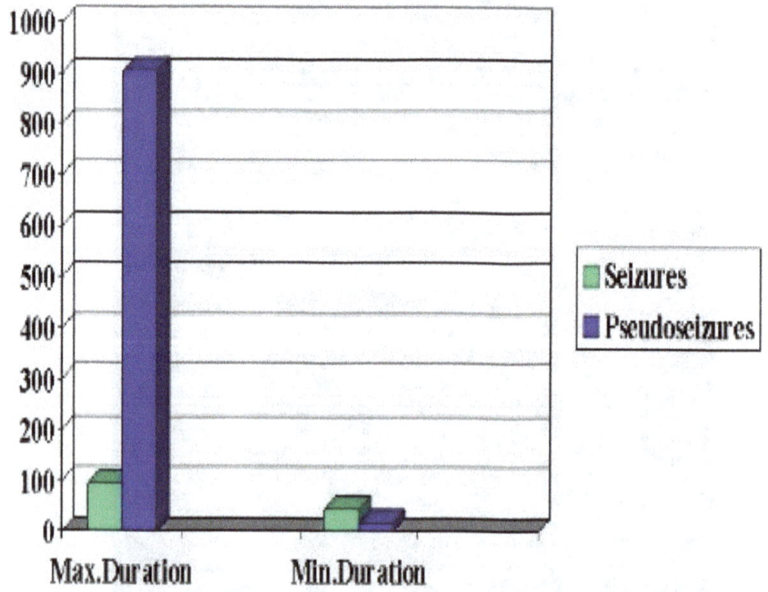

Table 1. Duration of the events in seconds.

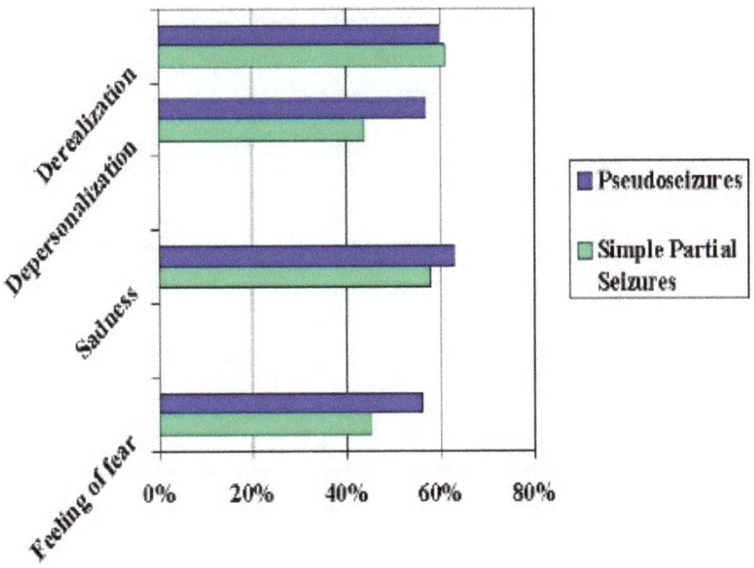

Table 2. Psychic manifestations in both groups.

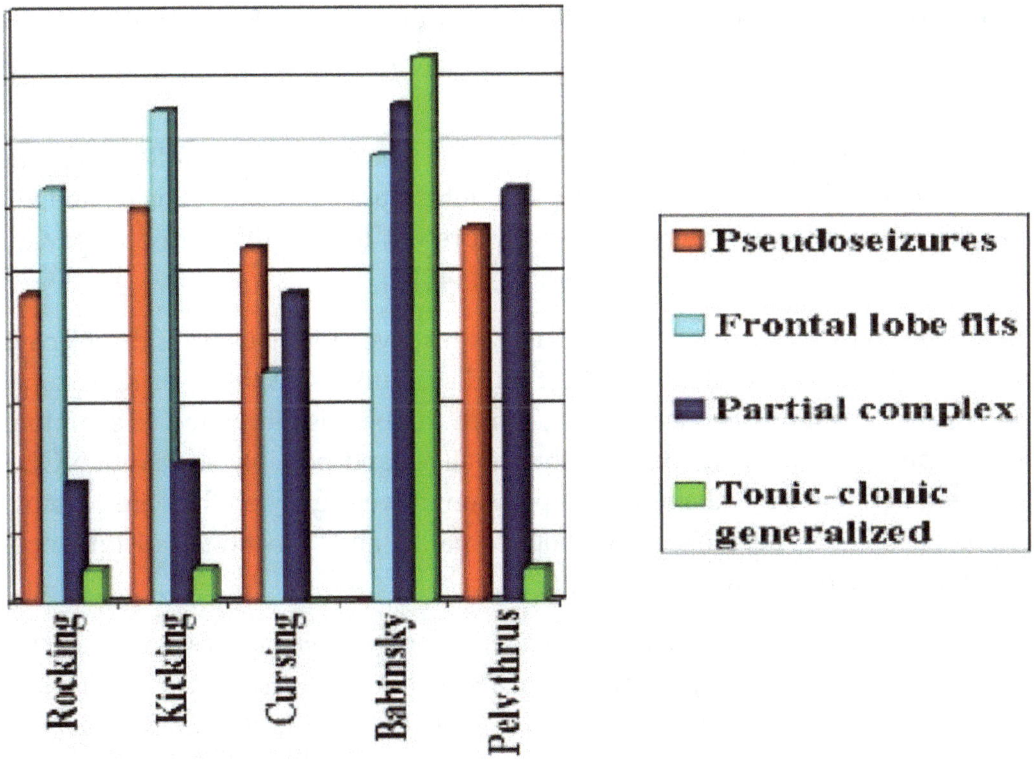

Table 3. Frequency of clinical signs during the event.

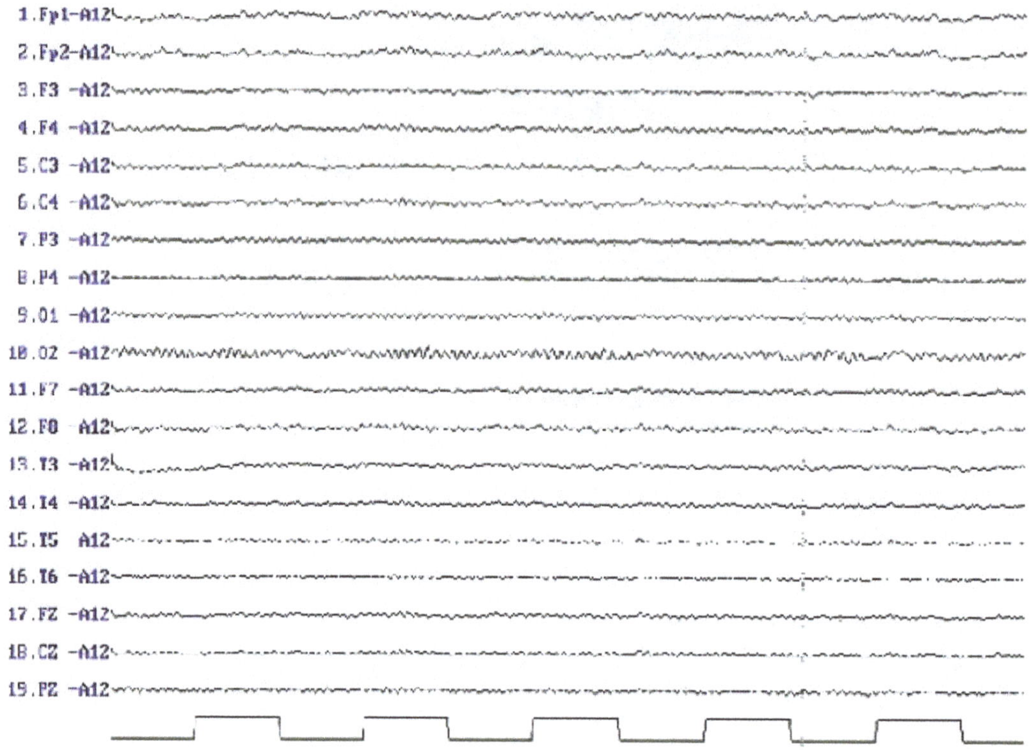

Figure 2. No changes of the background activity on the EEG during provocative saline infusion and the occurrence of PNES.

In Transkei, ES are the commonest clinical expression of calcified NCC followed by headache as it had been reported by us previously [19–40], but the associated PNES is related with other functional disturbances which were not usually present in patients with epilepsy and NCC alone, although some cases have been reported [41–43].

In temporal lobe epilepsy, some symptoms such as reactive automatisms and subjective abnormal sensations are difficult to differentiate from dissociative symptoms of depersonalization, derealisation, and alteration of consciousness, which can be misinterpreted as symptoms of ES; for the other hand, some nonspecific EEG abnormalities and possibly structural NCC findings can contribute to reinforce this diagnostic impression; therefore, when they are present, despite the absent of other reliable diagnostic tools, both "organic" and "functional" disturbances should be treated at the same time [13].

> *"Bilateral motor seizures with retained consciousness are rare and often mistaken for PNES* [42]. *When a realistic threat of physical or sexual assault to a member of their family involved in the problem is revealed, is important the role for family therapy skills in the evaluation and treatment of PNES"* [43].

Some patients did not improve from the occurrence of PNES probably because of lack of more specialized treatment, and others did not discontinue their treatment including AED, in spite of our personal agreement, probable because of fear to loss their disability grant among other reasons and also because of ignorance, superstitions, and poor health education. Many patients found solace in becoming and remaining neurological ill; thus, defense mechanism of denial, dissociation, introjections, identification, and symbolization contributed to the patient's symptom picture and to their adaptation to traumatic life events.

> *"Bringing the unconscious psychotic elements into conscious awareness is an important aspect of the treatment of dissociative disorders* [44] *and may be assayed by family physician if there is no other choice".*

Using AED in patients with PNES before its confirmation was a common problem in other series [45] but not for us because all patients from our series also presented ES and then were treated accordingly.

> *"Auditory hallucinations, are paradigmatic symptoms of the schizophrenic patients, and can be present in disorders such as: Alzheimer's disease, epilepsy, deafness, tumors of the temporal lobe, and toxic psychosis, usually due to disturbances of the left temporal lobe, limbic, and paralimbic areas. We could not have demonstrated the source of the hallucinations in our series but based on our observations we have hypothesized that hallucinations could be secondary to hyperactivity of the basal ganglia (thalamus and striatum) since that mechanism was before-published"* [46].

Malingering is an accusation, and the people have intentional and obvious goals, such as to get financial benefits or avoidance of duty or school, to reach better position in penitentiary, evasion of criminal prosecution, obtaining of drugs or compaction among other. These goals may resemble secondary gain in conversion symptoms but with the distinguishing feature being the conscious intent in the production of the symptoms.

Why more ladies than gentlemen in our series? Because there are more females than males living in Transkei (due to temporal migratory reasons) and also because women are more susceptible than men to develop this kind of somatoform disorder therefore increased incidence and prevalence of PNES is expected. Charcot and Freud [47] *emphasized the sexual aspects of the seizure as has the current interest in childhood sexual abuse.* Major mood disorders and severe environmental stress, especially sexual abuse, were common problems among our patients and they were considered in every case. From case studies and review of the medical literature, we believe that PNES in women express rage, fear, and helplessness against the dominant and abusive male rather than sexual conflicts. *Emphasizing the aggressive component of seizures does not minimize the traumatic effects of sexual abuse but rather includes it as leading to rage and helplessness* [13].

We performed EEG under provocative suggestion and intravenous (IV) normal saline solution in a small number of patients only because we consider that deceptive diagnostic tests are justified only in exceptional situations [13]. The use of provocative IV normal saline solution in that way is fundamentally deceptive, requiring the physician to intentionally and directly lie to the patient and causing the patient to believe that the administered solution caused his seizures, provocative saline infusion compromises the fiduciary obligation of truthfulness, is inimical to patient autonomy, is undignified, and risks grave harm to patient trust in physicians; however, if no deceptive alternatives are not available and the difficulty of distinguishing malingerers cannot be solved, then we have not choice and deceptive diagnostic testing should be implemented. Without such deception, the test might be useless [48].

From our personal experience, sometimes those patients have to be treated by family physicians. Under those circumstances, we strongly recommended being very patient, very kind, and also very gentle, we advise do not accuse anybody of malingering or deliberately faking the seizures under any circumstances and always advised to get counseling. We suggest do not forget they inability for controlling their PNES and for proper socialization and its impact on their families, friends, and other members of the community. We learned that it is a good practice to understand their disabilities and frustrations and to identify their hopes. It is very important to define the underlying causes and the triggering factors for PNES such as rage, fear, and panic among others and to contribute in the healing process of emotional hurts and their emotional control; to provide an ideal psychological support and to address an adequate management of stress, emotional upset, or physical illness are also recommended; do not named those patient as hypochondriac and to explain clearly why they are unaware of the source contributing to the events, when it will be appropriated [13].

> *"When patients are having PNES to keep them safe, just as would be done when they are having ES is strong recommended, if the diagnosis of PNES is clear-cut then leaving the patient alone until it is over, keeping the environment calmed and free of starling noises is the best choice".*

When the clinical event of PNES is over, try to elicit some kind of respond from the patient. Never use suggestions by hypnotic procedures if you have not enough expertise.

Physical abuse on patients having PNES must be damned forever. It is very successful to encourage patients for exploring their own feelings and assisted in learning to cope with the feelings in new ways. Patients with history of attend to suicide were not suitable for this group. If there is not a good response in a due time, the diagnosis must be revised.

The clinical differentiation of PNES from epileptic attacks in patients with NCC is particularly difficult and sometimes almost impossible, if 24-hour video-EEG monitoring techniques are not available, but duration of events, history of sexual abuse in females, focal neurological signs, vocalization in the middle of the seizures, and lack of postictal symptoms can be very useful for its differential diagnosis. However, if the patient presents PNES, temporal lobe epilepsy, other types of epileptic seizures because of NCC, and some associated conditions such as factitious disorder and malingering, then confirmation PNES cannot be reached. *Under exceptional circumstances those patients can be treated by their family physician if some specialized advices are adjusted.*

In summary, we review the commonest clinical features in PLNCC presenting PNES and epileptic seizures in our series of patients. To differentiate ES from PNES or vice versa, clinical psychiatric and neurological knowledge are mandatory; however, if both manifestations are present on the same patient other diagnostic tool should be required. We conclude that:

> *"Some features are more or less likely to suggest PNES but they are not conclusive and should be considered within the broader clinical picture. Features that are common in PNES but rare*

> *in epilepsy include: biting the tip of the tongue, seizures lasting more than 2 minutes (easiest factor to distinguish), seizures having a gradual onset, a fluctuating course of disease severity, the eyes being closed during a seizure, and side to side head movements. Features that are uncommon in PNES include automatisms (automatic complex movements during the seizure), severe tongue biting, biting the inside of the mouth, and incontinence. If a patient with suspected PNES has an episode during a clinical examination, there are a number of signs that can be elicited to help support or refute the diagnosis of PNES such as: normal size of the pupils, pupillary reflexes, cutaneous plantar reflexes, and caloric test"* [13].

2. PNES at the present moment

2.1. Definition

Despite the terminology of "*pseudo seizures*" is obsolete, some authors still using that at the present moment and define PNES, as paroxysmal episodes that can be similar to ES and can be misdiagnosed very often by general physician and medical officers. It is important to highlight that PNES are psychological disorders such as emotional or stress-related events

> *"Paroxysmal nonepileptic episodes can be either organic or psychogenic. Good examples of organic nonepileptic paroxysmal symptoms are migraine, syncope and transient ischemic attack (TIA). The terminology on the topic has been variable and, at times, confusing. Various terms are used, and apart from pseudo seizures, another such as: nonepileptic seizures, nonepileptic events, and psychogenic seizures"* [49],

and PNES, followed by nonepileptic event(s), psychogenic attack(s), nonepileptic attack(s), and psychogenic nonepileptic attack(s) in Google and PubMed Google and in PubMed using multiple search terms (https://www.google.com and http://www.ncbi.nlm.nih.gov/pubmed). The broad spectrum of synonyms used to refer to PNES in the medical literature reflects a lack of internationally accepted and uniform terminology for PNES. In addition to "seizure(s)," lay people use the word "attack(s)" to describe PNES [49, 50].

PNES has been the preferred term in the literature, but in practice, the term "seizures" is confusing to patients and families [49]. Other authors consider that PNESs are the most common paroxysmal event misdiagnosed as epilepsy, and they significantly affect quality of life, functional status and use of medical resources [51, 52].

By definition, PNES is a psychiatric disorder; more specifically, it is a conversion disorder, which falls under the diagnostic category of somatic symptom disorders in the Diagnostic and Statistical Manual of Mental Disorders, Fifth Edition (DSM-5). The specific *DSM-5* criteria for conversion disorder are:

One or more symptoms of altered voluntary motor or sensory function:

- Clinical findings provide evidence of incompatibility between the symptom and recognized neurological or medical conditions.

- The symptom or deficit is not better explained by another medical or mental disorder.
- The symptom or deficit causes clinically significant distress or impairment in social, occupational, or other important areas of functioning or warrants medical evaluation.

According to the *DSM-5* classification, neurological symptoms that are found, after appropriate neurological assessment, to be incompatible with neurological pathophysiology can fall under conversion disorder, factitious disorder, or malingering [49].

The immobility, loss of independence, and anxiety that occurs during the monitoring process using vEEG can be difficult for older adults [53]. PNES is also a remarkably challenging and complex medical condition that gives rise to a number of ethical issues with which even the most skilled clinician struggles [54].

> *"Seizures can be divided into three major categories: epileptic seizures (ES), PNES, or physiologic nonepileptic events"* [55].

Like epileptic seizures, PNES present as paroxysmal time-limited, alterations in motor, sensory, autonomic, and/or cognitive signs and symptoms, but unlike epilepsy, PNES are not caused by ictal epileptiform activity. In contrast to ES, which are a manifestation of excessive and hypersynchronous discharges in the brain, PNES have psychologic underpinnings and causes. Physiologic non-epileptic evoked seizures are neither epileptic nor psychogenic, rather they are events associated with systemic alterations that produce an ictus (e.g., convulsive syncope or hypoglycemic seizure) [56, 57]. PNES occur across cultures worldwide. Events described as PNES and occurring in a similar context to PNES seen in industrially developed countries are reported from threshold or developing countries, as well. PNES therefore seem to represent a fairly universal human condition. The semiology is described similarly across ethnicities and cultures [57].

As is very well known, functional neurological disorder (conversion disorder) is a neurobehavioral condition frequently encountered by epileptologist, neurologists, and family physicians.

> *Observational research studies "suggest that PNES and Functional Movement Disorders may represent variants of similar (or the same) conditions given that both groups exhibit a female predominance, have increased prevalence of mood-anxiety disorders, frequently endorse prior abuse, and share phenotypic characteristics"* [55].

Physical and neurologic findings are usually normal, but the examination can also uncover suggestive features. For example, overly dramatic behaviors, give-way weakness, and a weak voice or stuttering can be useful predictors. Psychological features suggestive of psychogenic episodes include anxiety, depression, inappropriate affect or lack of concern (*la belle indifference*), and multiple and vague somatic complaints suggestive of somatization disorder, and abnormal interaction with family members [49].

2.2. Gender

PNES are more prevalent among women worldwide and we also find similar results in our series. However, Asadi-Pooya et al. [57] investigated the potential differences in demographic and clinical characteristics of PNES between women and men from Iran in 2013 and they did not observe any significant differences between women and men with PNES with regard to demographic, clinical, and semiological characteristics. Likewise, seizure characteristics and semiology were very similar in both genders. It appears that an Islamic lifestyle (in Iran) has little influence on the sex ratio and clinical manifestations of PNES compared with the Western studies. For the other hand,

> *Gale et al.* [58] *compare males with PNES to females with PNES and to males with epilepsy and they concluded that gender difference in PNES seizure semiology was associated with whether or not clinically significant somatic symptoms were present; males with elevated somatic symptoms were much more likely to have motor PNES.*

However, they did not find evidence of greater psychopathology in males with PNES compared to females. Gender differences in the behavioral manifestation of PNES in the context of presence or absence of somatization may have implications for diagnosis and treatment.

2.3. Epidemiology

PNES is by far the most frequent nonepileptic condition seen in general hospital, neurological institutions, and epilepsy clinic, where they represent 20–30% of referrals. About 50–70% of patients become seizure free after diagnosis, and about 15% also have epilepsy [49]. Similar to conversion disorders, PNES typically begin in young adulthood and occur more frequently in women (approximately 70% of cases) than in men as we found in our study. Although very rare, PNES can also occur in elderly peoples. According to most authors (ourselves included), the combination of ES and PNES occurs in around 10% of patients with PNES. Some cautious should be taken in diagnosing PNES when the onset is in early childhood or elderly peoples. In young age groups, nonepileptic physiologic events may be more common than other organic conditions. Recurrent hospital admissions with apparent seizure status or daily convulsive events suggest PNES, especially when reported by a well and fully conscious patient [59].

> *Studies on the prevalence of PNES show variable but clinically significant results, from 5 to 33% of outpatients receiving treatment for epilepsy, and from 10 to 58% of inpatients treated for refractory epilepsy present PNES* [60].

According to Gates [55] such *a significant difference in results may be explained by differences in diagnostic criteria for PNES. A female preponderance of up to 80% has been observed in studies of patients with PNES* [50–62]. PNES is present in children and elderly people, but many patients' ages range between the 1920s and 1930s [62–64].

The incidence of PNES in our population was 6.45/100,000/year higher than in previous studies.

Duncan et al. [65] found an incidence of 4.90/100,000/year which is also high and the median diagnostic delay was 0.6±0.2 year. About 50% of their patients diagnosed early became spell free immediately or soon after diagnosis. There were high rates of psychological morbidity, medically unexplained symptoms, and economic dependence before or at the time of onset, and the early outcome was predicted by employment status.Other authors consider that

PNESs are diagnosed in at least 10–40% of the patients seen for long-term monitoring of epilepsy, and it is no surprise that patients with PNES are often treated for epilepsy [66].

PNES and psychogenic movement disorders (PMD) are among the most common psychogenic neurologic disorders.

PNES are common at neurological institutions and epilepsy clinics, where they are seen in 20–30% of patients referred for refractory seizures. PNES are probably also common in the general population, with an estimated prevalence of 2–33 cases per 100,000 population, which makes PNES nearly as prevalent as multiple sclerosis or trigeminal neuralgia [49].

2.4. Sexual abuse

Chen et al. [67] performed a systematic review and meta-analysis in some series of patients about sexual abuse and lifetime diagnosis of psychiatric disorders.

> *The search yielded 37 eligible studies, 17 case-controls, and 20 cohorts, with 3,162,318 participants. There was a statistically significant association between sexual abuse and a lifetime diagnosis of anxiety disorder (OR, 3.09; 95% CI, 2.43–3.94), depression (OR, 2.66; 95% CI, 2.14–3.30), eating disorders (OR, 2.72; 95% CI, 2.04–3.63), posttraumatic stress disorder (OR, 2.34; 95% CI, 1.59–3.43), sleep disorders (OR, 16.17; 95% CI, 2.06–126.76), and suicide attempts (OR, 4.14; 95% CI, 2.98–5.76).*

Therefore, a history of sexual abuse is associated with an increased risk of a lifetime diagnosis of multiple psychiatric disorders [67]. Patients having PNES present a high prevalence of traumatic life events; therefore, psychosocial factors are thought to play an important role in the etiology. Neurobiological factors may also contribute to the development of seizures, as a subgroup of patients is characterized by cognitive impairment and subtle structural and functional brain abnormalities [68].

Antecedent sexual trauma or abuse is thought to be important in the psychopathology of psychogenic seizures and psychogenic symptoms in general. A history of abuse may be more frequent in convulsive rather than limp type of PNES [49].

2.5. Psychogenic nonsyncopal collapse vs. PNESs

> *Heyer et al.* [69] *characterized the clinical features of tilt-induced psychogenic non-syncopal collapse (PNSC) from a cohort of young patients and to compare the semiology between PNSC and EEG-confirmed PNES and concluded that PNSC events were briefer than PNES events (median: 45 versus 201.5s, p<.001). Negative motor signs (head drop, body limpness) predominated in PNSC (85% versus 20%, p<.001), while the positive motor signs of convulsion occurred more often with PNES (90% versus 30%, p<.001). Behavioral arrest (25% versus 32.5%, p=.46) and eye closure (85% versus 72.5%, p=.21) did not differ between PNSC and PNES. Patients with PNSC were more likely to be tearful before (30% versus 7.5%, p=.02) and after (62.5% versus 7.5%, p<.001) an event.*

In spite of overlap exists, the features of PNSC generally appear similar to neutrally mediated syncope, while the features of PNES generally appear similar to ES.

2.6. Diagnosis

The patient's history may suggest the diagnosis. Several clues are useful in clinical practice and should raise the suspicion that seizures may be psychogenic rather than epileptic. Misdiagnosis of epilepsy is frequent and occurs in approximately 25% of patients with a previous diagnosis that does not respond to AED. Therefore, many cases of misdiagnosed epilepsy are eventually shown to be PNES.

> *Other paroxysmal conditions are occasionally misdiagnosed as epilepsy, but PNES is by far the most commonly misdiagnosed condition, accounting for >90% of misdiagnoses at epilepsy centers* [49].
>
> *Despite the ability to diagnose PNES with near certainty by using vEEG monitoring, the time to diagnosis is long, about 7–10 years. This delay indicates that neurologists may have an insufficiently high enough index of suspicion for PNES* [49, 70].

Approximately 80% of patients with PNES have been treated with AEDs before the correct diagnosis is made. A psychogenic etiology should be considered when AEDs have no effect whatsoever on the reported frequency of seizures [49].

> *Given the substantial economic costs and mental health burden of misdiagnosis, it is imperative to establish early identification, correct diagnosis, and effective treatment of PNES in order to provide the greatest opportunity for remission of events, improved psychological functioning, and social-vocational outcome* [65].
>
> *The great majority of PNES are classified as mental disorders in the current medical nosologies (only malingered seizures are not considered a mental disorder).*
>
> *The average delay from first seizure to diagnosis of psychogenic non-epileptic seizures (PNES) is over 7 years. The reason for this delay is not well understood. We hypothesized that a perceived decrease in seizure frequency after starting an anti-seizure medication (ASM) may contribute to longer delays, but the frequency of such a response has not been well established* [3].

Earlier diagnosis also reduces unnecessary doctor's visits and missed school/working days. The implementation of continuous education programmers for healthcare providers in particular could contribute positively to the diagnostic process of PNES for patients [71, 72].

> *In 2014 Elliot and Chariton* [73] *studied 689 patients presenting some events leading to a diagnosis, 47% (n=324) with PNES only, 12% (n=84) with PNES & Epilepsy and 41% (n=281) with Epilepsy only. Five biological predictors of a PNES only diagnosis was found; number of years with events (OR=1.10), history of head injury (OR=1.91), asthma (OR=2.94), gastro-esophageal reflux disease (OR=1.72) and pain (OR=2.25). One psychological predictor; anxiety (OR=1.72) and two social predictors; being married (OR=1.81) and history of physical/*

> *sexual abuse (OR=3.35). Two significant biological predictors of a PNES & Epilepsy diagnosis were found; migraine (OR=1.83) and gastro-esophageal reflux disease (OR=2.17).*

The importance of considering the biopsychosocial model for the diagnosis and treatment of PNES or PNES with concomitant epilepsy based on these finding is certain.

Clinicians need to take a detailed time-consuming history from parents and when possible from the patient to identify warning signs suggestive of PNES. Such as: *an inconsistent seizure history, gradual and slow onset, as well as long duration of seizures and lack of seizure occurrence when the patient is alone. Recognizing signs suggestive of PNES is particularly difficult in the 35–44% of patients that have comorbid epilepsy* [73, 74]. The diagnosis and management of PNES is often challenging and fraught with discord and disagreement between patients, parents, and physicians [70].

In neuropsychiatric diseases, disturbances of the autonomic nervous system (ANS) are common. Heart rate variability (HRV) is useful to assess for disturbances of both sympathetic and parasympathetic activity, whereas electrodermal activity (EDA) can assess sympathetic activity. Parasympathetic HRV parameters are typically decreased in posttraumatic stress disorder (PTSD), while EDA is increased. Nevertheless, in major depressive disorder (MDD) and dissociation, both parasympathetic and sympathetic markers are decreased. Using HRV, ANS abnormalities have also been identified in PNES, indicating lower parasympathetic activity at baseline [75]. Other authors also use HRV in order to compare maximum autonomic activity of ES and PNES as biomarkers for distinguishing these types of clinical episodes. However, the great variation of autonomic response within both groups makes it difficult to use these HRV measures as a sole measurement in distinguishing epileptic seizures from PNES [76].

PNES can be suspected in patients with a psychosocial history with evidence of maladaptive behaviors or associated psychiatric diagnoses. To pay special attention during mental status assessment, especially to the patient's general demeanor, the appropriateness of his or her level of concern, over dramatization, and hysterical features is strong recommended. Certain symptoms and signs suggest ES. These include significant physical injuries, in particular, tongue biting on the lateral side, the duration of the seizures, and an ictal cry are highly specific to generalized tonic-clonic seizures and are helpful signs when present [49].

> *Once the PNES diagnosis and underlying psychological problems have been ascertained by the neurologist and mental health professional, a communication process relaying the diagnosis in a manner that promotes early acceptance of PNES and the treatment plan is imperative to preserve the best outcome possible for the patient* [72].

Conducting the vEEG and mental health evaluation during the current hospitalization prevents additional delays in diagnosis. In areas where EEG video monitoring is not available, clinicians can be used a staged approach for diagnosis developed by the task force of the International League Against Epilepsy, these included: history, EEG, ambulatory EEG, vEEG/monitoring, neurophysiologic, neurohumoral, neuroimaging, neuropsychological testing, hypnosis, and conversation analysis [6, 77]. The task force proposed the following four categories of certainty for PNES diagnosis:

- Documented PNES – confirmed by clinical history plus EEG video monitoring.
- Clinically established PNES – defined by clinical history, clinician witness, and EEG recording of habitual events without video.
- Probable PNES – determined by clinical history, clinician witness of video or live events, and a normal EEG.
- Possible PNES – relies on patient's self-report of clinical events and a normal EEG.

As is done with PMD diagnosis, levels of diagnostic certainty are ranked based on what data are available from history, witnessed event, and diagnostic testing, with levels of Possible, Probable, Clinically Established, and Documented diagnosis.

The roles of the specialists involved in the patient's care, how the information is communicated, and subsequent follow-up needs to be carefully considered in the values trade-offs that occur [72]. The issues of communicating the diagnosis to the patient and making treatment recommendations which should ideally be coordinated using a multidisciplinary team approach, involving the disciplines of neurology, psychiatry, psychology, social work, nursing, and anyone else necessary for this process [65]. The language to be used in this communication requires special attention and dedication, selecting the best descriptor for patients and families that highlights transparency and honesty, with avoidance of stigma and negative emotional response. We argue for providing parents and the patient initial diagnostic feedback separately. We also recommend that after communicating a diagnosis of PNES, neurologist/epileptologist with independent prescriptive authority, in addition to physicians, and families may struggle with the choice of withdrawing AEDs for the treatment of young patients for whom the AEDs have been taken for a long time.

> *Although the* DSM-5 *classification is simple in theory, knowing whether a given patient is faking it is nearly impossible. In some circumstances, intentional faking can be diagnosed only by catching a person in the act of faking (e.g., self-inflicting injuries, ingesting medications or eye drops to cause signs, putting blood in the urine to simulate hematuria)* [49].

When the patient is purposely deceiving the physician (i.e., faking the symptoms), factitious disorder and malingering must to be taken into account. To distinguish factious disorder and malingering from PNES just consider that, in malingering, the reason for the deception is tangible and rationally understandable (albeit possibly reprehensible) such as avoiding military duty, avoiding work, obtaining financial compensation, evading criminal prosecution, or obtaining drugs. In factitious disorder, the motivation is a pathologic need for the sick role [49].

An important corollary is that malingering is not considered a mental illness, whereas factitious disorder is. As such there are no specific diagnostic criteria for malingering. A generally accepted view is that most patients with PNES have conversion disorder, rather than malingering or factitious disorder [49].

Dacrystic seizures are rare clinical occurrences characterized by sudden lacrimation, grimacing, sobbing, sad facial expression, and yelling, with a special challenging differential diagnosis with PNES. To differentiate dacrystic seizures from PNES can be very difficult from the point of view of symptomatology of psychiatric symptoms but if vEEG monitoring captures a prolonged seizure compatible with a dacrystic seizure its final diagnosis. The presentation of dacrystic seizures has common elements with PNES, and it is possible that the patient has both types of crisis. Apart from that there are a few medical reports in the literature about this matter [6, 78–80].

> *Laboratory studies are useful in excluding metabolic or toxic causes of seizures (e.g., hyponatremia, hypoglycemia, drugs). Prolactin and creatine kinase (CK) levels rise after generalized tonic-clonic seizures and not after other types of episodes. However, sensitivity is too low to be of any practical value (i.e., lack of elevation does not exclude epileptic seizures)* [49].

2.6.1. Electroencephalogram and provocative techniques, activation or inductions

The "gold standard" for proper diagnosis of PNES is vEEG [77]. During vEEG assessment, behavior and EEG activity are registered at the same time. A spontaneous or elicited event is defined as a PNES, when there is no spike/slow waves EEG activity, during or after the ictus, and semiology is consistent with PNES and not ES.

Jedrzejczak et al. [81] reported a clinical and electrophysiological analysis of type and duration of seizures recorded by means of long-term vEEG monitoring, a method which enables accurate diagnosis of PNES occurring with or without ES. Analysis is based on 1083 patients, hospitalized at their department between 1990 and 1997, with a preliminary diagnosis of epilepsy. A total of 85 patients (7.8%) were diagnosed as PNES. Long-term video-EEG monitoring was performed in 70 patients. In 55 (79%) of these patients, 230 seizures (221 pseudo epilepsy and nine epileptic) were recorded. In 30 patients (32%), the diagnosis was based on clinical observation of the seizures and on the number of EEG recordings, including activating procedures such as sleep deprivation, photo stimulation, hyperventilation, and AED withdrawal. The authors proved the difficulties involved in the diagnosis of psychogenic pseudoepileptic seizures and the negligible value of neuroimaging techniques and interictal EEG recordings in the differential diagnosis of epileptic versus nonepileptic seizures.

We review the influence of gender on psychogenic nonepileptic seizures (PNES) diagnosis and another author did the same.

> *Noe KH et al.* [80] *in 439 subjects undergoing video-EEG (vEEG) for spell classification, of which 142 women and 42 men had confirmed PNES. The epileptologist predicted diagnosis was correct in 72% overall. Confirmed epilepsy was correctly predicted in 94% men and 88% women. In contrast, confirmed PNES was accurately predicted in 86% women versus 61% men (p=0.003). Sex-based differences in likelihood of an indeterminate admission were not observed for predicted epilepsy or physiologic events, but were for predicted PNES (39% men, 12% women, p=0.0002).*

vEEG monitoring refers to continuous EEG recorded for a more or less prolonged period with simultaneous video recording of the clinical manifestations. Having a correlation of the recorded behavior (video) and the EEG cortical activity, the diagnosis of ES or PNES attacks can be made definitely in nearly all cases [81, 82].

> *Using vEEG of patients, Hubsch et al.* [83] *conducted multiple correspondence analysis and hierarchical cluster analysis to construct a practical and useful semiological classification of PNES, which identified five clusters of signs: dystonic attack with primitive gestural activity, pauci-kinetic attack with preserved responsiveness, pseudo syncope, hyperkinetic prolonged attack with hyperventilation and auras, and axial dystonic prolonged attack.*

The ability to diagnose PNES when vEEG is not available may open opportunities to lower and middle income countries, where monitoring is not available.

Provocative procedures, such as saline provocation, hypnosis, simple suggestions, suggestive interview, or a mixture of them, have been used to obtain a typical event; however, the ethics of provocative procedures has been raised.

Activation maneuver, inductions, or provocative techniques can be remarkably useful for the diagnosis of PNES, mainly when the diagnosis is uncertain and no spontaneous episodes occur during assessment. In many epilepsy centers, to use a provocative technique to aid in the diagnosis of PNES is allowed. For example, an intravenous injection of normal saline is traditionally and most commonly used, but other techniques such as hypnosis, among others, can be used. The use of suggestion techniques ranging from simple verbal suggestion to injection of saline may improve rate of seizure capture; at the present moment, an important number of authors are in favor [6, 77, 84–89], while others do not approve these procedures [90, 91]. Some authors support use of simple suggestion techniques, if the patient is clearly informed of what is being done and why (this does not seem to prevent patients from having events during recording) [92].

The recent use of hypnosis in the diagnostic process of PNES includes its use in seizure provocation, which was tested in samples in the recent literature.

2.6.2. Neuroimaging

Excepting lesions with epileptogenic potential (such as mesial temporal sclerosis) neuroimaging findings are of modest differential diagnostic value for ES and PNES at present, but it is diagnostic for patients PLNCC.

All patients presenting epileptic seizures secondary to NCC have abnormalities on CT scan or magnetic resonance imaging (MRI) scan of the brain characterized by calcified edema surrounding or not by perilesional edema and or active cysticerci at different stage [1, 2, 13, 19–40]. However, most patients with idiopathic epilepsy have normal MRI studies [62], and a significant number of patients with lone PNES have abnormalities [61, 77]. More recently, structural and functional imaging studies in patients with PNES have documented changes in cortical and cerebellar regions at group level [92]; in functional connectivity between emotional, cognitive, and motor regions [93–95] and between structural and functional connectivity network coupling [95]. More studies are needed to determine whether there are actual conversion/dissociation networks [93].

Lesions with epileptogenic potential (such as mesial temporal sclerosis) are more commonly found in patients with epilepsy but have also been described in patients with PNES and are clearly not sufficient for a diagnosis of epilepsy.

Convergent neuroimaging findings implicate alterations in brain circuits mediating emotional expression, regulation and awareness (anterior cingulate and ventromedial prefrontal cortices, insula, amygdala, vermis), cognitive control and motor inhibition (dorsal anterior cingulate, dorsolateral prefrontal, inferior frontal cortices), self-referential processing and perceptual awareness (posterior parietal cortex, temporoparietal junction), and motor planning and coordination (supplementary motor area, cerebellum). Striatal-thalamic components of prefrontal-parietal networks may also play a role in pathophysiology. Aberrant medial prefrontal and amygdala neuroplastic changes mediated by chronic stress may facilitate the development of functional neurological symptoms in a subset of patients [94–96].

Neuroimaging studies have demonstrated that PNES are characterized by unstable cognitive-emotional and motor system, which is engaged in hyperactivity of limbic regions and sensorimotor area. The insula, which is a part of the limbic system, includes various sub regions with some distinct connectivity patterns separately, whether these insular sub regions show different connectivity patterns respectively in PNES remains largely unknown according with the investigations done by Rong et al. [97].

They investigated the functional connectivity (FC) of insular sub regions in PNES and extend the understanding of the complex pathophysiological mechanisms of this disease. A resting state FC based on the insular sub regions was conducted in 18 patients and 20 healthy controls. They examined the differences in FC values between PNES patients and controls using two sample t tests, and their results showed that patients had significantly stronger FC between insular sub regions and sensorimotor network, lingual gyrus, superior parietal gyrus and putamen, which suggested a hyperlink pattern of insular sub regions involved in abnormal emotion regulation, cognitive processes, and motor function in PNES. Pearson correlation analysis between the mean FC values within abnormal regions and the frequency of PNES further indicated that PNES exhibited abnormal functional organization whose stressful emotion of patients has great direct influence on their motor functions.

They concluded that *differentially impaired functional connectivity patterns of insular sub regions might provide new insights into the complex neurological mechanism of PNES* [97].

Functional neuroimaging data in various functional neurological disorders increasingly support specific neurobiological dysfunction. However, to date, only one study has been reported on positron emission tomography (PET) in patients presenting with PNES.

Arthuis et al. [98] *reported sixteen patients being evaluated in a specialist epilepsy centre underwent PET with 2-deoxy-2-[fluorine-18] fluoro-d-glucose (18) FDG-PET) because of suspected intractable epileptic seizures. However, in all patients, the diagnosis was subsequently confirmed to be PNES with no coexisting epilepsy. (18) FDG-PET was also performed in 16 healthy controls. A voxel by voxel intergroup analysis was performed to look for significant differences in interictal (resting state) cerebral metabolism. In addition, metabolic connectivity was studied using voxel-wise inter-regional correlation analysis.*

They found that patients with PNES exhibited significant PET hypometabolism within the right inferior parietal and central region and within the bilateral anterior cingulate cortex. A significant increase in metabolic correlation was found in patients with PNES, in comparison to healthy participants, between the right inferior parietal/central region and the bilateral cerebellum and between the bilateral anterior cingulate cortex and the left parahippocampal gyrus. Although they cannot exclude that their data reflect changes due to comorbidities, they may indicate a dysfunction of neural systems in patients with PNES. Hypometabolism regions might relate to two of the pathophysiological mechanisms that may be involved in PNES, that is, emotional dysregulation (anterior cingulate hypometabolism) and dysfunctional processes underlying the consciousness of the self and the environment (right parietal hypometabolism) [97].

2.7. Treatment

The first treatment phase in PNES is patient engagement. Treatment is complex, requiring multidisciplinary care and patients, and their families must understand the diagnosis to comply with the recommendations of the psychiatric caregiver [49]. The next phase of treatment is acute interventions, and most research studies focus on short-term evidence-based interventions. It seems to be that the cognitive-behavioral therapy is supported by most of randomized controlled pilot trials. However, psychotherapeutic and psychopharmacological interventions have been less well-studied using controlled and uncontrolled trials [98].

Treatment of PNES varies and can include psychotherapy and use of adjunctive medications to treat coexisting anxiety or depression. Psychogenic symptoms are, by definition, a psychiatric disease, and a mental health professional should manage them. The main obstacle to effective treatment is effective delivery of the diagnosis. The physician delivering the diagnosis must be compassionate, remembering that most patients are not faking, but also firm and confident to avoid the use of ambiguous and confusing terms. Patients who accept their diagnosis and follow through with therapy are more likely to experience a successful outcome; therefore, patient education is critical and is the first step in treatment [49].

LaFrance Jr et al. [6] found that a cognitive behavior therapy-informed psychotherapy significantly reduces the seizures in patients with PNES.

> *"Cognitive behavioral therapy has evidence of efficacy, including one pilot randomized, controlled trial where cognitive behavioral therapy was compared with standard medical care. The antidepressant sertraline did not show a significant difference in event frequency change when compared to placebo in a pilot randomized, double-blind, controlled trial, but it did show a significant pre- versus post treatment decrease in the active arm."*
>
> *"Other interventions that have shown efficacy in uncontrolled trials include augmented psychodynamic interpersonal psychotherapy, group psychodynamic psychotherapy, group psycho education, and the antidepressant venlafaxine"* [6].

Some investigations done in 2010 and 2013 suggested serotonin selective reuptake inhibitors (SSRIs) and sertraline may be helpful in reducing seizures in PNES, respectively [49].

> *Carlson and Nicholson Perry* [99] *"evaluated and synthesized the available evidence from the previous 20 years regarding the utility of psychological interventions in the management of*

psychogenic non-epileptic seizures (PNES) and found that 82% of people with PNES who complete psychological treatment experience a reduction in seizures of at least 50%."

Hilmarsdóttir et al. [100] *"addressed the current research on psychotherapeutic treatment for PNES by discussing recent reviews and six randomized controlled trials (RCTs) on the subject and concluded that, larger well-designed randomized controlled trials are needed in order to support the evidence of psychological interventions for their patient group".*

Duncan et al. [101] *"reported that half of their patients informed being free of seizures following intervention. Being employed predicted good outcome, but the best predictor of being seizure free at 6 months was having an internal locus of control. This may be useful practically and requires further study".*

"No good predictors of long-term outcome were found, possibly because of loss to follow up. PNES may manifest themselves in very different ways and usually have complex root causes". Optimal treatment of persons experiencing PNES requires close cooperation between the neurologist and the psychiatrist [102].

The delivery of brief manualized psycho-educational intervention for PNES by health professionals with minimal training in psychological treatment was feasible. The intervention was associated with higher rates of PNES cessation than those observed in previous studies [103].

Some authors investigated whether initial adherence to treatment in PNES differed on the basis of mental health treatment modality and which subject characteristics were predictive of adherence. Initial adherence rates were 54% for combined treatment conducted in the same institution (integrated intervention) and 31% for psychotherapy and psychiatric management offered in different settings (divided intervention). Cognitive complaints and current exposure to antiepileptic drugs (AEDs) were more common among nonadherent patients, and being married (or having a live-in partner) was more common among adherent patients. A predictive model using the mentioned variables (intervention type, marital status, cognitive complaints, and concurrent use of AEDs) showed that this set of variables was predictive of adherence [104].

While PNES is treated by mental health professionals, continued involvement by a neurologist or epileptologist is associated with better outcomes, regardless of the limited direct care provided. Moreover, parents of children with PNES are expected to discuss the diagnosis with the pediatric epileptologist/neurologist, and this expectation should be respected [72].

Plioplys [105] *suggests that "professionals in epilepsy care that lack sufficient knowledge about PNES may be more likely to continue AEDs at a parent's request. These professionals may also be more likely to continue AEDs in order to facilitate acceptance of the diagnosis and/or to prevent a delay in psychological treatment. A clinician may be concerned that refusing a request to continue AED treatment will result in the family seeking out a clinician who would unquestioningly supply them with requested medicines, i.e. "doctor-shopping." This risk may be heightened if parents observe their child's non-epileptic episodes becoming worse. Parents may also wish to continue AEDs as a means to avoid social stigma associated with PNES, particularly at school".*

It is clear-cut defined that clinicians are under obligation to provide medical treatment deemed to be inappropriate or ineffective [106, 107]. Instead of continuing to prescribe AEDs, exploring the underlying reasons for why the parents want to continue AEDs despite the PNES diagnosis allows the physician to directly address parents' concerns regarding discontinuation. PNES patient and their relatives may turn to clinicians for advice regarding disclosure of PNES diagnosis to third-parties, including school nurses, school administrators, teachers, classmate, day care providers, and peers. The clinicians' obligation is to counsel patients and their parents on the conflicting values that are at stake: preserving the patient's and family's privacy, protecting the patient from social stigma and physical harms, and promoting continuity of therapeutic care.

Neurologist and epileptologist should educate the patient and their relatives that these values are not easily reconcilable and deciding whether to disclose the diagnosis involves an inherent trade-off, and the prognosis of these patients is still relatively poor, and a good outcome seems dependent on a young age at diagnosis, early diagnosis, less severe psychological comorbidities, and continued follow-up and management by the diagnosing neurologist, epileptologist, or clinician [8, 49, 105, 108–116].

The arguments for disclosing with both parents and child together would be primarily based on cultivating trust with patient and parents and between patient and parents through maximal transparency [72].

2.8. PNES vs. epileptic seizures

Impairment of consciousness and reduced self-control are key features of most psychogenic nonepileptic seizures (PNESs), although, compared with patients with epilepsy, those with PNESs demonstrate greater conscious awareness during their seizures.

> *Some authors* [117, 118] *"suggest that an understanding of conscious experiences and discrepancies between subjective impairment of consciousness and the lack of objectifiable neurobiological changes in PNESs may benefit from an examination of emotion processing, including understanding sensory, situational, and emotional triggers of PNESs; emotional and physiological changes during the attacks; and styles of emotional reactivity and regulatory capacity* [117] *reported allergies helps distinguish epilepsy from psychogenic nonepileptic seizures"* [118].

Psychopathology levels are elevated in patients with PNES and those with epilepsy. However, patients with PNES report higher rates of trauma and neglect, poorer health-related quality of life (HRQoL), and an increased prevalence of insecure attachment. In this study, patients with PNES reported higher levels of anxiety and depression and lower HRQoL than those with epilepsy. PNES: No significant correlations were found with HRQoL but depression correlated positively with attachment avoidance, attachment anxiety, and relationship conflict. Anxiety correlated positively with attachment avoidance, attachment anxiety, and relationship conflict, and negatively with relationship depth and support. Epilepsy: HRQoL correlated negatively with seizure severity, depression, anxiety, attachment avoidance, and attachment anxiety. Depression correlated positively with attachment avoidance, attachment anxiety, and relationship conflict. Anxiety correlated positively with seizure severity, attachment avoidance, and attachment anxiety. Correlations between measures of relationship quality and anxiety were stronger in patients with PNES versus those with epilepsy (zs = 2.66 to 2.97, $p < 0.004$). Attachment style and relationship quality explained larger amounts of variance in depression (45%) and anxiety (60%) in the patients with PNES than those with epilepsy (16 and 13%). In conclusion, levels of anxiety and depression were higher in patients with PNES than those with epilepsy. Interpersonal problems were much more closely associated with anxiety and depression in patients with PNES than those with epilepsy. The findings support the use of therapeutic interventions for PNES focusing on attachment and relationship issues [119].

Some investigations have attempted to compare patients affected by PNES to patients affected by functional motor symptoms from a demographic, clinical, and psychological perspective. Nevertheless, results are quite controversial, and significant conclusions have not been reached. Therefore, some authors evaluated the phenomenology of psychology of the two groups assessing levels of dissociation and its subcomponents, alexithymia and interceptive sensitivity in patients with PNES and in patients with FMS, and the investigation showed different psychological mechanisms underlying patients with PNES and patients with FMS [120].

> *Some authors* [121] *"studied eligible patients (n = 51) that were divided into those with PNES + ES (n = 24) and those with PNES alone (n = 27). The follow-up period was 4.8 ± 0.3 and 4.3 ± 0.3 years, respectively. Both groups had similar female predominance and similar age at admission to the vEEG unit. Time from PNES onset to hospitalization was longer in PNES patients compared to those with PNES + ES. The majority of subjects in each group reported a history of at least one major stressful life event. Opisthotonus was significantly more frequently observed in PNES patients, and they had more events during vEEG hospitalization. Psychogenic events ceased during the follow-up period in 22% of the PNES patients and in 58% of the PNES + EPI patients (P > 0.001)".*
>
> *Their results indicate that following vEEG-based diagnosis of PNES, the long-term outcome of PNES cessation may be more favorable for patients with concomitant epilepsy than for patients without epilepsy.*

Neuropsychological tests do not distinguish ES from PNES at the individual level. Clinical features that favor PNES are:

Fluctuating course.

Asynchronous movements (frontal lobe partial seizures excluded).

Pelvic thrusting (frontal lobe partial seizures excluded).

Side to side head or body movement (convulsive events only).

Closed eyes during the episode.

Long duration.

Other signs that can help are gradual onset, no stereotyped events, flailing or thrashing movements, opisthotonus "arc en cercle", tongue biting, urinary incontinence, and "swoon" type events should raise suspicion of PNES if prolonged over a minute, atonic ESs are much shorter and typically occur in the epilepsies with other seizure types, for example, Lennox–Gastaut syndrome.

Signs that favor ES.

Occurrence from EEG-confirmed sleep.

Postictal confusion.

Stertorous breathing.

Occurrence during sleep only (*EEG-confirmed sleep).*

2.9. Associated minor or major injuries

Ictal injuries in PNES have been reported previously and history of any minor (e.g., tongue biting, bruises, and lacerations) or major (e.g., burns and fractures) physical injuries associated with their seizures, since their disease started is well known. In our region, one of the most common type of reported injury was burning lesions that happened in patients fitting close to the fire used to heat the room apart from tongue biting, lacerations, bruises, limb fractures, and dental injury. Therefore, PNES is also associated with physical injuries. Despite the shibboleth that injuries rarely occur during PNES, mild injuries commonly happen and even severe injuries such as fractures and burns are not uncommonly reported in these patients. *Patients with more dramatic seizure manifestations (e.g., urinary incontinence) were more likely to report ictal injuries* [121].

Tongue biting (TB) may occur both in seizures and in PNES. A systematic review to determine sensitivity, specificity, and likelihood ratios (LR) of TB was done.

> *"Five studies (222 epilepsy patients and 181 subjects with PNES) were included. There was a statistically significant higher prevalence of TB (both without further specifications on site of lesions and lateral TB) in patients with seizures. Pooled accuracy measures of TB (no further specifications) were sensitivity 38%, specificity 75%, pLR 1.479 (95% CI 1.117-1.957), and nLR 0.837 (95% CI 0.736-0.951). Pooled measures of lateral TB were sensitivity 22%, specificity 100%, pLR 21.386 (95% CI 1.325-345.169), and nLR 0.785 (95% CI 0.705-0.875). Only a pooled analysis of data demonstrated a statistically significant pLR for lateral TB. Lateral TB but not 'any' TB has diagnostic significance in distinguishing seizures from PNES, supporting the diagnosis of seizures. Tongue biting without further specifications has, therefore, no value in the differential diagnosis between seizures and PNES"* [122].

3. Ethics

> *Currently, only a very narrow window of ethical dilemmas in PNES has been explored.*
>
> *Numerous distinct ethical dilemmas arise in diagnosing and treating pediatric and adolescent patients with PNES. Important ethical values at stake include trust, transparency, confidentiality, professionalism, autonomy of all stakeholders and justice* [122].

In 2003, we had not video-EEG facilities and then a procedure to provoke and to distinguish PNES from ES in our setting is introduced. At that time, we got IRB number, an approval by the Ethical Advisory Board (A0;012-2000) and written informed consent from selected patients. However, today, we have no doubt that it was a nonethical procedure, and in spite of that we did not afford any problem, we deeply regret about that procedure.

Confirming a PNES diagnosis and disclosure this information to the child, parents and other interested people build up a special challenge related to the values of justice professionalism, human resource utilization, and trust for health care providers in relation to patients, families, and other colleagues. The preservation of an adequate therapeutic relationship plays strongly in the values at stake. Most of neurologists felt confident about discontinuing the medical treatment when diagnosis of PNES is confirmed, but ethical dilemma arises when the prescribing clinician faces is discontinuing AEDs in a timely manner without losing the trust and confidence of the patient and/or the patient's relatives. Sometimes some patients and relatives decide to seek for a second medical opinion and we have to respect that.

Elements often taken into account during ethical dilemmas include the patient and family's treatment preferences, developmental stage, psychosocial background, quality of life, applicable laws, institutional policies, professional duties, and other practical stakeholder obligations and responsibilities. Even the most skilled attending doctor struggles with ethical dilemmas that arise during diagnosis and management of PNES patients. These relationships coupled with the uncertainty and stigma surrounding PNES result in complex dilemmas for treating clinicians. Significant mental health, social, and community resources are frequently necessary to effectively treat this patient population, but these resources are scarce. To ensure a successful management of PNES, all ethical values should be taken in to consideration from the first clinic [122–126].

Acknowledgements

We would like to thanks to Prof. Olivier Wenker, CEO of Internet Journal of Publications to granted permission for including in this chapter some figures and tables published online by the before-mentioned editorial house.

Parts of this chapter are taken from the authors' former work. In this regards we also want to acknowledge to following sources:

1. Foyaca-Sibat and Ibañez-Valdés [13].

2. Cole et al. [123].

3. Benbadis [49].

One of the article was published by IJN and co-authored by Prof. H Foyaca who is also an Editor-in-Chief of the IJN. The other two sources were properly cited in the body of this chapter and the reference list. We also declare that we have not conflict of interest.

Author details

Lourdes de Fátima Ibañez-Valdés* and Humberto Foyaca-Sibat

*Address all correspondence to: lourdesfibanezvaldes@gmail.com

Department of Neurology, Nelson Mandela Academic Central Hospital, Walter Sisulu University, Mthatha, South Africa

References

[1] Foyaca-Sibat H, Ibañez-Valdés LdeF. Neurocysticercosis in HIV-positive patients. The Internet Journal of Infectious Diseases. 2003:**2**(2):15-23. Available from: http://www.ispub.com/ostia/index.php?xmlFilePath=journals/ijn/current.xml

[2] Sibat HF, Ibañez Valdés LdeF. Uncommon clinical manifestations of cysticercosis. In: Sibat HF, editor. Novel Aspects on Cysticercosis and Neurocysticercosis. InTech; 2013. DOI: 10.5772/53078. Available from: http://www.intechopen.com/books/novel-aspects-on-cysticercosis-and-neurocysticercosis/uncommon-clinical-manifestations-of-cysticercosis

[3] Hingray C, Biberon J, El-Hage W, de Toffol B. Psychogenic non-epileptic seizures (PNES).Revue Neurologique (Paris). Apr–May 2016;**172**(4–5):263-269. DOI: 10.1016/j.neurol.2015.12.011 [Epub Apr 23, 2016]

[4] Brown R, Markus R. Psychogenic Non-epileptic Seizures. Available from: https//www.ncbi.nlm.nih.gov/pubmed/27084446 [Accessed: Mar 3, 2017]

[5] Kanaan R, Duncan R, Goldstein L, Jankovic J, Cavanna A. Are Psychogenic Non-epileptic Seizures Just Another Symptom of Conversion Disorder? DOI: http://dx.doi.org/10.1136/jnnp-2017-315639 [Accessed: Mar 3, 2017]

[6] LaFrance Jr WC, Baker GA, Duncan R, Goldstein LH, Reuber M. Minimum requirements for the diagnosis of psychogenic nonepileptic seizures: A staged approach: A report from the international league against epilepsy nonepileptic seizures task force. Epilepsia. 2013;**54**(11):2005-2018. DOI: http://dx.doi.org/10.1111/epi.12356

[7] Baslet G, Dworetzky B, Perez DL, Oser M. Treatment of psychogenic nonepileptic seizures: Updated review and findings from a mindfulness-based intervention case series. Clinical EEG and Neuroscience. Jan 2015;**46**(1):54-64. DOI: 10.1177/1550059414557025 [Epub Dec, 2014]

[8] Baslet G. Psychogenic nonepileptic seizures: A treatment review. What have we learned since the beginning of the millennium?. Neuropsychiatric Disease and Treatment. 2012; **8**:585-598. DOI: 10.2147/NDT.S32301. [Epub Dec 10, 2012]

[9] Gul A, Ahmad H. Cognitive deficits and emotion regulation strategies in patients with psychogenic nonepileptic seizures: A Task-switching study.Epilepsy & Behavior. Mar 2014;**32**:108-113. DOI: 10.1016/j.yebeh.2014.01.015. [Epub Feb 13, 2014]

[10] Robbins NM, Larimer P, Bourgeois JA, Lowenstein DH. Number of patient-reported allergies helps distinguish epilepsy from psychogenic nonepileptic seizures. Epilepsy & Behavior Feb 2016;**55**:174-177. DOI: 10.1016/j.yebeh.2015.12.022. [Epub Feb 1, 2016]

[11] Marsh P, Benbadis S, Fernandez F. Psychogenic nonepileptic seizures: Ways to win over skeptical patients. Current Psychiatry. Jan 2008;**7**(1):21-34

[12] Beghi M, Negrini P, Perin C, Peroni F, Magaudda A, Cerri C, Cornaggia CM. Psychogenic Non-epileptic Seizures: So-called Psychiatric Comorbidity and Underlying Defense Mechanisms. Available from: https//www.ncbi.nlm.nih.gov/pubmed/4594147 [Accessed: Mar 5, 2017]

[13] Foyaca-Sibat H, Ibañez-Valdés L. Pseudoseizures and epilepsy in neurocysiticercosis: Some advice for family doctors. The Internet Journal of Neurology. 2003;**2**(2):27-33. Available from: https://ispub.com/IJN/2/2/3786 [Accessed: Mar 6, 2017]

[14] Bowman ES. Pseudoseizure. The Psychiatric Clinics of North America. 1968;**21**(3):649-657

[15] Bowman E, Markand O. The contribution of life events to pseudoseizure occurrence in adults. Bulletin of the Menninger Clinic. 1999;**63**(1):70-88

[16] Bowman ES, Coons PM. The differential diagnosis of epilepsy, pseudoseizures, dissociative identity disorder, and dissociative disorder not otherwise specified. Bulletin of the Menninger Clinic. 2000;**64**(2):164-180

[17] Fleisher W, Staley D, Krawetz P, Pillay N, Arnett JL, Maher J. Comparative study of trauma-related phenomena in subjects with pseudoseizures and subjects with epilepsy. The American Journal of Psychiatry. 2002;**159**(4):660-663

[18] Harden CL. Pseudoseizures and dissociative disorders: A common mechanism involving traumatic experiences. Seizure. 1997;**6**(2):151-155

[19] Foyaca-Sibat H, Ibañez-Valdés LdeF. Treatment of epilepsy secondary to neurocysticercosis. In: Foyaca-Sibat H, editor. Novel Treatment of Epilepsy. InTech; 2011. DOI: 10.5772/31465. Available from: http://www.intechopen.com/books/novel-treatment-of-epilepsy/treatment-of-epilepsy-secondary-to-neurocysticercosis

[20] Foyaca SH, Ibañez Valdés LdeF. Clinical trial of praziquantel and prednisone in rural patients with neurocysticercosis presenting recurrent epileptic attacks. The Internet Journal of Neurology. 2002;**1**(2):19-24. Available from: http://www.ispub.com/ostia/index.php?xmlFilePath=Journals/ijn/vol1n2/ncc.xml [Accessed: Mar 3, 2017]

[21] Foyaca-Sibat H, Ibañez Valdés LdeF. Clinical features of epilepsy secondary to neurocysticercosis at the insular lobe. In: Foyaca-Sibat H, editor. Novel Aspects on Epilepsy. InTech; 2011. DOI: 10.5772/19476. Available from: http://www.intechopen.com/books/novel-aspects-on-epilepsy/clinical-features-of-epilepsy-secondary-to-neurocysticercosis-at-the-insular-lobe

[22] Foyaca Sibat H, Ibañez Valdés LdeF. Introduction to cysticercosis and its historical background. In: Foyaca Sibat H, editor. Novel Aspects on Cysticercosis and Neurocysticercosis. InTech; 2013. DOI: 10.5772/50318. Available from: http://www.intechopen.com/books/novel-aspects-on-cysticercosis-and-neurocysticercosis/introduction-to-cysticercosis-and-its-historical-background

[23] Foyaca SH, Ibanez-Valdes LdeF. Intraventricular neurocysticercosis in HIV positive patients. The Internet Journal of Neurology. 2003;**2**(1):37-42. Available from: http://www.ispub.com/ostia/index.php?xmlFilePath=journals/ijn/vol2n1/ncc.xml [Accessed: Mar 7, 2017]

[24] Foyaca SH, Ibanez-Valdes LdeF. Vascular dementia type Binswanger's disease in patients with active neurocysticercosis. Electronic Journal of Biomedicine. 2002;**1**(1):1-12. Available from: http://www.uninet.edu/biomed/rebio/reb/2002/n1/foyaca.html [Accessed: Mar 7, 2017]

[25] Foyaca Sibat H, Ibañez Valdés LdeF. What is a low frequency of the disseminated cysticercosis suggests that neurocysticercosis is going to disappear? In: Foyaca Sibat H, editor. Novel Aspects on Cysticercosis and Neurocysticercosis. InTech; 2013. DOI: 10.5772/51395. Available from: http://www.intechopen.com/books/novel-aspects-on-cysticercosis-and-neurocysticercosis/what-is-a-low-frequency-of-the-disseminated-cysticercosis-suggests-that-neurocysticercosis-is-going-to-disappear?

[26] Foyaca-Sibat H. Epilepsy secondary to parasitic zoonoses of the brain. In: Foyaca-Sibat H, editor. Novel Aspects on Epilepsy. InTech; 2011. DOI: 10.5772/31463. Available from: http://www.intechopen.com/books/novel-aspects-on-epilepsy/epilepsy-secondary-to-parasitic-zoonoses-of-the-brain

[27] Foyaca-Sibat H, Del Rio AR, Ibañez-Valdés LdeF, Vega-Novoa EC, Awotedu A. Neuroepidemiological survey for Epilepsy and knowledge about neurocysticercosis at Sidwadweni location, South Africa. Electronic Journal of Biomedicine. 2004;**2**(1):40-48 Available from: http://www.biomed.edu/2004/n1/foyaca.html

[28] Foyaca Sibat H, Salazar Campos MC, Ibañez Valdés LdeF. Orbital cysticercosis. a challenger for neurologists, ophthalmologists, neuro-ophthalmologists, and general practitioners. In: Foyaca Sibat H, editor. Novel Aspects on Cysticercosis and Neurocysticercosis. InTech; 2013. DOI: 10.5772/52515. Available from: http://www.intechopen.com/books/novel-aspects-on-cysticercosis-and-neurocysticercosis/orbital-cisticercosis-a-challenger-for-neurologists-ophthalmologists-neuro-opthalmologists-and-general-practitioner

[29] Foyaca-Sibat H, Del Rio-Romero AH, Ibañez-Valdés LdeF, Vega-Novoa E. Neuroepidemiological survey for epilepsy and knowledge about neurocysticercosis at Ngqwala Location, South Africa. The Internet Journal of Neurology. 2005;**3**(2):11-16. Available from: http://www.ispub.com/journal/the_internet_journal_of_neurology/volume_3_number_2_31/article/neuroepidemiological_survey_for_epilepsy_and_knowledge_about_neurocysticiercosis_at_ngqwala_location_south_africa.html [Accessed: Mar 7, 2017]

[30] Foyaca-Sibat H, Del Rio-Romero AH, Ibañez-Valdés LdeF. Neuroepidemiological survey for epilepsy and knowledge about neurocysticercosis at Tsolo Location, South Africa. The Internet Journal of Neurology. 2005;**3**(3):41-44. Available from: http://www.ispub.com/

journal/the_internet_journal_of_neurology/volume_3_number_2_31/article/neuroepidemiological_survey_for_epilepsy_and_knowledge_about_neurocysticiercosis_at_tsolo_location_south_africa.html [Accessed: Mar 7, 2017]

[31] Foyaca-Sibat H, Del Rio-Romero AH, Ibañez-Valdés LdeF. Prevalence of epilepsy and general knowledge about neurocysticercosis at Ngangelizwe Location, South Africa. The Internet Journal of Neurology. 2005;**4**(1):30-36. [cited Mar 7, 2017]. Available from: http://www.ispub.com/journal/the_internet_journal_of_neurology/volume_4_number_1_30/article/prevalence_of_epilepsy_and_general_knowledge_about_neurocysticercosis_at_ngangelizwe_location_south_africa.html [Accessed: 2017-March-10]

[32] Del Rio A, Foyaca-Sibat H, Ibañez-Valdés LdeF. Epidemiological survey about socio-economic characteristic of Mpindweni Location, South Africa. The Internet Journal of Neurology. 2005;**4**(2):18-26. [cited Mar 10, 2017]. Available from: http://www.ispub.com/journal/the_internet_journal_of_neurology/volume_4_number_2_27/article/epidemiological_survey_about_socio_economic_characteristic_of_mpindweni_location_south_africa.html [Accessed: Mar 2017, 10]

[33] Ibañez-Valdés LdeF, Foyaca-Sibat H. Refractory epilepsy in neurocysticercosis. The Internet Journal of Neurology. 2006;**5**(2):34-41. Available from: http://www.ispub.com/journal/the_internet_journal_of_neurology/volume_5_number_2_19/article/refractory_epilepsy_in_neurocysticercosis.html [Accessed: Mar 10, 2017]

[34] Foyaca-Sibat H Ibañez-Valdés LdeF. Insular neurocysticercosis: Our finding and review of the medical literature. The Internet Journal of Neurology. 2006;**5**(2):31-35. Available from: http://www.ispub.com/journal/the_internet_journal_of_neurology/volume_5_number_2_19/article/insular_neurocysticercosis_our_findings_and_review_of_the_medical_literature.html [Accessed: Mar 10, 2017]

[35] Foyaca-Sibat H, Ibañez-Valdés LdeF, Del Rio IA. Prevalence of epilepsy and general knowledge about neurocysticercosis at Ngangelizwe Location, South Africa. The Internet Journal of Neurology. 2005;**4**(1):23-37 [cited Mar 10, 2017]. Available from: http://www.ispub.com/journal/the_internet_journal_of_neurology/volume_4_number_1_30/article/prevalence_of_epilepsy_and_general_knowledge_about_neurocysticercosis_at_ngangelizwe_location_south_africa.html [Accessed: 2017-March-10]

[36] Del Rio AR, Foyaca-Sibat H, Ibañez-Valdés LdeF: Neuroepidemiological Survey For Epilepsy, Knowledge About Epilepsy, Neurocysticercosis And HIV/Aids At The Makaula Village In South Africa. The Internet Journal of Neurology. 2007;**7**(3):41-49. ISSN: 1531-295X. Available from: http://www.ispub.com/journal/the_internet_journal_of_neurology/volume_7_number_2_5/article/neuroepidemiological_survey_for_epilepsy_knowledge_about_epilepsy_neurocysticercosis_and_hiv_aids_at_the_makaula_village_in_south_africa.html [Accessed: Mar 10, 2017]

[37] Del Rio-Romero AI, Foyaca-Sibat H, Ibañez-Valdés LdeF. Neuroepidemiology findings as contributors for epilepsy due to neurocysticercosis at Mngceleni Location, South Africa. The Internet Journal of Neurology. 2008;**9**(1):33-40. ISSN: 1531-295X. Available form: http://www.ispub.com/journal/the_internet_journal_of_neurology/volume_9_number_1_6/article/

neuroepidemiology_findings_as_contributors_for_epilepsy_due_to_neurocysticercosis_at_mngceleni_location_south_africa.html [Accessed: Mar 12, 2017]

[38] Foyaca-Sibat H, Ibañez-Valdés LdeF, Moré-Rodríguez J. Parasitic zoonoses of the brain: Another challenger? The Internet Journal of Neurology. 2010;**12**(2):9-14. Available from: http://www.ispub.com/journal/the_internet_journal_of_neurology/volume_12_number_2_4/article/parasitic-zoonoses-of-the-brain-another-challenger.html [Accessed: Mar 12, 2017]

[39] Foyaca Sibat H, Ibañez Valdés LdeF. Chapter V: Treatment of epilepsy secondary to neurocysticercosis. In: Foyaca Sibat H, editor. Treatment Approach to Epilepsy. Text Book I. Rijeka: InTech Open Access; 2011. pp. 213-236. ISBN: 978-953-307-887-6. Available from: http://www.intechweb.org/

[40] Foyaca Sibat H, Ibañez Valdés LdeF. Chapter III: Clinical features of Epilepsy Secondary to Neurocysticercosis at the Insular Lobe. In: Foyaca Sibat H, editor. Novel Aspect on Epilepsy. Text Book II. Rijeka: InTech Open Access; Jun 2011. pp. 173-193. ISBN: 978-953-307-678-2. Available from: http://www.intechweb.org/ [Accessed: Mar 15, 2017]

[41] Ashkenazi A, Kaufman Y, Ben-Hur T. Bilateral focal motor status epilepticus with retained consciousness after stroke. Neurology. 2000;**54**(4):976-978

[42] Kamaşak T, Türedi S, Serin HM, Menteşe A, Gündüz A, Alver A, Cansu A. Can ischemia-modified albumin be used to differentiate between generalized seizures and pseudoseizures? Turkish Journal Of Medical Sciences Feb 27 2017;**47**(1):282-286. DOI: 10.3906/sag-1504-105

[43] Griffith JL, Polles A, Griffith ME. Pseudoseizures, families, and unspeakable dilemmas. Psychosomatics. 1998;**39**(2):144-153

[44] Nemiah JC. Dissociation, conversion and somatization. In: Tasman A, Goldinger SM, editors. American Psychiatry Press Review of Psychiatry. Washington, DC: American Psychiatric Press; 1991;**10**:248-260

[45] Gunatilake SB, De Silva HJ, Ranasinghe G. Twenty-seven venous cutdowns to treat pseudostatus epilepticus. Seizure. Feb 1997;**6**(1):71-72

[46] Benbadis SR, Stern E, Frith C, Cahill C, Holmes A, Grootoonk S, Seanward J, Mckenna P, Chua SE, et al. A functional neuroanatomy of hallucinations in schizophrenia. Nature. 1995;**378**:176-179

[47] Rosenbaum M. Why women? Psychosomatics. 2000;**41**:147-149

[48] Burack JH, Back AL. Provoking nonepileptic seizures: The ethic of deceptive diagnostic testing. Hasting Center Report. 1997;**27**(4):24-34

[49] Benbadis S. Psychogenic Nonepileptic Seizures. 2016. Available form: http://emedicine.medscape.com/article/1184694-workup#c9 [Accessed: Mar 14, 2017]

[50] Brigo F, Igwe SC, Ausserer H, Nardone R, Tezzon F, Bongiovanni LG, Tinazzi M, Trinka E. Terminology of psychogenic nonepileptic seizures. Epilepsia Mar 2015;**56**(3):e21-e25. DOI: 10.1111/epi.12911. [Epub Jan 29, 2015]

[51] Baslet G, Seshadri A, Bermeo-Ovalle A, Willment K, Myers L.Psychogenic non-epileptic seizures: An updated primer. Psychosomatics Jan–Feb, 2016;**57**(1):1-17. DOI: 10.1016/j.psym.2015.10.004. [Epub Oct 22, 2015]

[52] Perez DL, Dworetzky BA, Dickerson BC, Leung L, Cohn R, Baslet G, Silbersweig DA. An integrative neurocircuit perspective on psychogenic non-epileptic seizures and functional movement disorders: Neural Functional Unawareness. 2014;**22**:23-34

[53] Yates E. Psychogenic non-epileptic seizures in the older adult. Journal of Psychosocial Nursing and Mental Health Services. May 2014;**52**(5):17-20. DOI: 10.3928/02793695-20140423-01

[54] Nguyen ML, Shapiro MA, Demetree JM, White KA. When non-epileptic seizures fool the experts. International Journal of Psychiatry in Medicine. 2011;**42**(3):331-338

[55] Gates JR. Epidemiology and classification of non-epileptic events. In: Gates JR, Rowan AJ, editors. Non-epileptic Seizures. 2th ed. Boston: Butterworth-Heinemann; 2000. pp. 3-14

[56] Kerr AL et al. Minimum requirements for the diagnosis of psychogenic nonepileptic seizures: A staged approach Epilepsia,2013;**54**(11):2005-2018

[57] Asadi-Pooya AA, Emami M, Emami Y. Gender differences in manifestations of psychogenic non-epileptic seizures in Iran. Journal of the Neurological Sciences Sep 15, 2013; **332**(1–2):66-68. DOI: 10.1016/j.jns.2013.06.016. [Epub Jun 30, 2013]

[58] Gale SD, Hill SW, Pearson C. Seizure semiology in males with psychogenic nonepileptic seizures is associated with somatic complaints. Epilepsy Research Sep 2015;**115**:153-157. DOI: 10.1016/j.eplepsyres.2015.06.011. [Epub Jun 21, 2015]

[59] De Paola L, Marchetti RL, Ghizoni Teive HA, Curt LaFrance WC. Psychogenic nonepileptic seizures and psychogenic movement disorders: Two sides of the same coin? Arquivos de Neuro-Psiquiatria. 2014;**72**(10):x-x. DOI: http://dx.doi.org/10.1590/0004-282X20140111

[60] Benbadis SR, Hauser AW. An estimate of the prevalence of psychogenic non-epileptic seizures. Seizure. 2000;**9**(4):280-281. DOI: http://dx.doi.org/10.1053/seiz.2000.0409

[61] Rowan AJ. An introduction to current practice in the diagnosis of non-epileptic seizures. In: Gates JR, Rowan AJ, editors. Non-epileptic Seizures. Boston: Butteworth-Heinemann; 1993. pp. 1-8

[62] LaFrance Jr WC, Bjornaes H. Designing treatment plans based on etiology of psychogenic nonepileptic seizures. In: Schachter SC, LaFrance Jr WC, editors. Gates & Rowan's Nonepileptic Seizures. 3rd ed. New York: Cambridge University Press; 2010. pp. 266-280

[63] Reuber M, Pukrop R, Bauer J, Helmstaedter C, Tessendorf N, Elger CE. Outcome in psychogenic nonepileptic seizures: 1 to 10-year follow-up in 164 patients. Annals of Neurology. 2003;**53**(3):305-311. DOI: http://dx.doi.org/10.1002/ana.3000

[64] Brown RJ, Syed TU, Benbadis S, LaFrance Jr WC, Reuber M. Psychogenic nonepileptic seizures. Epilepsy & Behavior. 2011;**22**(1):85-93. DOI: http://dx.doi.org/10.1016/j.yebeh.2011.02.016

[65] Duncan R, Razvi S, Mulhern S. Psychogenic non-epileptic seizures. Epilepsy & Behavior. Feb 2011;**20**(2):308-311

[66] Doss RC, LaFrance Jr WC. Psychogenic non-epileptic seizures. Epileptic Disorders. Dec 1, 2016;**18**(4):337-343. DOI: 10.1684/epd.2016.0873

[67] Chen LPMurad H, ParasColbenson BSK, Sattler AL, Goranson EN, et al. Sexual abuse and lifetime diagnosis of psychiatric disorders: Systematic review and meta-analysis. Mayo Clinic Proceedings Jul 2010;**85**(7):618-629. DOI: http://dx.doi.org/10.4065/mcp.2009.0583

[68] Bernadett S, Zoltán H. Psychogenic Nonepileptic Seizures: Overview and Implications for Practice. Oct 2016. Available from: https//www.ncbi.nlm.nih.gov/pubmed/27156524 [Accessed: Mar 12, 2017]

[69] Heyer GL, Dara V F, Weber A, Gedela S, Vidaurre J. Comparison of Semiologies between Tilt-induced Psychogenic Nonsyncopal Collapse and Psychogenic Nonepileptic Seizures. Nov 2014. Available from: https//www.ncbi.nlm.nih.gov/pubmed/27486953 [Accessed: Mar 16, 2017]

[70] Takasaki K, Diaz Stransky A, Miller G. Psychogenic nonepileptic seizures: Diagnosis, management, and bioethics. Pediatric Neurology. Sep 2016;**62**:3-8. DOI: 10.1016/j.pediatrneurol.2016.04.011 [Epub Apr 27, 2016]

[71] Pretorius C. Barriers and facilitators to reaching a diagnosis of PNES from the patients' perspective: Preliminary findings. Seizure. May 2016;**38**:1-6. DOI: 10.1016/j.seizure.2016.03.007 [Epub Mar 24, 2016]

[72] Reilly C, Menlove L, Fenton V, Das KB. Psychogenic nonepileptic seizures in children: A review. Epilepsia Oct 2013;**54**(10):1715-1724. DOI: 10.1111/epi.12336. [Epub Aug 14, 2013]

[73] Elliott JO, Charyton C. Biopsychosocial predictors of psychogenic non-epileptic seizures. Epilepsy Research. Nov 2014;**108**(9):1543-1553. DOI: 10.1016/j.eplepsyres.2014.09.003. [Epub Sep 16, 2014]

[74] Patel H, Dunn DW, Austin JK, Doss JL, LaFrance Jr WC, Plioplys S, Caplan R. Psychogenic nonepileptic seizures (pseudoseizures). Pediatrics in Review. Jun 2011;**32**(6):e66-e72. DOI: 10.1542/pir.32-6-e66

[75] Reinsberger C, Sarkis R, Papadelis C, Doshi C, Perez DL, Baslet G, Loddenkemper T, Dworetzky BA. Autonomic Changes in Psychogenic Nonepileptic Seizures: Toward a Potential Diagnostic Biomarker? Mar 2016. Available from: https//www.ncbi.nlm.nih.gov/pubmed/25780264 [Accessed: Mar 17, 2017]

[76] Jeppesen J, Beniczky S, Johansen P, Sidenius P, Fuglsang-Frederiksen A. Comparing maximum autonomic activity of psychogenic non-epileptic seizures and epileptic seizures using heart rate variability. Seizure. Apr 2016;**37**:13-19. DOI: 10.1016/j.seizure.2016.02.005 [Epub Feb 15, 2016]

[77] LaFrance Jr WC. Psychogenic nonepileptic "seizures" or "attacks"? It's not just semantics: seizures. Neurology. 2010;**75**(1):87-88

[78] Blumberg J, Fernández IS, Vendrame M, Oehl B, Tatum WO, et al. Dacrystic seizures: Demographic, semiologic, and etiologic insights from a multicenter study in long-term video-EEG monitoring units. Epilepsia. 2012;**53**:1810-1819

[79] Teche SP, Laporte P, Medeiros F, Bragatti JA, Gomes F. Dacrystic seizures and psychogenic non-epileptic seizures: A case report. Journal of Neurological Disorders. 2015;**3**: 249. DOI: 10.4172/2329-6895.1000249

[80] Noe KH ,Grade M, Stonnington CM, Driver-Dunckley E, Locke DE. Confirming psychogenic nonepileptic seizures with video-EEG: Sex matters. Epilepsy & Behavior 2012 Mar; **23**(3):220-223. DOI: 10.1016/j.yebeh.2011.12.015. [Epub Feb 15, 2012]

[81] Jedrzejczak J, Owczarek K, Majkowski J. Psychogenic Pseudoepileptic Seizures: Clinical and Electroencephalogram (EEG) Video-tape Recordings.1999. Available form: https// www.ncbi.nlm.nih.gov/pubmed/10362902 [Accessed: Mar 17, 2017]

[82] Noe KH, Grade M, Stonnington CM, Driver-Dunckley E, Locke DEC. Confirming Psychogenic Nonepileptic Seizures with Video-EEG: Sex Matters. Nov 2014. Available form: https//www.ncbi.nlm.nih.gov/pubmed/22341181 [Accessed: Mar 17, 2017]

[83] Hubsch H et al. An integrative neurocircuit perspective on psychogenic nonepileptic seizures and functional movement disorders: Neural functional unawareness. Clinical EEG and Neuroscience. 2015;**46**:4-15. DOI: 10.1177/1550059414555905

[84] Devinsky O, Fisher R. Ethical use of placebos and provocative testing in diagnosis nonepileptic seizures. Neurology. 1996;**47**(4):866-870

[85] Stagno SJ, Smith ML. Use of induction procedures in diagnosing psychogenic seizures. Journal of Epilepsy. 1996;**9**(3):153-158

[86] Burak JH, Back AL, Pearlman RA. Provoking nonepileptic seizures: The ethics of deceptive diagnostic testing. The Hastings Center Report. 1997;**27**(4):24-33

[87] Stagno SJ, Smith ML. The use of placebo in diagnosing psychogenic seizures: Who is being deceived? Seminars in Neurology. 1997;**17**(3):213-218

[88] Benbadis S. Provactive techniques should be used for the diagnosis of psychogenic nonepileptic seizures. Archives of Neurology. 2001;**58**(1):2063-2065

[89] Smith ML, Stagno SJ, Dolske M, et al. Induction procedures for psychogenic seizures: Ethical and clinical considerations. The Journal of Clinical Ethics. 1997;**8**(3):217-229

[90] Leeman BA. Provocative techniques should not be used for the diagnosis of psychogenic nonepileptic seizures. Epilepsy & Behavior. 2009;**15**(2):110-114

[91] Gates JR. Provocative testing should not be used for nonepileptic seizures. Archives of Neurology. 2001;**58**(12):2065-2066

[92] McGonigal A, Russell A, Oto M, Duncan R. Use of suggestion methods to induce psychogenic non-epileptic seizures. Seizure. Nov 2015;**32**:47-48. DOI: 10.1016/j.seizure.2015.09.004. [Epub Sep 16, 2015]

[93] Labate WW et al. Psychogenic seizures and psychogenic movement disorders: Are they the same patients? Epilepsy & Behavior. 2012;**25**:666-669. DOI: 10.1016/j.yebeh.2012.10.007

[94] van der Kruijs L et al. Are psychogenic non-epileptic seizures and psychogenic movement disorders two different entities? When even neurologists stop talking to each other. Epilepsy & Behavior. 2013;**26**(1):100. DOI: 10.1016/j.yebeh.2012.07.024

[95] Ding P et al. Emotional dysregulation, alexithymia, and attachment in psychogenic nonepileptic seizures. Epilepsy & Behavior. 2013;**29**:178-183. DOI: 10.1016/j.yebeh.2013.07.019

[96] Perez DL, Dworetzky BA, Dickerson BC, Leung L, Cohn R, Baslet G, Silbersweig DA. An integrative neurocircuit perspective on psychogenic non-epileptic seizures and functional movement disorders: Neural functional unawareness. Epilepsia. 2013;**54**(Suppl 1): 53-67. DOI: 10.1111/epi.12106

[97] Li R, Liu K, Ma X, Li Z, Duan X, An D, Gong Q, Zhou D, Chen H. Altered Functional Connectivity Patterns of the Insular Subregions in Psychogenic Nonepileptic Seizures. Aug 2015. Available from: https//www.ncbi.nlm.nih.gov/pubmed/25352166 [Accessed: Mar 19, 2017]

[98] Arthuis M, Micoulaud-Franchi JA, Bartolomei F, McGonigal A, Guedj E. Resting cortical PET metabolic changes in psychogenic non-epileptic seizures (PNES). Journal of Neurology, Neurosurgery, and Psychiatry. Oct 2015;**86**(10):1106-1112. DOI; 10.1136/jnnp-2014-309390. [Epub Dec 2, 2014]

[99] Carlson P, Nicholson Perry K. Psychological interventions for psychogenic non-epileptic seizures: A meta-analysis. Seizure. Feb 2017;**45**:142-150. DOI: 10.1016/j.seizure.2016.12.007. [Epub Dec 21, 2016]

[100] Hilmarsdóttir D, Birk S, Rask CU. Psychotherapeutic treatment of psychogenic non-epileptic seizures. Ugeskr Laeger. Nov 28, 2016;**178**(48):14-18. pii: V04160303

[101] Duncan R, Anderson J, Cullen B, Meldrum S. Predictors of 6-month and 3-year outcomes after psychological intervention for psychogenic non-epileptic seizures. Seizure. Mar 2016;**36**:22-26. DOI: 10.1016/j.seizure.2015.12.016 [Epub Feb 3, 2016]

[102] Tuft M, Karterud HN, Villagran A, Nakken KO.Treatment for psychogenic non-epileptic seizures. Tidsskrift for den Norske Lægeforening. Sep 8, 2015;**135**(16):1449-1451. DOI: 10.4045/tidsskr.14.1361. eCollection 2015

[103] Mayor R, Brown RJ, Cock H, House A, Howlett S, Smith P, Reuber M. A feasibility study of a brief psycho-educational intervention for psychogenic nonepileptic seizures. Seizure. Nov 2013;**22**(9):760-765. DOI: 10.1016/j.seizure.2013.06.008. [Epub Aug 2, 2013]

[104] Baslet G, Prensky E. Initial treatment retention in psychogenic non-epileptic seizures. The Journal of Neuropsychiatry and Clinical Neurosciences. Winter 2013;**25**(1):63-67. DOI: 10.1176/appi.neuropsych.11090223

[105] Plioplys S, Siddarth P, Asato MR, Caplan R. Clinicians' views on antiepileptic medication management in nonepileptic seizures. Journal of Child Neurology Jun 2014;**29**(6): 746-750. DOI: 10.1177/0883073813488679. [Epub May 10, 2013]

[106] American Medical Association Code of Medical Ethics. Opinion 2.035 Futile Care [Internet]. 1994. [cited Feb 22, 2014]. Available from: http://www.ama-assn.org/ama/pub/physician-resources/medical-ethics/code-medical-ethics/opinion2035.page? [Accessed: Mar 19, 2017]

[107] American Medical Association Code of Medical Ethics. Opinion 8.20 Invalid Treatment [Internet]. 1998. Available from: http://www.ama-assn.org/ama/pub/physician-resources/-medical-thics/code-medical-ethics/opinion802.page? [Accessed: Mar 22, 2017]

[108] LaFrance WC, Reuber M, Goldstein LH. Management of psychogenic non-epileptic seizures. Epilepsia. 2013;**54**(Suppl. 1):53-67

[109] Goldstein LH, Chalder T, Chigwedere C, et al. Cognitive-behavioral therapy for psychogenic nonepileptic seizures. A pilot RCT. Neurology. 2010;**74**:1986-1994

[110] Plioplys S, Asato AR, Bursch B, et al. Multidisciplinary management of pediatric nonepileptic seizures. Journal of the American Academy of Child and Adolescent Psychiatry. 2007;**46**(11):1491-1495

[111] Kanner AM. More controversies on the treatment of psychogenic pseudoseizures: An addendum. Epilepsy & Behavior. 2003;**4**(3):360-364

[112] LaFrance Jr WC, Devinsky O. The treatment of psychogenic nonepileptic seizures: Historical perspectives and future directions. Epilepsia. 2004;**45**(Suppl. s2):15-21. DOI: http://dx.doi.org/10.1111/j.0013-9580.2004.452002.x

[113] LaFrance Jr WC, Alper K, Babcock D, Barry JJ, Benbadis S, Caplan R et al. Nonepileptic seizures treatment workshop summary. Epilepsy & Behavior. 2006;**8**(3):451-461. DOI: http://dx.doi.org/10.1016/j.yebeh.2006.02.004

[114] LaFrance Jr WC, Marinis AJ, Webb AF, Machan JT, Rusch MD, Kanner AM. Comparing standard medical care for nonepileptic seizures in Chile and the United States. Epilepsy & Behavior. 2012;**25**(2):224-229. DOI: http://dx.doi.org/10.1016/j.yebeh.2012.07.028

[115] LaFrance Jr WC, Miller IW, Ryan CE, Blum AS, Solomon DA, Kelley JE et al. Cognitive behavioral therapy for psychogenic nonepileptic seizures. Epilepsy & Behavior. 2009; **14**(4):591-596. DOI: http://dx.doi.org/10.1016/j.yebeh.2009.02.016

[116] LaFrance Jr WC, Baird GB, Barry JJ, Blum AS, Webb FA, Keitner GL et al. Multicenter pilot pre-treatment trial for psychogenic nonepileptic seizures. JAMA Psychiatry. 2014; **71**(9):997-1005. DOI: http://dx.doi.org/10.1001/jamapsychiatry.2014.817

[117] Roberts NA, Reuber M. Alterations of Consciousness in Psychogenic Nonepileptic Seizures: Emotion, Emotion Regulation and Dissociation. Available from: https//www.ncbi.nlm.nih.gov/pubmed/24196398 [Accessed: Mar 19, 2017]

[118] Gul A, Ahmad H. Number of Patient-reported Allergies Helps Distinguish Epilepsy from Psychogenic Nonepileptic Seizures. Jun 2016. Available from: https//www.ncbi.nlm.nih.gov/pubmed/26803428 [Accessed: Mar 29, 2017]

[119] Green B, Norman P, Reuber M. Attachment style, relationship quality, and psychological distress in patients with psychogenic non-epileptic seizures versus epilepsy. Epilepsy & Behavior. Jan 2017;**66**:120-126. DOI: 10.1016/j.yebeh.2016.10.015 [Epub Dec 28, 2016]

[120] Demartini B, Goeta D, Barbieri V, Ricciardi L, Canevini MP, Turner K, D'Agostino A, Romito L, Gambini O. Psychogenic non-epileptic seizures and functional motor symptoms: A common phenomenology? Journal of the Neurological Sciences. Sep 15, 2016; **368**:49-54. DOI: 10.1016/j.jns.2016.06.045 [Epub Jun 23, 2016]

[121] Karterud HN, Knizek BL, Nakken KO. Changing the diagnosis from epilepsy to PNES: Patients' experiences and understanding of their new diagnosis. Seizure. 2009;**19**(1):40-46

[122] Brigo F, Storti M, Lochner P, Tezzon F, Fiaschi A, Bongiovanni LG, Nardone R. Tongue biting in epileptic seizures and psychogenic events: An evidence-based perspective. Epilepsy & Behavior. Oct 2012;**25**(2):251-255. DOI: 10.1016/j.yebeh.2012.06.020. [Epub Oct 2, 2012]

[123] Cole CM, Falcone T, Caplan R, Timmons-Mitchell J, Jares K, Ford PJ. Ethical dilemmas in pediatric and adolescent psychogenic non-epileptic seizures. Epilepsy & Behavior. Aug 2014;**37**:145-150. DOI: 10.1016/j.yebeh.2014.06.019

[124] DeMarco JP, Ford PJ. Balancing in ethical deliberation: Superior to specification and casuistry. The Journal of Medicine and Philosophy. 2006;**31**(5):483-497

[125] American Medical Association Code of Medical Ethics. Opinion 2.035 Futile Care [Internet]. 1994 [cited Mar 12, 2017]. Available from: http://www.ama-assn.org/ama/pub/physician-resources/medical-ethics/code-medical-ethics/opinion2035.page? [Accessed: Mar 26, 2017]

[126] American Medical Association Code of Medical Ethics. Opinion 8.20 Invalid Treatment [Internet]. 1998 [cited March 12, 2017]. Available from: http://www.ama-assn.org/ama/pub/physician-resources/medical-thics/code-medical-ethics/opinion802.page? [Accessed: Mar 29, 2017]

2

Seizures in Children with Brain Tumours — Epidemiology, Significance, Management, and Outcomes

Adrianna Ranger and David Diosy

1. Introduction

Cancer is the most frequently diagnosed disease-related cause of death among children and adolescents [1], and malignancies involving the brain are collectively the most common solid tumour [2, 3]. They are also either first or second in incidence overall (second only to leukaemia) in the United States (USA) [1, 4,7], Canada [8], and Mexico [9]. The *American Brain Tumour Association* has estimated that approximately 4,200 American children younger than age 20 would be diagnosed with a primary brain tumour in the year 2012, of whom three in four would be under the age of 15 years [10]. However, the overall prognosis for brain malignancies is much better in children than in adults, with up to half of paediatric brain cancer patients surviving long-term [11]. The reason for this enhanced survival in youths is that children and adolescents are much more likely than adults to have low-grade astrocytomas, in particular pilocytic astrocytomas and other low-grade gliomas that are almost never fatal and often cured, depending upon their location and surgical accessibility, rather than the grade III and IV astrocytomas that account for the majority of tumours among adults [12-14].

Long-term survival, even in the setting of cure, is not without problems, however, with empirical evidence accumulating that paediatric brain cancer survivors continue to suffer from significant morbidity [15-20] and, sometimes, early death [15]. Among the more common long-term sequelae of brain cancer and brain cancer treatment in children are seizures, which can be quite disabling and, at times, life-threatening in themselves [15, 21-30]. In one study, seizures were the number one predictor of disability in long-term brain cancer survivors [24, 25]. Seizures even increase a paediatric survivor's risk of suicide into adulthood [31]. In addition, there is a subset of children, up to 50% [32], whose low-grade brain cancer presents as seizures [26, 32-42]. Though the vast majority of epileptogenic tumours are supratentorial, some are not, especially among children in whom infratentorial tumours generally comprise the majority [43, 44], and in less typical locations like the thalamus and hypothalamus [38, 45-47]. Among thalamic tumours, for example, up to one third of paediatric patients present with seizures [38]. As such, and because even low-grade gliomas can nonetheless be infiltrative into high-function brain tissue [19, 48-50], while some of these lesions are totally resectable, others are not [51-54]. This creates dilemmas as to how aggressive to be, and therefore how much risk to take in their resection [55]. As well, the return of seizures at some distant time post-operatively may indicate tumour growth or relapse [28, 30, 56-66], transformation into a more aggressive lesion [28, 60, 65, 67, 68], or even the emergence of a secondary (e.g., radiation-induced) tumour [64].

Why seizures occur in patients with brain tumours is not entirely clear [27, 69-71], and several conjectures have been made, including alterations in regional metabolism and pH, immunologic activity, disordered neuronal function, altered vascular supply and permeability, the release of altered tumoral amino acids, proteins and enzymes, and abnormal protein transport and binding to receptors [27, 44, 69, 71-74]. Even genetic predispositions for tumour-related seizures have been postulated [71, 75]. A recent excellent review of current theories and empirical evidence on the pathogenesis of tumour-related epilepsy has been published by You et al. [74] Discussing the relative merits of each theory is a paper in itself, and beyond the scope of the current review.

Interestingly, tumour size has a somewhat paradoxical relationship with seizure occurrence, in that, though the opposite is true of low-grade lesions, high-grade gliomas that present with seizures tend to be smaller than those that present with other symptoms [76]. Moreover, high-grade lesions that present with seizures tend to have a better prognosis than lesions of the same size that present otherwise [77]. What this suggests is that the aggressiveness of the tumour might have an effect upon seizure development. This being said, low-grade lesions comprise the majority of epileptogenic tumours, both in children and adults [78]; and some tumour types — like gangliogliomas and dysembryoplastic neuroepithelial tumours (DNET) — are more likely to induce seizures than others [28].

In this chapter, we will thoroughly review the literature on seizures in paediatric brain cancer patients, looking at them (1) as a presenting symptom; (2) in the early tumour management/ peri-operative period; and (3) long-term. Specific questions to be addressed in each of these sections are: How common are they? What is their history? How do they impact patients' lives, both short-and long-term, and in terms of management and prognosis? How do they effect management of the underlying tumour? How are seizures managed themselves? As much as possible, these questions will be answered by examining empirical evidence across a number of studies to provide, if not definitive answers, at least conclusions that are supported by published research.

2. Seizures as a presenting symptom of a brain tumour

2.1. How seizures present

A brain tumour is ultimately discovered in between one and three percent of children who present with new-onset seizures [40, 42], though a slightly higher percentage has been reported in children presenting with partial versus generalized seizures [79], and percentages as high as 20% have been reported in children undergoing epilepsy surgery [80]. From the reverse perspective, somewhere between 10 and 50% of brain tumours present with seizures as a symptom [69, 74, 81-83], and sometimes as the only symptom [32, 41, 84-86], with supratentorial and especially temporal lesions the most likely to be epileptogenic [44, 66, 78, 86-88]. In one study that compared children with supra-and infratentorial tumours, for example, among those with supratentorial lesions, 42% experienced vomiting as their first symptom, followed by seizures in 37%, and headache in 31% [43]. Meanwhile, 62% of children with an infratentorial lesion experienced headaches as their first symptom, with vomiting and ataxia accounting for most of the remainder, and seizures not observed in a single case.

Because children are more likely than adults to have infra-versus supratentorial lesions, the percentage of children presenting with seizures may be somewhat less than among adults, closer to the 10-20% than the 30-50% range [51, 89, 90], though 50% or more has been reported in some series [32, 35]. As in adults, of these epileptic tumours, the vast majority are supratentorial. For example, in their series of 157 children presenting to the hospital with brain tumour-related seizures, of mean age 3.3 years, Khan et al. found that 81% of the tumours were supratentorial and just 19% within the posterior fossa [82]. Meanwhile, Ianelli et al. reported that 80% of their 37 paediatric patients presenting with a temporal lobe malignancy had seizures as a presenting symptom [86]. Another excellent study on new-onset seizures presenting in children with brain cancers was published by Shady et al. [32] who analyzed 98 paediatric brain tumour patients and found that 50% percent of the children had seizures as part of their presentation, and 30% as their only presenting phenomenon; complex (55%) and simple (28%) partial seizures were the most common types, accounting for more than three quarters of all cases. Pre-operative electroencephalography (EEG) accurately lateralized to the tumour side in 88% of the cases and to the correct lobe in 56%. In addition, tumours involving cerebral cortex were much more likely than non-cortical lesions to present with seizures (59% vs. 15% of patients, respectively), with temporal and frontal lobe lesions exhibiting the highest incidence of seizures. Moreover, whereas 88% of gangliogliomas and 86% of oligoastrocytomas were associated with seizures, seizures were noted in just 21% of the patients with an anaplastic astrocytoma. Finally, as described elsewhere [32, 77], patients with seizures at presentation had a better prognosis than those without ($p=0.02$) [32].

Virtually every possible tumour type has been reported presenting as seizures, especially low-grade gliomas [27, 30, 32, 34, 37, 39, 70-72, 75, 76, 78, 91-93] and glioneuronal tumours like ganglioglioma and dysembryoplastic neuroepithelial tumour [28, 44, 62, 73, 88, 89, 91, 94, 95]; but including oligodendroglioma [77, 96, 97], cortical ependymoma [98], medulloblastoma

[47], subependymal giant cell astrocytoma (SEGA) [99], meningioma [10]^{0}, thalamic and cerebellar glioma [38, 46], and a variety of atypical, systemic and metastatic tumours, like primary meningeal osteosarcoma [84], acute lymphoblastic leukemia [101], anaplastic large cell lymphoma [102], neuroblastoma [103], melanoma [104], various sarcomas [105, 106], Ewing's sarcoma [107], malignant germ cell tumours [108], and others [16, 109].

There is no stereotypical seizure presenting as an early symptom of a brain tumour. Early seizures may be generalized, simple partial, complex partial, or mixed, depending upon the tumour's size, location, level of aggressiveness, and other factors [24, 26, 27, 33, 34, 37, 70, 74, 77, 82, 87, 110-115]. This being said, among children, seizures as a presenting symptom of brain tumour are most commonly complex or simple partial, versus generalized, with complex partial seizures generally accounting for from 50% to as high as 85% of all new-onset seizures [32, 63, 69, 86, 115-117]. The lone series in which this was not true was that reported by Hirsch et al., in which complex and simple partial seizures together only accounted for half of all cases [118]. The percentages generally reported for children and adolescents are somewhat different than for adults, in whom tumour-associated seizures tend to be more evenly distributed across the four most typical seizure types [58]. Other atypical and, therefore, less well recognized forms of seizure have been described in children as well, including gelastic seizures, characterized by uncontrolled fits of inappropriate laughter [45], tics and Tourrette-like symptoms [119], and sympathetic storms in a 7-year old with a midbrain glioma [120]. In addition, especially in the paediatric population, tumors may arise in the setting of a variety of familial syndromes such as neurofibromatosis types 1 [121] and 2 [122], and tuberous sclerosis [123]. Seizures in these conditions are often blong-standing, frequent, and intractable because of the numerous non-neoplastic lesions that can involve the CNS [55, 124, 125]. In such patients, the diagnosis of a new neoplastic lesion can be especially challenging [124, 126].

The diagnosis of brain tumour does not always quickly follow the onset of seizures. In one study reported by Ibrahim et al., for example, the time from seizure onset to tumour diagnosis among ten children presenting with seizures ranged from two weeks to two years, averaging six months [37]. A wide range of opinions and practices exist regarding how aggressive to pursue diagnostic imaging in children presenting with seizures [36, 41, 51, 79, 80, 100, 127-133]. For example, in one series of eighteen patients between the ages of 1 month and 13 years who presented with seizures and were discovered to have DNETs between January 1992 and December 2004, the preoperative evaluation included magnetic resonance (MR) imaging and interictal scalp electro-encephalography (EEG) in all patients, but functional MR imaging also was performed in eight patients, video monitoring with scalp EEG during seizures in 12 patients, interictal single-photon emission computerized tomography (SPECT) scanning in one patient, and ictal SPECT scanning in two patients [132]. Meanwhile, in their 2010 review of eleven clinical trials for anti-epileptic drugs (AEDs) conducted over the preceding two years, Jansky et al. noted that none of the trials required MRI as part of the patient enrollment protocol [128]. Increasingly, with advances in imaging and the recognition that the resection of epileptogenic lesions is both safe and effective for many patients, there seems to be growing opinion that the initial work-up of new-onset non-febrile seizures in children should include both an EEG and MRI, despite the likelihood that the majority of imaging studies will be either normal or inconclusive [134, 135]. As discussed in the next section, mounting evidence suggests that new-onset seizures in the setting of a tumour, and conversely, tumours in the setting of new-onset seizures both have therapeutic and prognostic implications.

2.2. Implications of brain-tumour induced seizures

Having a child's brain tumour present as seizures adds therapeutic complexity with respect to how the patient is initially managed, since peri-operative control of seizures is obviously considered of extreme clinical importance. The type of seizure a patient has also may have prognostic significance, both in terms of patient survival [65, 136] and how easily the seizures are controlled with anti-epilepsy drugs (AED), both peri-operatively and long-term. How well AEDs work, in turn, may have implications relating to how aggressive surgical resection should be.

Although no reliable data have been published for children, adults who present with seizures as their sole symptom tend to have less aggressive or advanced lesions than those who present with symptoms or signs of increased intracranial pressure like papilloedema, headaches [65], neurological or cognitive deficits [65, 136]. Although this intrinsically makes sense — the fewer the symptoms, the less aggressive or advanced the disease — extrapolating these findings to children must be done with caution, because a disproportionate number of paediatric lesions tend to be brainstem tumours that, though usually low-grade and non-epileptogenic, often are non-resectable because of their location and proximity to function-rich neural tissue [2, 3, 137-139]. Nonetheless, especially among supratentorial lesions, it makes sense that having seizures present before all other symptoms develop is a hopeful prognostic sign, given that low-grade gliomas and other so-called benign lesions tend to be associated with much higher seizure rates than high-grade lesions [32, 87, 91, 113, 140, 141].

Having seizures in the presence of a tumour has implications with respect to management of the seizures as well, in that studies have shown that such seizures tend to be more resistant to AEDs than idiopathic seizures [133, 142]. This appears to be especially true for patients who present with a history of numerous seizures [142]. This likelihood of *drug resistance*, which has been formally defined as *"the failure of adequate trials of two tolerated, appropriately-chosen and used antiepileptic drug schedules (whether as monotherapies or in combination) to achieve sustained seizure freedom"* [143], may play a role in determining the aggressiveness of surgery for tumour resection. For example, given the clear superiority of epilepsy surgery over medical management alone, in terms of achieving freedom from seizures in patients with intractable seizures (65% vs. 8% in one relatively recent meta-analysis [144]), a decision might be made to pursue more aggressive resection in a patient with repeated new-onset seizures upon initial work-up of seizures and diagnosis of their brain tumour, versus the patient who presents with a single seizure prior to tumour detection. Moreover, for many epileptogenic lesions, surgical resection often leads to either complete resolution of seizures, sometimes without the need for continued AEDs, or to a marked reduction in their frequency, as will be elaborated upon next.

2.3. General principles of management

How tumor-induced seizures are managed largely depends upon the aggressiveness and location, and therefore, the prognosis of the underlying tumour. In patients with invariably terminal forms of cancer, including primary brain neoplasms like glioblastoma multiforme (GBM), and metastatic spread to brain, the goal usually is to prolong life over months to, at most, a few years, while preserving as high a quality of life as possible. In both adult and paediatric patients with high-grade astrocytomas like GBM, even partial resection of terminal lesions has been shown both to prolong life and reduce the frequency and severity of seizures [145-147]. Clearly, such surgery needs to be performed as soon after diagnosis of the lesion as possible to have any effect upon outcome. Such is not the case in many patients with low-grade tumours like stage I and II gliomas and gangliogliomas, in whom progression of the tumour may be so slow as to be virtually undetectable, and patients can live for years without apparent disease progression, so that any decision to surgically remove the offending lesion may be delayed for years [58, 93, 148, 149]. This being said, there has been increasing emphasis on surgically resecting low-grade tumours early in the course of disease [131] for a multiplicity of reasons. Among these reasons are that anywhere from 20% to roughly one third of low-grade gliomas (LGG) fail to respond to anti-epileptic medications [72, 150], and many that do respond require more than a single AED [150], placing patients, and especially children, at risk for long-term drug toxicities [23, 24, 59, 71, 151-153]. Among the various documented toxicities of AEDs are wide-ranging adverse effects on cognitive function [23, 153], which already may be impaired because of the tumour itself and the radiation therapy sometimes administered to treat it [18, 20, 154-156]. Moreover, surgical resection of LGG has been shown to enhance long-term survival [19] and to significantly improve the likelihood of seizure control [27, 70].

Though the data are not definitive, there is some evidence suggesting that, among the various seizure types, partial seizures, either simple or complex, may be less likely to respond to anti-epileptic drugs than generalized or mixed seizures [93, 157, 158]. This resistance may be noted initially, so that seizure control is never achieved; but it also may develop over time, so that seizure control is lost and never regained [158, 159]. In such patients, therefore, there may even be an increased incentive to pursue surgical resection of the tumour+/-any adjacent epileptogenic foci, if the lesion can be accessed with no undue risk.

Several studies have shown that radical removal of an epileptogenic brain tumour is a strong, and likely the strongest, predictor of seizure freedom [127]. However, additional predictors include the type of seizure, the histopathology of the tumour, the age of the patient at the time of surgery, and the duration of epilepsy [127]. Among the various tumour histologies, tumours that are non-resectable due to infiltration, like high-grade astrocytomas, can be problematic over the patient's relatively brief period of survival [160]. However, as stated earlier, such high-grade lesions tend to be less often epileptogenic than their low-grade counterparts [32, 87, 91, 113, 140, 141]. In long-term brain cancer survivors, glioneuronal tumours, and particularly low-grade gliomas, gangliogliomas and dysembryoplastic neuroepithelial tumours (DNETs), often produce quite drug-resistant epilepsy in children, so that complete surgical resection of the tumour is typically considered the primary focus of treatment [28, 61-63, 88, 94, 116, 132].

In such patients, post-operative seizure-freedom rates often approach or exceed 80% [35, 48, 51, 58, 66, 86, 88, 90, 93, 115, 157, 161-169].

Traditionally, there has been some concern about being too aggressive with younger children with brain tumours, because of the risk of long-term adverse effects on neurological development, the risk of secondary neoplasms, and other neurological sequelae [155]. That such risks exist is certainly true of radiation therapy [18, 20, 64, 153-156], but it also is true of surgery [170]. However, recent studies have shown that surgery to resect epileptogenic brain tumours is both effective and safe for the vast majority of infants and toddlers [35, 55, 171]. In one large survey, for example, data were collected retrospectively on 116 patients less than 3-years old from eight centers across Canada from January 1987 to September 2005 who had undergone epilepsy surgery [171]. Among the various seizure aetiologies were malformations of cortical development (n=57), tumours (22), Sturge-Weber syndrome (19), and infarcts (8), with 10 cases either of unknown or some other cause. Seizure onset was in the first year of life in 82%, and the mean age at the time of the initial surgery was 15.8 months (range: 1-35 months). Second surgeries were performed in 27 patients, with six patients requiring a third surgical procedure. Among the initial 116 procedures performed were 40 hemispheric operations, 33 cortical resections, 35 lesionectomies, 7 temporal lobectomies, and one callosotomy. Of the 151 operations, including the 27 second and six third procedures, only one resulted in a surgery-related death. The most common surgical complications were infection, in 17 patients, and aseptic meningitis in 13. Of 107 patients assessed more than one year postoperatively, 72 (67.3%) were seizure free (Engel I), 15(14%) had experienced at least a 90% reduction in seizures (Engel II), and 12 had at least a 50% reduction (Engel III), with only eight exhibiting no benefit (Engel IV). Moreover, 55.3% of the children exhibited signs of improved development post-operatively [171].

Consequently, regardless of patient age, the focus for most patients with low-grade lesions has become, whenever possible without the undue risk of peri-operative death or long-term adverse neurological sequelae, to attempt total or at least subtotal tumor resection earlier rather than later in the course of disease. Debate rages, however, as to how aggressive to be achieving this goal, whether or not resecting the lesion alone is enough, and what intra-operative technologies to use to aid in identifying tumour margins and other epileptogenic foci. Moreover, not all patients will be eligible for surgery and will have to rely on non-neurosurgical treatments alone, most notably anti-epileptic drugs (AEDs) and radiation therapy. The next section briefly discusses the benefits, risks and utilization of AEDs both prior to and in lieu of surgery.

3. Anti-Epileptic Drugs (AEDs)

An extensive review paper could be written discussing the various advantages and disadvantages, indications and contra-indications, and drug-drug interactions that exist for the extensive list of anti-epileptic drugs that now are available for use in patients with brain tumour-induced epilepsy, all of which is beyond the scope of the current review. Here, we briefly describe the roles of AEDs, both in prophylaxis against and control of tumour-induced seizures, some of the risks of prolonged use, and at least the theoretical advantages of the new class of non-enzyme inducing drugs.

3.1. AEDs for seizure prophylaxis

In three recent surveys of neurosurgeons, including one survey specifically of members of the *American Association of Neurologic Surgeons* (AANS), the majority (up to 70%) of respondents reported prophylactically initiating AEDs in brain tumour patients who had not yet experienced a seizure [172-174]. This practice of prescribing AEDs prophylactically in brain tumour patients with no seizure history persists, even though empirical evidence addressing this practice is inconclusive at best [78, 81, 127, 140, 172]. Moreover, many authors and the most current *American Association of Neurology* practice parameters argue against it [113, 140, 172, 175, 176]. The argument of AED detractors is that both meta-analyses published since 2000 to address this issue failed to provide sufficient evidence to promote their prophylactic use in brain-tumour patients without seizures [173, 177]. The first meta-analysis, published in 2000 by Glantz et al. [173], analyzed 12 studies, of which four were randomized controlled trials and eight were considered to be "well-designed observational studies with concurrent controls", sufficient to be classified as class II evidence. Not one of these twelve studies demonstrated a statistical advantage of the AED being studied (phenytoin, depakote, or phenobarbital) over placebo [173]. The second, somewhat more stringent meta-analysis, published in 2004 by Sirven et al [177], only included five RCTs, assessing the prophylactic use of either phenobarbital, phenytoin, or valproic acid. Of the five trials, four identified no statistical benefit of AED use for peri-operative seizure prophylaxis. The one exception was a 1983 study published by North et al [178], in which not only patients with brain tumours, but patients who had undergone craniotomies for aneurisms and head injuries were included. A closer, empirical look at these data reveals no advantage at all when brain tumours are considered alone: seizures occurred in 9/42 on phenytoin, and in 5/39 on placebo (OR=1.11, 95% CI=0.58, 2.12). Further considering just those patients with glial tumours (versus meningiomas, sellar tumours, and metastases), seizures occurred in three of 16 on phenytoin versus just one of 16 on placebo (1.15; 0.42, 3.19) [178]. Overall meta-analysis across the five RCT confirmed the lack of any AED benefit at both one week (OR, 0.91; 95% confidence interval [CI], 0.45-1.83) and six months (OR, 1.01; 95% CI, 0.51-1.98) of follow-up. The AEDs also exhibited no effect on seizure prevention for specific tumours, including primary glial tumors (OR, 3.46; 95% CI, 0.32-37.47), cerebral metastases (OR, 2.50; 95% CI, 0.25-24.72), and meningiomas (OR, 0.62; 95% CI, 0.10-3.85) [177].

More recently, in a review published in 2011, Kargiotis et al. non-statistically examined published evidence on more currently-used AED, including the newer non-enzyme inducing drugs, and concluded that, among patients with either brain metastases or primary brain tumors who have never experienced seizures, prophylactic anticonvulsant treatment might be justified, but only for up to six months postoperatively after surgical excision of the cerebral tumour, since most of these patients will never experience seizures, and the anti-epileptic drugs may cause toxicity and adverse interactions with chemotherapeutic treatments administered to control the neoplasm itself [109]. For such prophylaxis, the authors argued that newer antiepileptic drugs like levetiracetam and oxcarbazepine are preferable to older agents like phenytoin and carbamazepine [109]. To date, however, no hard evidence supports any of these recommendations, and certainly not in children.

In a study by Hardesty et al., only 7.4% of 223 paediatric patients with brain tumours but no history of seizures experienced even a single seizure during their surgical admission, even though only 4.4% of patients had been started on a prophylactic AED [179]. This percentage is similar to the 8.0% observed among those on placebo in a controlled study in which 127 patients awaiting brain tumour surgery, ranging in age from 16 to 84 years, were randomized to receive either phenytoin 15mg/kg intravenously in the operating room, followed by 100 mg three times daily, either by mouth or intravenously, for seven days or placebo [180]. Thereafter, the dose of each was tapered. The 30-day incidence of seizures actually was higher in the phenytoin group (10.0%) than in controls (8.0%), albeit not statistically so. Moreover, the rate of complications was 18.0% versus 0% in the treatment versus placebo group, respectively ($p < 0.001$).

In the Hardesty study on youths [179], dependent factors associated with peri-operative seizures included a supratentorial tumour, patient age less than two years, and the presence of post-operative hyponatraemia due to either the syndrome of inappropriate antidiuretic hormone (SIADH) or cerebral salt wasting. No other factor was independently predictive of incident seizures, including tumour type, the lobe of the brain affected, the amount of operative blood loss, and the length of surgery [179]. Consequently, though children and adolescents who are awaiting brain-tumour resection and have recurrent seizures might warrant the initiation of an AED pre-operatively, and perhaps also children under age two years with a supratentorial tumour and those with highly-epileptogenic tumours like DNETs, even in the absence of seizures, the prophylactic use of these drugs is far from empirically justified. What is more prudent is to monitor all patients carefully throughout the peri-operative period to identify clinical factors that might place the child at risk, like electrolyte imbalances and fever.

3.2. AEDs for seizure control

Although in some small series of patients, seizures have been found to occur in up to 50% of paediatric patients with a brain tumour [170], in most populations, the overall incidence of seizures in this patient population is considerably lower, in the 10-20% range [51, 89, 90]. This is largely due to the infratentorial location of the majority of paediatric tumours, where very few are epileptogenic [37]. As such, only a small minority of children and adolescents with a brain tumour will likely ever require an AED, and almost all will have a supratentorial lesion. For example, from a database of 334 patients up to 21-years old, Sogawa et al. only identified 32 (10%) who had been started on an AED [83]; 94% of these 32 tumours were supratentorial, and 78% were glial [83]. Similarly, in their series of 280 patients between the ages of two months and 18 years of age, Khan et al. identified only 55 (20%) patients who had required an AED, among whom 49 (89%) had a supratentorial lesion [90]. This being said, over a 20-year period at a single institution, Khan et al. followed 157 patients who had presented with seizures and a brain tumour during childhood or adolescence, all of whom had been on at least one AED at some point [82]. Of these patients, phenytoin was the first AED used for 52 patients, carbamazepine for 38 patients, gabapentin for 31, and phenobarbitol for 14. Sixty-two of these patients ultimately were taken off all AEDs; but 17 of these 62 (27%) suffered seizure recurrence [181].

DNETs and gangliogliomas, which typically become manifest during childhood, adolescence or young adulthood, represent only a small percentage of CNS tumours in either youths or adults [6]. However, these tumours are almost always associated with seizures. Consequently, they comprise a disproportionate percentage of tumour-associated epilepsy cases [28, 44, 62, 73, 88, 89, 91, 94, 95]. Moreover, DNETs tend to be extremely resistant to AED therapy [62, 182-186]. Consequently, though AEDs generally are initiated in such patients, the majority ultimately will require surgical resection.

There is virtually no debate that AEDs are of use in treating brain tumour patients with seizures, in patients with repeated seizures awaiting surgery, in patients in whom tumour resection is infeasible, and in those whose seizures remain refractory despite surgery. However, there is concern about the risks of their long-term use, especially in patients who require on-going chemotherapy for their brain malignancy due to drug interactions and mutually-shared toxicities [81, 83, 127, 140, 151, 159, 172, 176], 187]; and significant debate regarding when and how AEDs should be discontinued post-operatively.

One of the biggest issues relating to AEDs is their potential interactions with anti-neoplastic drugs administered to control tumours and prolong survival. In a paper reviewing anti-epileptic drugs, Kargiotis et al. [109] listed 25 chemotherapeutic medications that interact with AEDs, most commonly carbamazepine, phenobarbitol, phenytoin and primidone, but also valproic acid. Common interactions are the AED accelerating metabolism of the chemotherapeutic drug, and the chemotherapeutic drug reducing serum levels of the AED [109], two results that potentially accentuate each other — when AED levels fall, AED doses must be increased to achieve seizure control, which will further increase metabolism of the chemotherapeutic drug, resulting in its doses needing to be increased, and so on. Included on their list of 25 drugs were 13 drugs often selected for the treatment of brain metastases, as well as nine drugs currently used to treat glioblastomas, six drugs to treat medulloblastomas, and five to treat malignant meningiomas.

In the current paper, Table 1 lists these interactions in reverse, indicating those anti-neoplastic drugs used for CNS malignancies that have had documented interactions with each of the five AEDs listed above. What is clear from this table is that all but valproic acid interacts with almost all of the chemo-therapeutic drugs typically used for CNS cancers.

The only drug on the list published by Kargiotis et al. [109] this is not considered to interact with AEDs is temozolomide (TMZ), a less toxic and more-easily tolerated orally-administered drug that effectively crosses the blood-brain barrier [188] and is now commonly used for both high-grade [189] and low-grade [190, 191] gliomas, as well as for brain metastases [192] and melanomas, often in combination with radiation therapy. There also is evidence that TMZ itself reduces the frequency of seizures, independent of AED dose. In one study in which 39 patients receiving TMZ (mean age 46.0 years) were followed for a mean 39 months and compared with 30 patients not on TMZ (mean age 41.5 years), patients on TMZ experienced a 59% reduction in seizure frequency versus just 13% in controls ($p < 0.001$) [150]. However, for reasons that are not entirely understood, TMZ appears to be less effective in children [193]. For this reason, other anti-neoplastic drugs typically are prescribed in children and adolescents, particularly multiple-drug regimens that include carboplatin and vincristine [193-195], two drugs both documented to interact with the older, cytochrome P450-inducing anti-eptileptics [109] (Table 1).

Meanwhile, evidence continues to mount documenting both the effectiveness and safety of newer-generation AEDS, like levetiracetam, oxcarbazepine and pregabalin [152, 196-204]. Though direct comparisons against the older drugs are generally lacking, theoretical advantages include the lack of any effect on cytochrome P450, and the fact that these drugs generally target specific risk factors for tumour-induced seizures [81]. Recently, in a survey of 32 paediatric brain-tumour patients requiring AEDs for seizure control, Sogawa et al. found that patients who had been started on any the newer–generation drugs (levetiracetam, oxcarbazepine and lamotrigine) were three times as likely to remain on these drugs than those started on one of the older drugs like valproic acid, phenytoin, and phenobarbitol (73% vs. 28%, respectively, $p=0.04$) [83]. Although the sample was small, there also was evidence of increased toxicity with the older drugs, with five versus just two adverse events resulting in drug discontinuation [83].

Of course, the treatment of brain tumours is anything but a static field. In attempts to reduce tumour progression and prolong survival, newer chemotherapeutic drugs are continuously being tested. Some, like nimotuzumab [205]and bevacizumab [206], both of them antibodies against epithelial growth factor receptors (EGFR), have been demonstrating considerable promise, and this may have implications for which AEDs are best tolerated as interactions and mutual toxicities become clearer. What is evident is that AEDs, in themselves, are usually inadequate to control seizures in most patients with epileptogenic brain tumours. And while novel treatments like stereotactic radiosurgery [154], vagus nerve stimulation [207], and ionizing radiation [208] are emerging, at this time optimal management of a child or adolescent with epilepsy caused by a brain tumour almost always necessitates resection of the lesion itself.

4. Surgical resection of epileptogenic brain tumours

4.1. The benefits and risks of surgery

In recent years, there has been a trend towards earlier surgical intervention in young patients with low-grade epileptogenic tumours; but is this justified? One potential justification is the risk of malignant transformation of low-grade tumours which, even though uncommon, has been described for virtually all tumour types and often is catastrophic [60, 64, 65, 67, 68, 97, 112, 131, 209-213]. A second justification pertains to improved seizure control and the decreased reliance on AEDs, with some patients potentially able to discontinue anti-epileptic medications altogether[59], [61, 181, 185]. But how successful is tumour resection in terms of controlling or eliminating seizures?

Table 2 lists 26 studies [35, 51, [61-63, 86, 90, 94, 96, 132, 148, 149, 168, 182, 184, 185, 214-223] published over the past two decades in which seizure outcomes in children and adolescents undergoing surgery to remove epileptogenic brain neoplasms were examined. Across these 26 studies are 741 patients, ranging in age from one month to 21 years of age, with a mean age of 9.1 years and a mean duration of post-operative follow-up of more than four years (overall mean=52 months, with individual study means ranging from 12 to 148 months). Though one study [86] included six paediatric patients with high-grade gliomas (either GBM or grade III astrocytoma), and another indicated 11 patients with either grade III or grade IV lesions [35], almost all of the remaining 724 patients had low-grade (grade I or II) lesions, including various low-grade gliomas and glioneuronal tumours, and less typically epileptogenic tumours like craniopharyngiomas and a dysplastic cyst. Spanning these studies, surgical approaches clearly differed, with some surgeons either largely or exclusively performing lesionectomies alone, others performing further procedures like partial lobectomies [86, 148] and amygdylohypocampectomies [182], and still others using various intra-operative mapping technologies like electrocortography (ECoG) [63, 132, 184, 214] to identify and ultimately resect extra-tumoral epileptogenic tissue. However, the ubiquitous goal was total tumour resection, whenever possible, an objective that was achieved in roughly two-thirds of cases.

Overall, the series with the lowest total resection rates were those that included a number of oligodendrogliomas (ODG), with resection rates ranging from 30% in a study exclusively of ODG and ODG-mixed lesions [96] and 40% in an older study in which half the patients had ODG [219], to 58% and 61% in studies in which the proportion of ODG was considerably lower [90, 220]. This discovery is not unexpected, given the highly infiltrative nature of these tumours [77, 96, 97, 191].

The outcomes of surgery otherwise were impressive, with almost four out of every five patients (77.7%) seizure free at the time of the final follow-up assessment, and 92.6% experiencing a significant improvement in their seizures from baseline, to Engel class 1, 2 or 3. Examining these data further reveals moderately strong, borderline statistically-significant correlations between the percentage of total resections achieved within any given series and the rate of seizure freedom ($r=0.37$, $p=0.08$), and between the percentage of total resections and the percentage of patients whose seizures were improved post-operatively ($r=0.36$, $p=0.09$). However, no correlation is apparent between the duration of follow-up and either outcome ($r=0.06$, $p=0.78$ and $r=0.26$, $p=0.22$, respectively), suggesting that it was the surgical procedure, rather than post-operative management, that influenced seizure outcomes.

There also were no peri-operative deaths among the 741 patients, some of whom even underwent second procedures to resect residual tumour detected by imaging after the first procedure. The overall operative complication rate, adjusted for missing data, was 11.7%, with the vast majority of complications and new neurological deficits transient and completely resolved within weeks to months of the procedure. As stated above, a small number of patients required repeat surgeries to achieve seizure control, sometimes associated with total tumour resection. For example, in one series a second surgery was required in three of 29 paediatric patients with supratentorial gangliogliomas, and all became seizure free after the second operation [216].

The studies by Jo et al. [223] and Gaggero et al. [35] are of special note because all the patients were infants, under the age of 5 and 3 years, respectively. In the first small series of 14 patients of mean age 2.7 years (32 months) [223], total resection of the epileptogenic lesion was achieved in 71%, as was total seizure freedom an average of 35 months post-operatively. In addition, all 14 infants experienced a significant reduction in seizure frequency, either being totally seizure free or having seizures limited to auras alone [223]. There also were no deaths and no reported operative complications. In the second study, which included 20 infants under age 3 years (mean age 1.5 years), eleven of the 20 children had either a grade III or grade IV neoplasm, including four choroid plexus carcinomas, one anaplastic oligodendroglioma, one anaplastic ependymoma, one immature teratoma, two glioblastoma multiforme, one PNET and one neuroblastoma [35]. Despite this, total resection was achieved in 70% of the children, seizure freedom beyond four years in 55%, and seizure improvement in 90%. Interestingly, all 20 patients lived beyond four years, and 17 remained alive at eight years of follow-up [35]. These two studies that imply both the effectiveness and safety of aggressive brain tumour resection in infants is counter to another study on 18 infants under one year of age who had a variety of grade I through IV lesions [170]. In this series, there was only one peri-operative death, due to massive brain haemorrhage in an 8-month old child with a deep, right parieto-occipital ganglioglioma. However, three patients had new-onset seizures following surgery, and an additional three had worsened neurological deficits. Of the nine patients who had pre-operative seizures, three improved, five did not improve, and one died. Overall, as of the paper's publication, only eight of the twenty patients had survived beyond infancy, with five now into adulthood (ages 18 – 26) [170]; two of the adult survivors were severely disabled at the time of the report, both having a Karnofsky score [224] of just 40%.

Also worth noting from Table 2 are the six studies in which only patients with dysembryoplastic neuroepithelial tumours (DNETs) were included (Table 3) [61, 62, 94, 132, 182, 184]. These six studies encompass 132 patients, of mean age 9.7 years, amongst whom total tumour resection was achieved in almost 82%, seizure freedom in 87%, and seizure improvement in all but a single patient (99%). However, the adjusted surgical complication rate was slightly higher than that noted across all 26 studies.

Table 4 lists four additional studies of note. Among these four additional studies, three were excluded from the previous table and its summation totals because vascular and other non-neoplastic lesions were intermingled with non-vascular lesions, with no data provided to distinguish between them; and the fourth was excluded because all the patients had tuberous sclerosis, in which brain tubors often cause uncontrolled seizures [225, 226]. The fifteen patients in this fourth study all had subependymal giant cell astrocytomas (SEGA), a tumour that is found in between five and fifteen percent of TS patients [123], typically developing in the region of the foramen of Monro, where it frequently causes obstructive hydrocephalus. Seizures primarily result from a broad array of intra-cerebral tumors, which include the cortical tubers mentioned above, and subependymal nodules, in addition to SEGA [225, 226]. The long-term prognosis therefore is poor, with death primarily resulting from intractable seizures or SEGA-induced obstructive hydrocephalus [225, 226]. As such, it is not unexpected that Cuccia et al. [99] failed to achieve either seizure freedom or any meaningful clinical improvement in seizure frequency in any of their patients. The inherent complexities of SEGA removal, given the relative inaccessibility of these tumours, also could account for the high complication rate (6 of 15, 40%).

The three remaining studies [117, 227, 228] involved a high proportion of non-neoplastic lesions that were not analyzed distinctly from neoplastic cases. Mean seizure free rates across the three studies ranged from a low of 56% to a high of 81%, with seizure improvement noted in 81.3% and 92.4% in the two studies in which this outcome was reported [117, 227]. Although no deaths were reported, almost one in four patients (73 of 320, 22.8%) had a significant post-operative complication, likely due to the highly vascular nature of many of the lesions and the increased risk of intracranial bleeding.

4.2. Post-operative management

According to the 30 studies (26+4) analysed above, the rate of post-operative complications among patients with epileptogenic brain tumours is low, likely somewhere between 10 and 20 percent, depending upon the nature of the tumour resected, its location, and perhaps other factors as well. The risk of peri-operative mortality also appears to be exceedingly low, with not a single surgery-related death reported among those 873 patients.

Few papers have been published on the post-operative management of paediatric brain tumour patients. What has been reported is that youths tend to experience different intra-operative and post-operative complications than adults, and that these complications affect both short and long-term outcomes, including disability, mortality and hospital and PICU lengths of stay and, hence, direct health care costs [229, 230]. Among the various risk factors for complications are fluid and electrolyte imbalances, which may be especially significant in children. One also must consider that volume of blood loss is all relative to the age and size of the child, given that a human's total blood volume varies dramatically relative to their age and size: falling from roughly 85 to 90 ml per kg in term neonates, to roughly 85 ml/kg in infants, 80 ml/kg in children under age 10, 70-75 ml in children > 10 and adolescents, and 70ml/kg in adults [231, 232]. Clearly then, 100 ml of blood loss may mean nothing to an adult, but may represent 25% or more of the total blood volume of a newborn.

In general, the most common fluid and electrolyte abnormalities observed after brain surgery in children relate to serum sodium levels, with hyponatraemia secondary to either the syndrome of inappropriate diuretic hormone (SIADH) secretion or cerebral salt wasting syndrome, and hypernatraemia caused by diabetes insipidis (DI) [233-236]. In one series of 79 children, for example, water and sodium disorders were noted in 36 (46%): 23 (29%) with DI, 12 (15%) with SIADH, and a single patient with cerebral salt wasting [236]. Why this is especially important in the paediatric patient in whom an epileptogenic brain tumour has been resected is that sodium disturbances are a significant risk factor for seizures. In one study involving 223 paediatric patients with epileptic brain tumours undergoing 229 surgical procedures, post-operative hyponatraemia — due to either SIADH or cerebral salt wasting — was one of just three independent factors associated with peri-operative seizures, the other two being a supratentorial tumour and patient age less than two years [179].

In another study of 105 paediatric patients post brain tumor resection admitted to the PICU, patients required an average of 0.7 unexpected intensive care unit interventions, mostly secondary to sodium abnormalities, followed by new neurologic deficits, paresis, and seizures

[237]. Interestingly, however, 68% of the patients were stable enough to be transferred out of the PICI within 24 hours of surgery.

With respect to anti-epileptic drugs, the same applies post-operatively as pre-operatively, in that there is generally no need to initiate AEDs in patients who have not yet experienced seizures, given the lack of evidence documenting any benefit of prophylaxis [180, 238]. This being said, there are no clear guidelines as to when and how to discontinue AEDs if they have been initiated pre-operatively, and there is always the potential risk of withdrawal-induced seizures [59]. In one study of 332 mostly adult patients, but including some as young as age 16, among those with AEDs that had been initiated to treat seizures pre-operatively, patients with a longer history of seizures ($p<0.001$) and those with simple partial seizures ($p=0.004$) were found to be especially likely to continue to have seizures in the immediate post-operative period, as well as poorer control long-term [58]. If AEDs are started post-operatively to reduce the risk of seizures following the trauma of surgery in a patient who otherwise has not had seizures, they generally should be administered short-term [239].

5. When seizures persist or recur

In virtually every series we have reviewed, patients were described who underwent resection of their epileptogenic brain tumour, with apparently successful removal of the tumour, yet no achieved control of seizures. Additional patients were noted to suffer from the post-operative onset of new seizures [170]. And still others had complete control of their seizures, only to relapse later, either while still on an anti-epileptic drug or after all AEDs had been withdrawn. Each of these three scenarios has implications with respect to patient prognosis and management.

5.1. Implications of post-operative seizures

The clinical implications of seizures that either start or re-start months or years after the initial resection of tumour are somewhat different than seizures that start immediately post-operatively or that started pre-operatively and failed to resolve with surgery. The major concern with the latter two scenarios is that tumour resection either was incomplete, or that extra-tumoral epileptogenic tissue was not removed. Over the years, attempts have been made to optimize the resection of epileptogenic lesions by both better delineating their margins and identifying extra-tumoral epileptogenic tissue, using intra-operative tools like electrocorticography (ECoG) to identify potential seizure-inducing tissue irregularities like cortical dysplasia [63, 77, 93, 132, [1] [6][3], 184, 214, 216, 240, 241]. This has led to debate regarding the relative benefits and safety of performing epilepsy surgery rather than just lesionectomies in patients with tumour-triggered seizures [242]; though, in fact, many surgeons have been utilizing additional surgical steps like lobectomies, amygdylohypocampectomies and, in extreme cases, hemispherectomies for decades [63, 86, 94, 117, 132, 148, 149, 168, 182, 185, 214, 217, 218, 222, 227, 243]. To date, almost no direct empirical comparisons have been undertaken. In perhaps the most methodologically sound study, Gelinas et al. retrospectively compared

34 patients who underwent ECoG-aided epilepsy surgery and 33 patients who had undergone simple lesionectomies without ECoG, all between the ages of 3 months and 16 years, in Vancouver, Canada [214]. One year post-operatively, the two treatment arms were virtually identical, with roughly 80% of patients in each group seizure free. However, at a mean follow-up of 5.8 years, there was a trend towards improved seizure freedom in patients in the ECoG group, with 79% versus 61% patients still seizure free (p=0.08). The investigators also noted no increase in neurological morbidity among patients who had undergone the more extensive ECoG-guided cortical resection, and that these patients were less likely to require repeat epilepsy surgery [214]. Why this has implications post-operatively relates to the potential need for re-operation, as discussed in the next section.

If the major concern of continued seizures is residual tumour or other epileptogenic tissue, the major concerns with later tumour recurrence are multiple. They include the possibility: (1) that the tumour itself is re-growing, having never been fully resected; (2) that the tumour has undergone malignant transformation; or (3) that some secondary tumour has started to develop, perhaps as a consequence of brain irradiation, chemotherapy, or some other cause. The risk of second brain malignancies is especially high in patients with CNS tumour-associated familial syndromes like neurofibromatosis types 1 [121] and 2 [122], tuberous sclerosis [123], von Hippel Lindau disease [244, 245], and basal cell nevus syndrome [246], with some of these tumours originating within the brain and others the result of metastatic spread from some extra-cranial site. All of the above-mentioned scenarios warrant investigation, which will include diagnostic imaging, due to their potentially dire consequences

Re-growth of tumour is anticipated among children with high-grade lesions, especially glioblastomas [81, 146, 247]. However, although long-term prognoses remain dismal, small improvements in survival times are being reported even among patients with GBMs, relating to advanced surgical techniques, the introduction of real-time, intra-operative imaging and brain mapping, and combining TMZ with radiation therapy [147, 189, 247-250]. Recall that in one study in which eleven of the 20 children had either a grade III or grade IV lesion, including two GBMs, a grade IV PNET, and a grade IV neuroblastoma, all 20 patients lived beyond four years [35]. Nonetheless, when the return of seizures leads to the discovery of grade IV tumour progression, surgery is almost never indicated. Instead, radiation therapy, chemotherapy, or both can be used and may be effective at reducing seizures [81, 208]. The recurrence of seizures does not necessarily indicate tumour progression, however. Sometimes, intrinsic changes within the tumour itself render AEDs less effective, so that switching or combining drugs may be beneficial [72]. As mentioned in Section 3, in such cases, care must be taken to avoid interactions between chemotherapeutic and anti-epileptic drugs [109].

Tumour re-growth also in anticipated in many low-grade gliomas and other neuroglial tumours when total resection is not achieved, and this can be manifested by the recurrence or worsening of seizures. This being said, malignant transformation has been documented with virtually every form of low-grade brain tumour, especially low-grade gliomas [65, 68, 112, 131], but also traditionally-benign lesions like DNETS [64, 67, 209-211], gangliogliomas [209, 212], meningiomas [251, 252], vestibular schwannomas [251], pituitary adenomas [251], and haemangioblastomas [251], among others. Glioblastomas have even been documented to arise at the site of previously totally-resected tumours [253]. Previously-controlled seizures generally are harder to control once malignant-transformation has occurred, even independent of tumour size or rate of progression [78]. Identification of such transformation therefore has implications in terms of patient prognosis, and management of both the tumour and the seizures.

Finally, the late recurrence of seizures can represent the formation of a secondary tumour, perhaps induced by brain irradiation or chemotherapy [251].

5.2. Surgical management of persistent and recurrent seizures

Whether seizures start immediately after surgery, later along in follow-up, or never fully remit, in all three scenarios, some patients will have seizures that remain uncontrolled despite the use of AEDs. In our review of the 26 studies listed in Table 2, as well as in various other case series and case studies, we found that, occasionally, patients undergo second or even third resections to remove either residual tumour that is now identified on post-operative imaging, or a residual or newly-identified epileptogenic focus. Though sometimes prolonged attempts are made to control the seizures with medication prior to the second surgery, in some cases, surgery is almost immediate, even within a few days of the initial procedure [254]. In one multi-centre survey that involved 116 children under age 3 undergoing epilepsy surgery for a variety of causes, 27 children were brought into the operating room for a second procedure, and six of these for a third procedure to control seizures [171]. Both the approaches and results of these second operations are mixed. In terms of the former, attempts are usually made to resect any residual or newly-discovered tumour, as well as to identify and resect other epileptogenic foci. Approaches range from simple lesionectomies to lobectomies and, in the most severe cases, hemispherectomies [243].

Table 5 summarizes ten studies we identified, published over the past two decades, in which second operative procedures were performed [46, 77, 157, [1] [6][2], 171, 216, 242, 254-256]. Half of these studies were exclusive to paediatric patients, while the other half included children, adolescents and adults. The study by Steinbok et al. was restricted to infants under the age of 3 years at the time of their initial surgery [171]. In this study, six of the patients required a third surgical procedure prior to achieving their final seizure outcome. Follow-up for most of these studies was approximately two years, but sometimes not reported. Overall, slightly less than half of the patients (46%) achieved seizure freedom, with roughly half the remainder (where reported) achieving at least a significant reduction in seizures. As with the first procedures, operative mortality was low, with only one death in 132 patients and 138 procedures.

6. Conclusions

A brain tumour is identified in one to three percent of non-febrile seizures that occur in a child. Meanwhile, seizures occur in between one in ten and one in five paediatric patients with a brain tumour, often as a presenting symptom. Most are associated with low-grade gliomas, like pilocytic astrocytoma, or with neuroglial tumours like ganglioglioma or dysembryoplastic neuroectodermal tumour (DNET). There is no empirical justification for initiating an anti-epileptic drug in a brain tumour patient without seizures, and some would restrict their use to those patients who experience at least two ictal episodes.

The cornerstone of management in most patients with a low-grade lesion is surgical resection, both because doing so often prolongs survival and reduces or eliminates seizures. Overall, almost 80% of children who undergo surgery to for resection of an epileptogenic brain tumour will attain prolonged seizure-freedom, and more than 90% will experience at least some meaningful clinical improvement, associated with a negligible risk of death in experienced surgical hands. Risks may be greater and results poorer in very small infants (under one year of age), but most-preschool children can undergo epilepsy-lesion resections safely and with benefit. Significant surgical complications occur in 10-20% of patients and include fluid and electrolyte imbalances, as well as typically short-lived neurological deficits in most patients, so that vigilant post-operative monitoring is essential.

Late post-operative seizure recurrence is an ominous sign that can be a harbinger of tumour recurrence, progression, or malignant transformation, as well as the appearance of new tumours, especially in patients with familial tumour syndromes like neurofibromatosis and tuberous sclerosis, and those who have received brain irradiation. When low-grade tumours recur and cause seizures, second resections may be effective at again controlling seizures.

These claims must be interpreted with caution, however, given that many essential questions remain unanswered — like whether more extensive epilepsy surgery is more effective or as safe as lesionectomy alone; and what factors best predict outcomes. In addition, with the emergence of new anti-epileptics, new anti-neoplastic treatments, and new surgical technologies, the management of epilepsy in children and adolescents with brain tumours appears to be rapidly changing.

AED	Interactions with
Phenytoin	carboplain, cisplatin, cyclophosphamide, dacarbazine, erlotinib, etoposide, fluorouracil, ifosfamide, imatanib, irinotecan, carmustine, lomustine, paclitaxel, procarbazine, tegafur, teniposide, thiotepa, topotecan, vincristine
Carbamazepine	cisplatin, cyclophosphamide, erlotinib, etoposide, ifosfamide, imatinib, irinotecan, carmustine, lomustine, palitaxel, procarbazine*, teniposide, thiotepa, topotecan, vincristine
Phenobarbitol	cyclophosphamide, erlotinib, etoposide, ifosfamide, imatinib, irinotecan, carmustine, lomustine, paclitaxel, procarbazine, teniposide, thiotepa, topotecan, vincristine
Primidone	cyclophosphamide, erlotinib, etoposide, ifosfamide, imatinib, irinotecan, carmustine, lomustine, paclitaxel, procarbazine, teniposide, thiotepa, topotecan, vincristine
Valproic Acid	cisplatin, cyclophosphamide, vorinostat

*Carbamazepine is contraindicated in patients on procarbazine

Table 1. Anti-epileptic drugs (AED) and their interactions with CNS anti-neoplastic drugs

First Author	Year Published	# Subjects	Mean Age (y)	Age Range	Tumour Types	Surgical Procedure	# Total Resection	% Total Resection	Mean FU (mo)	# Seizure Free	% Seizure Free	# Improved	% Improved	# Peri-Op Deaths	# Surgical Compl.
Ramantani	2014	29	11.7	2y - 17y	GG, DNET	L+E	16	55.2%	148	22	75.9%	29	100.0%	0	2
Consales	2013	22	6.5	10m - 16y	GG, DNET	L	15	68.2%	12	20	90.9%	22	100.0%	0	0
Babini	2013	30	12.1	3y - 18y	GG, DNET, PGNT	L, L+E	30	100.0%	85	26	86.7%	30	100.0%	0	1
Fattal-Valevski*	2013	54	7.1	1m - 19y	LGG, DNET	?	?	?	24	38	77.6%	51	94.4%	0	4
Jo	2013	9	2.7	6m - 5y	GG(2), AC(2), ODG, DNT, PNET, CPP, CP	L	7	77.8%	63	7	77.8%	9	100.0%	0	0
Uliel-Sibony	2011	41	8.2	1y - 18y	LGG, DNET	L, L+A	35	85.4%	62	34	82.9%	36	87.8%	0	2
Gelinas	2011	67	9.1	3m - 16y	43 LGG, 11 DNET; 14 other	L vs. L=ECoG	65	97.0%	12	52	77.6%	?	?	0	13
Spalice	2010	13	6.7	1y - 14y	DNET	L+E	12	92.3%	78	13	100.0%	13	100.0%	0	1
Ogiwara	2010	30	8.6	9m - 16y	GG	L, L+E	29	96.7%	62	27	90.0%	30	100.0%	0	2
Bilginer	2009	29	10.7	3y - 21y	DNET	TL ± AHC	?	?	52	27	93.1%	29	100.0%	0	?
Lee	2009	22	12.4	3y - 18y	DNET	L ± L	22	100.0%	44	20	90.9%	22	100.0%	0	1
Gaggero	2009	20	1.5	1m - 3y	Grade I(5), II(4), III(7), IV(4)	L	14	70.0%	48	11	55.0%	18	90.0%	0	?
Minkin	2008	24	8.9	1y - 15y	DNET	L	21	87.5%	80	20	83.3%	24	100.0%	0	9
Kan***	2008	16	?	2y - 21y	GG, DNET, LGG	L+E	?	?	(1 - 8 y)	13	81.3%	15	93.8%	0	?
Khan	2006	55	9.3	2m - 18y	LGG, DNET, ODG	L	32	58.2%	54	46	83.6%	50	90.9%	0	?
Cataltepe	2005	29	10.5	2y - 18y	GG, DNET, AC (T)	L, L+L+A, L+L	18	62.1%	31	20	69.0%	24	82.8%	0	5
Sandberg	2005	18	9.6	1m - 13y	DNET	L ± mapping	18	100.0%	19	18	100.0%	18	100.0%	0	1
Giulioni	2005	15	12.6	3y - 18y	GG, DNET	L	13	86.7%	67	13	86.7%	15	100.0%	0	2
Nolan	2004	26	10.0	4y - 18y	DNET	?	11	42.3%	52	16	61.5%	25	96.2%	0	?
Im**	2002	18	9.2	1y - 16y	GG	L	14	77.8%	48	15	83.3%	18	100.0%	0	?
Kim	2001	23	7.9	8m - 15y	DNET, ODG, GG	L, L+E	14	60.9%	43	16	69.6%	21	91.3%	0	7
Ianelli*	2000	37	9.1	1y - 15y	LGG (31), HGG (6)	L, L+A, L+L	22	59.5%	72	26	81.3%	37	100.0%	0	3
Khajavi	1999	34	12.6	1.5y - 18y	GG, LGG, DNET	L, lobectomy	28	82.4%	43	25	73.5%	29	85.3%	0	5
Razach	1998	10	11.2	1y - 16y	ODG/mixed ODG/AC	L	3	30.0%	40	?	?	3	30.0%	0	?
Kim	1995	10	9.8	1y - 15y	5 ODG, 3 LGG, PNET, vasc	L	4	40.0%	40	6	60.0%	9	90.0%	0	?
Packer	1994	60	10.6	1y - 20y	LGG, GG	L, L+E	47	78.3%	24	45	75.0%	47	78.3%	0	?
TOTALS		741	9.1	1m - 19y			490	66.1%	51.9	576	77.7%	624	92.6%	0	58
														0.0%	7.8%
														Adjusted =	11.7%

* some patients died before final seizure assessment; ** three patients underwent a second resection; *** these 16 patients part of a larger series with other seizure aetiologies included

GG = ganglioglioma; DNET = dysembryoplastic neuroepithelial tumour; PGNT = papillary glioneuronal tumour; LGG = low-grade glioma; ODG = oligodendroglioma; AC = astrocytoma; CPP = choroid plexus papilloma; CP = craniopharyngioma

L = lesionectomy; L+E = lesionectomy + additional resection of adjacent epileptogenic tissue; L+A = lesionectomy + amygdylohypocampectomy; L+L = lesionectomy + lobectomy;

TL = temporal lobectomy; L+L+A = lesionectomy + lobectomy + amygdylohypocampectomy; AHC = amygdylohypocampectomy; (T) = all temporal lesions

? = missing data

* Some patients died before final seizure assessment; ** Three patients underwent a second reaction; *** These 16 patients part of a larger series with other seizure aetiologies included

GG=ganglioglioma; DNET=dysembryoplastic neuroepithelial tumor; PGNT=papillary glioneuronal tumor; LGG=low-grade glioma; ODG=oligodendroglioma; AC=astrocytoma; CPP=choroid plexus papilloma; CP=craniopharyngioma; L=lesionectomy; L+E=lesionectomy+additional resection of adjacent epileptogenic tissue; L+A=lesionectomy+amygdylohypocampectomy; L+L=lesionectomy+lobectomy; TL=temporal lobectomy; L+L+A=lesionectomy+lobectomy+amygdylohypocampectomy; AHC=amygdylohypocampectomy; (T)=all temporal lesions

Table 2. Seizure response to surgical resection of epileptogenic tumor

First Author	Year Published	# Subjects	Mean Age (y)	Age Range	Tumour Types	Surgical Procedure	# Total Resection	% Total Resection	Mean FU (mo)	# Seizure Free	% Seizure Free	# Improved	% Improved	# Peri-Op Deaths	# Surgical Compl.
Spalice	2010	13	6.7	1y - 14y	DNET	L+E	12	92.3%	78	13	100.0%	13	100.0%	0	1
Bilginer	2009	29	10.7	3y - 21y	DNET	TL ± AHC	?	?	52	27	93.1%	29	100.0%	0	?
Lee	2009	22	12.4	3y - 18y	DNET	L ± L	22	100.0%	44	20	90.9%	22	100.0%	0	1
Minkin	2008	24	8.9	1y - 15y	DNET	L	21	87.5%	80	20	83.3%	24	100.0%	0	9
Sandberg	2005	18	9.6	1m - 13y	DNET	L ± mapping	18	100.0%	19	18	100.0%	18	100.0%	0	1
Nolan	2004	26	10.0	4y - 18y	DNET	?	11	42.3%	52	16	61.5%	25	96.2%	0	?
		132	9.7				84	81.6%	54.2	114	86.4%	131	99.2%	0	12
															15.6%

Table 3. Seizure response to surgical resection of dysembroplastic neuroectodermal tumors

First Author	Year Published	# Subjects	Mean Age (y)	Age Range	Tumour Types	Surgical Procedure	# Total Resection	% Total Resection	Mean FU (mo)	# Seizure Free	% Seizure Free	# Improved	% Improved	# Peri-Op Deaths	# Surgical Compl.
Kim	2008	134	8.5	8m - 18y	various, incl. vasc.	various	?	?	62	93	69.4%	109	81.3%	0	23
Cuccia	2003	15	10.5	4.5y - 19y	SEGA (+TS)	L	12	80.0%	52	0	0.0%	0	0.0%	0	6
Sonderkaer	2003	18	?	?	various	?	?	#VALUE!	128	10	55.6%	?	?	?	?
Borgeois	1999	171	8.3	10m - 15y	~40 vascular, etc	various	?	?	62	139	81.3%	158	92.4%	0	44

vasc. = vascular lesion; SEGA = subependymal giant cell astrocytoma; TS = tuberous sclerosis; FU = follow-up

Vasc=vascular lesions; SEGA=subependymal cell astrocytoma; TS=tuberous sclerosis; FU=follow-up

Table 4. Seizure response to surgical resection of epileptogenic tumor – studies including vascular lesions

First	Year	#	Mean	#
Author	**Published**	**Subjects**	**Age (y)***	**Seizure Free**
Benifla	2006	12	13.5	7
Chae	2001	1	0.3	1
Gonzalez-Martinez	2007	57	24.7	22
Im	2002	3	16.5	3
Jooma	1995	8	24.0	5
Lombardi	1997	1	?	1
Ojemann	2012	4	8.5	2
Steinbok	2009	24	1.5	12
Tian	2011	9	13.7	3
Whittle	1995	4	36.0	0
Totals		123		56
Mean			15.4	
Percentages				45.5%

Table 5. Seizure response to a second surgical resection

Author details

Adrianna Ranger[1*] and David Diosy[2]

*Address all correspondence to: aranger@uwo.ca

1 Department of Clinical Neurological Sciences, Division of Neurosurgery, Children's Hospital-London Health Sciences Center, Western University, London, Ontario, Canada

2 Department of Clinical Neurological Sciences, Division of Neurology, London Health Sciences Center, Western University, London, Ontario, Canada

References

[1] Centers for Disease Control and Prevention (CDC). Trends in childhood cancer mortality--United States, 1990-2004. *MMWR Morb Mortal Wkly Rep*. 2007;56:1257-1261.

[2] Centers for Disease Control and Prevention (CDC): Trends in childhood cancer mortality--United States, 1990-2004. *MMWR Morb Mortal Wkly Rep*. 2007;56:1257-1261.

[3] Ellison LF, De P, Mery LS, Grundy PE. Canadian Cancer Society's Steering Committee for Canadian Cancer Statistics.: Canadian cancer statistics at a glance: cancer in children. *CMAJ*. 2009;180:422-424.

[4] Linet MS, Ries LA, Smith MA, Tarone RE, Devesa SS. Cancer surveillance series: recent trends in childhood cancer incidence and mortality in the United States. *J Natl Cancer Inst*. 1999;91:1051-1058.

[5] Bunin GR, Feuer EJ, Witman PA, Meadows AT. Increasing incidence of childhood cancer: report of 20 years experience from the greater Delaware Valley Pediatric Tumor Registry. *Paediatr Perinat Epidemiol*. 1996;10:319-338.

[6] Gurney, J. G., Smith, M. A., and Bunin, G. R. CNS and miscellaneous intra-cranial and intraspinal neoplasms. SEER Pediatric Monograph, National Cancer Institute, 51-63. 2001. Ref Type: Serial (Book,Monograph)

[7] National Cancer Institute. A Snapshot of Pediatric Cancers: Incidence on Mortality Rate Trends. 2011. Ref Type: Report

[8] Ellison LF, De P, Mery LS, Grundy PE, Canadian Cancer Society's Steering Committee for Canadian Cancer Statistics. Canadian cancer statistics at a glance: cancer in children. *CMAJ 2009 Feb 17;180(4):422-4*. 2009;180:422-424.

[9] Rendón-Macías ME, Ramos-Becerril C, Bernardez-Zapata I, Iglesias-Leboreiro J. [Cancer epidemiology in children and adolescents at private health care (1995-2004)] [Article in Spanish]. *Rev Med Inst Mex Seguro Soc*. 2008;46:353-360.

[10] Brain Tumor Facts. American Brain Tumor Association. 2012. Ref Type: Electronic Citation

[11] Dolecek TA, Propp JM, Stroup NE, Kruchko C. CBTRUS statistical report: primary brain and central nervous system tumors diagnosed in the United States in 2005-2009. *Neuro Oncol*. 2012;14:1-49.

[12] Sievert AJ, Fisher MJ. Pediatric low-grade gliomas. *J Child Neurol*. 2009;24:1397-1408.

[13] Qaddoumi I, Sultan I, Gajjar A. Outcome and prognostic features in pediatric gliomas: a review of 6212 cases from the Surveillance, Epidemiology, and End Results database. *Cancer*. 2009;115:5761-5770.

[14] Taylor MD, Sanford RA, Boop FA. Cerebellar pilocytic astrocytomas. In: Albright AL, Pollack IF, Adelson PD, eds. *Principles and Practice of Pediatric Neurosurgery*. New York: Thieme Medical pUBLISHERS, iNC.; 2008:655-67.

[15] Sato I, Higuchi A, Yanagisawa T et al. Impact of Late Effects on Health-Related Quality of Life in Survivors of Pediatric Brain Tumors: Motility Disturbance of Limb(s), Seizure, Ocular/Visual Impairment, Endocrine Abnormality, and Higher Brain Dysfunction. *Cancer Nurs 2014 Mar 13 [Epub ahead of print]*. 2014.

[16] Huang LT, Hsiao CC, Weng HH, Lui CC. Neurologic complications of pediatric systemic malignancies. *J Formos Med Assoc.* 1996;95:209-212.

[17] Lovely MP. Symptom management of brain tumor patients. *Semin Oncol Nurs.* 2004;20:273-283.

[18] Packer RJ, Gurney JG, Punyko JA et al. Long-term neurologic and neurosensory sequelae in adult survivors of a childhood brain tumor: childhood cancer survivor study. *J Clin Oncol.* 2003;21:3255-3261.

[19] Shields LB, Choucair AK. Management of Low-Grade Gliomas: A Review of Patient-Perceived Quality of Life and Neurocognitive Outcome. *World Neurosurg 2014 Feb 19 pii: S1878-8750(14)00164-8 doi: 10 1016/j wneu 2014 02 033 [Epub ahead of print].* 2014.

[20] Vargo M. Brain tumor rehabilitation. *Am J Phys Med Rehabil.* 2011;90:S50-S62.

[21] Sato I, Higuchi A, Yanagisawa T et al. Impact of Late Effects on Health-Related Quality of Life in Survivors of Pediatric Brain Tumors: Motility Disturbance of Limb(s), Seizure, Ocular/Visual Impairment, Endocrine Abnormality, and Higher Brain Dysfunction. *Cancer Nurs [Epub ahead of print].* 2014.

[22] Armstrong GT. Long-term survivors of childhood central nervous system malignancies: the experience of the Childhood Cancer Survivor Study. *Eur J Paediatr Neurol.* 2010;14:298-303.

[23] Klein M, Engelberts NH, van der Ploeg HM et al. Epilepsy in low-grade gliomas: the impact on cognitive function and quality of life. *Ann Neurol.* 2003;54:514-520.

[24] Maschio M, Dinapoli L. Patients with brain tumor-related epilepsy. *J Neurooncol.* 2012;109:1-6.

[25] Maschio M, Sperati F, Dinapoli L et al. Weight of epilepsy in brain tumor patients. *J Neurooncol.* 2014;118:385-393.

[26] Riva M. Brain tumoral epilepsy: a review. *Neurol Sci.* 2005;26 Suppl 1:S42.

[27] Ruda R, Trevisan E, Soffietti R. Epilepsy and brain tumors. *Curr Opin Oncol.* 2010;22:611-620.

[28] Thom M, Blumcke I, Aronica E. Long-term epilepsy-associated tumors. *Brain Pathol.* 2012;22:350-379.

[29] Ullrich NJ. Neurologic sequelae of brain tumors in children. *J Child Neurol.* 2009;24:1446-1454.

[30] Wells EM, Gaillard WD, Packer RJ. Pediatric brain tumors and epilepsy. *Semin Pediatr Neurol.* 2012;19:3-8.

[31] Brinkman TM, Liptak CC, Delaney BL, Chordas CA, Muriel AC, Manley PE. Suicide ideation in pediatric and adult survivors of childhood brain tumors. *J Neurooncol.* 2013;113:425-432.

[32] Shady JA, Black PM, Kupsky WJ et al. Seizures in children with supratentorial astroglial neoplasms. *Pediatr Neurosurg.* 1994;21:23-30.

[33] Backus RE, Millichap JP. The seizure as a manifestation of intracranial tumor in childhood. *Pediatrics.* 1962;29:978-984.

[34] Blume WT, Girvin JP, Kaufmann JC. Childhood brain tumors presenting as chronic uncontrolled focal seizure disorders. *Ann Neurol.* 1982;12:538-541.

[35] Gaggero R, Consales A, Fazzini F et al. Epilepsy associated with supratentorial brain tumors under 3 years of life. *Epilepsy Res.* 2009;87:184-189.

[36] Gaillard WD, Chiron C, Cross JH et al. Guidelines for imaging infants and children with recent-onset epilepsy. *Epilepsia.* 2009;50:2147-2153.

[37] Ibrahim K, Appleton R. Seizures as the presenting symptom of brain tumours in children. *Seizure.* 2004;13:108-112.

[38] Martinez-Lage JF, Perez-Espejo MA, Esteban JA, Poza M. Thalamic tumors: clinical presentation. *Childs Nerv Syst.* 2002;18:405-411.

[39] Rutledge SL, Snead OC3, Morawetz R, Chandra-Sekar B. Brain tumors presenting as a seizure disorder in infants. *J Child Neurol.* 1987;2:214-219.

[40] Sjors K, Blennow G, Lantz G. Seizures as the presenting symptom of brain tumors in children. *Acta Paediatr.* 1993;82:66-70.

[41] Sun DC, Shen EY, Wong TT. Epilepsy as the sole manifestation of brain tumor--report of two cases. *Zhonghua Min Guo Xiao Er Ke Yi Xue Hui Za Zhi.* 1995;36:142-145.

[42] Williams BA, Abbott KJ, Manson JI. Cerebral tumors in children presenting with epilepsy. *J Child Neurol.* 1992;7:291-294.

[43] Klitbo DM, Nielsen R, Illum NO, Wehner PS, Carlsen N. Symptoms and time to diagnosis in children with brain tumours. *Dan Med Bull.* 2011;58:A4285.

[44] Shamji MF, Fric-Shamji EC, Benoit BG. Brain tumors and epilepsy: pathophysiology of peritumoral changes. *Neurosurg Rev.* 2009;32:275-284.

[45] Coppola G, Spagnoli D, Sciscio N, Russo F, Villani RM. Gelastic seizures and low-grade hypothalamic astrocytoma: a case report. *Brain Dev.* 2002;24:183-186.

[46] Chae JH, Kim SK, Wang KC, Kim KJ, Hwang YS, Cho BK. Hemifacial seizure of cerebellar ganglioglioma origin: seizure control by tumor resection. *Epilepsia.* 2001;42:1204-1247.

[47] Ho CH, Chen SJ, Juan CJ, Lee HS, Tsai SH, Fan HC. Sudden death due to medulloblastoma: a case report. *Acta Neurol Taiwan.* 2013;22:76-80.

[48] Berger MS, Ghatan S, Geyer JR, Keles GE, Ojemann GA. Seizure outcome in children with hemispheric tumors and associated intractable epilepsy: the role of tumor removal combined with seizure foci resection. *Pediatr Neurosurg.* 1991;17:185-191.

[49] Berger MS. Functional mapping-guided resection of low-grade gliomas. *Clin Neurosurg.* 1995;42:437-452.

[50] Chang EF, Clark A, Smith JS et al. Functional mapping-guided resection of low-grade gliomas in eloquent areas of the brain: improvement of long-term survival. Clinical article. *J Neurosurg.* 2011;114:566-573.

[51] Fattal-Valevski A, Nissan N, Kramer U, Constantini S. Seizures as the clinical presenting symptom in children with brain tumors. *J Child Neurol.* 2013;28:292-296.

[52] Consales A, Striano P, Nozza P et al. Glioneuronal tumors and epilepsy in children: seizure outcome related to lesionectomy. *Minerva Pediatr.* 2013;65:609-616.

[53] Gump WC, Skjei KL, Karkare SN. Seizure control after subtotal lesional resection. *Neurosurg Focus.* 2013;34:E1.

[54] Babini M, Giulioni M, Galassi E et al. Seizure outcome of surgical treatment of focal epilepsy associated with low-grade tumors in children. *J Neurosurg Pediatr.* 2013;11:214-223.

[55] Jo KI, Shin HJ, Hong SC. Seizure outcomes of lesionectomy in pediatric lesional epilepsy with brain tumor--single institute experience. *Brain Dev.* 2013;35:810-815.

[56] Kim YH, Park CK, Kim TH et al. Seizures during the management of high-grade gliomas: clinical relevance to disease progression. *J Neurooncol.* 2013;113:101-109.

[57] Chaichana KL, Parker SL, Oliva A, Quinones-Hinojosa A. Long-term seizure outcomes in adult patients undergoing primary resection of malignant brain astrocytomas. Clinical article. *J Neurosurg.* 2009;111:282-292.

[58] Chang EF, Potts MB, Keles GE et al. Seizure characteristics and control following resection in 332 patients with low-grade gliomas. *J Neurosurg.* 2008;108:227-235.

[59] Das RR, Artsy E, Hurwitz S et al. Outcomes after discontinuation of antiepileptic drugs after surgery in patients with low grade brain tumors and meningiomas. *J Neurooncol.* 2012;107:565-570.

[60] Luyken C, Blumcke I, Fimmers R et al. The spectrum of long-term epilepsy-associated tumors: long-term seizure and tumor outcome and neurosurgical aspects. *Epilepsia.* 2003;44:822-830.

[61] Minkin K, Klein O, Mancini J, Lena G. Surgical strategies and seizure control in pediatric patients with dysembryoplastic neuroepithelial tumors: a single-institution experience. *J Neurosurg Pediatr.* 2008;1:206-210.

[62] Nolan MA, Sakuta R, Chuang N et al. Dysembryoplastic neuroepithelial tumors in childhood: long-term outcome and prognostic features. *Neurology.* 2004;62:2270-2276.

[63] Ogiwara H, Nordi DR, DiPatri AJ, Alden TD, Bowman RM, Tomita T. Pediatric epileptogenic gangliogliomas: seizure outcome and surgical results. *J Neurosurg Pediatr.* 2010;5:271-276.

[64] Ray WZ, Blackburn SL, Casavilca-Zambrano S et al. Clinicopathologic features of recurrent dysembryoplastic neuroepithelial tumor and rare malignant transformation: a report of 5 cases and review of the literature. *J Neurooncol.* 2009;94:283-292.

[65] Smits A, Duffau H. Seizures and the natural history of World Health Organization Grade II gliomas: a review. *Neurosurgery.* 2011;68:1326-1333.

[66] Tandon N, Esquenazi Y. Resection strategies in tumoral epilepsy: is a lesionectomy enough? *Epilepsia.* 2013;54:72-78.

[67] Hammond RR, Duggal N, Woulfe JM, Girvin JP. Malignant transformation of a dysembryoplastic neuroepithelial tumor. Case report. *J Neurosurg.* 2000;92:722-725.

[68] Unal E, Koksal Y, Cimen O, Paksoy Y, Tavli L. Malignant glioblastomatous transformation of a low-grade glioma in a child. *Childs Nerv Syst.* 2008;24:1385-1389.

[69] Schaller B, Ruegg SJ. Brain tumor and seizures: pathophysiology and its implications for treatment revisited. *Epilepsia.* 2003;44:1223-1232.

[70] Ruda R, Bello L, Duffau H, Soffietti R. Seizures in low-grade gliomas: natural history, pathogenesis, and outcome after treatments. *Neuro Oncol.* 2012;14:iv55-iv64.

[71] van Breemen M, Wilms EB, Vecht CJ. Epilepsy in patients with brain tumours: epidemiology, mechanisms, and management. *Lancet Neurol.* 2007;6:421-430.

[72] Calatozzolo C, Pollo B, Botturi A et al. Multidrug resistance proteins expression in glioma patients with epilepsy. *J Neurooncol.* 2012;110:129-135.

[73] Alkonyi B, Mittal S, Zitron I et al. Increased tryptophan transport in epileptogenic dysembryoplastic neuroepithelial tumors. *J Neurooncol.* 2012;107:365-372.

[74] You G, Sha Z, Jiang T. The pathogenesis of tumor-related epilepsy and its implications for clinical treatment. *Seizure.* 2012;21:153-159.

[75] Berntsson SG, Malmer B, Bondy ML, Qu M, Smits A. Tumor-associated epilepsy and glioma: are there common genetic pathways? *Acta Oncol.* 2009;48:955-963.

[76] Lee JW, Wen PY, Hurwitz S et al. Morphological characteristics of brain tumors causing seizures. *Arch Neurol.* 2010;67:336-342.

[77] Whittle IR, Beaumont A. Seizures in patients with supratentorial oligodendroglial tumours. Clinicopathological features and management considerations. *Acta Neurochir (Wien).* 1995;135:19-24.

[78] Rosati A, Tomassini A, Pollo B et al. Epilepsy in cerebral glioma: timing of appearance and histological correlations. *J Neurooncol.* 2009;93:395-400.

[79] Kramer U, Nevo Y, Reider-Groswasser I et al. Neuroimaging of children with partial seizures. *Seizure.* 1998;7:115-118.

[80] Harvey AS, Cross JH, Shinnar S, Mathern GW, ILAE Pediatric Epilepsy Surgery Survey Taskforce. Defining the spectrum of international practice in pediatric epilepsy surgery patients. *Epilepsia.* 2008;49:146-155.

[81] Perucca E. Optimizing antiepileptic drug treatment in tumoral epilepsy. *Epilepsia.* 2013;54:97-104.

[82] Khan RB, Hunt DL, Boop FA et al. Seizures in children with primary brain tumors: incidence and long-term outcome. *Epilepsy Res.* 2005;64:85-91.

[83] Sogawa Y, Kan L, Levy AS, Maytal J, Shinnar S. The use of antiepileptic drugs in pediatric brain tumor patients. *Pediatr Neurol.* 2009;41:192-194.

[84] Dagcinar A, Bayrakli F, Yapicier O, Ozek M. Primary meningeal osteosarcoma of the brain during childhood. Case report. *J Neurosurg Pediatr.* 2008;1:325-329.

[85] Fulton SP, Clarke DF, Wheless JW, Ellison DW, Ogg R, Boop FA. Angiocentric glioma-induced seizures in a 2-year-old child. *J Child Neurol.* 2009;24:852-856.

[86] Iannelli A, Guzzetta F, Battaglia D, Iuvone L, Di Rocco C. Surgical treatment of temporal tumors associated with epilepsy in children. *Pediatr Neurosurg.* 2000;32:248-254.

[87] Bromfield EB. Epilepsy in patients with brain tumors and other cancers. *Rev Neurol Dis.* 2004;1:S27-S33.

[88] Wallace D, Ruban D, Kanner A et al. Temporal lobe gangliogliomas associated with chronic epilepsy: long-term surgical outcomes. *Clin Neurol Neurosurg.* 2013;115:472-476.

[89] Shamji MF, Vassilyada M, Lam CH, Montes JL, Farmer JP. Congenital tumors of the central nervous system: the MCH experience. *Pediatr Neurosurg.* 2009;45:368-374.

[90] Khan RB, Boop FA, Onar A, Sanford RA. Seizures in children with low-grade tumors: outcome after tumor resection and risk factors for uncontrolled seizures. *J Neurosurg.* 2006;104:377-382.

[91] Lynam LM, Lyons MK, Drazkowski JF et al. Frequency of seizures in patients with newly diagnosed brain tumors: a retrospective review. *Clin Neurol Neurosurg.* 2007;109:634-638.

[92] Ruda R, Trevisan E, Soffietti R. Low-grade gliomas. *Handb Clin Neurol.* 2012;105:437-450.

[93] Englot DJ, Berger MS, Barbaro NM, Chang EF. Predictors of seizure freedom after resection of supratentorial low-grade gliomas. A review. *J Neurosurg.* 2011;115:240-244.

[94] Spalice A, Ruggieri M, Grosso S et al. Dysembryoplastic neuroepithelial tumors: a prospective clinicopathologic and outcome study of 13 children. *Pediatr Neurol.* 2010;43:395-402.

[95] Karremann M, Pietsch T, Janssen G, Kramm CM, Wolff JE. Anaplastic ganglioglioma in children. *J Neurooncol.* 2009;92:157-163.

[96] Razack N, Baumgartner J, Bruner J. Pediatric oligodendrogliomas. *Pediatr Neurosurg.* 1998;28:121-129.

[97] Wang KC, Chi JG, Cho BK. Oligodendroglioma in childhood. *J Korean Med Sci.* 1993;8:110-116.

[98] Lehman NL, Jordan MA, Huhn SL et al. Cortical ependymoma. A case report and review. *Pediatr Neurosurg.* 2003;39:50-54.

[99] Cuccia V, Zuccaro G, Sosa F, Monges J, Lubienieky F, Taratuto AL. Subependymal giant cell astrocytoma in children with tuberous sclerosis. *Childs Nerv Syst.* 2003;19:232-243.

[100] Amirjamshidi A, Mehrazin M, Abbassioun K. Meningiomas of the central nervous system occurring below the age of 17: report of 24 cases not associated with neurofibromatosis and review of literature. *Childs Nerv Syst.* 2000;16:406-416.

[101] Goldsby RE, Liu Q, Nathan PC et al. Late-occurring neurologic sequelae in adult survivors of childhood acute lymphoblastic leukemia: a report from the Childhood Cancer Survivor Study. *J Clin Oncol.* 2010;28:324-331.

[102] Karikari O, Thomas KK, Lagoo A, Cummings TJ, George TM. Primary cerebral ALK-1-positive anaplastic large cell lymphoma in a child. Case report and literature review. *Pediatr Neurosurg.* 2007;43:516-521.

[103] Astigarraga I, Lejarretta R, Navajas A, Fernandez-Teijeiro A, Imaz I, Bezanilla JL. Secondary central nervous system metastases in children with neuroblastoma. *Med Pediatr Oncol.* 1996;27:529-533.

[104] Lopez-Castilla J, Diaz-Fernandez F, Soult JA, Munoz M, Barriga R. Primary leptomeningeal melanoma in a child. *Pediatr Neurol.* 2001;24:390-392.

[105] Postovsky S, Ash S, Ramu IN et al. Central nervous system involvement in children with sarcoma. *Oncology.* 2003;65:118-124.

[106] Postovsky S, Moaed B, Krivoy E, Ofir R, Ben Arush MW. Practice of palliative sedation in children with brain tumors and sarcomas at the end of life. *Pediatr Hematol Oncol.* 2007;24:409-415.

[107] Shuper A, Cohen IJ, Mor C, Ash S, Kornreich L, Zaizov R. Metastatic brain involvement in Ewing family of tumors in children. *Neurology.* 1998;51:1336-1338.

[108] Spunt SL, Walsh MF, Krasin MJ et al. Brain metastases of malignant germ cell tumors in children and adolescents. *Cancer.* 2004;101:620-626.

[109] Kargiotis O, Markoula S, Kyritsis AP. Epilepsy in the cancer patient. *Cancer Chemother Pharmacol.* 2011;67:489-501.

[110] Hughlings-Jackson J. Localised convulsions from tumour of the brain. *Brain.* 1882;5:364-374.

[111] Jackson JH. Localized convulsions from tumors of the brain. *Brain.* 1882;36:4-374.

[112] Loiacono G, Cirillo C, Chiarelli F, Verrotti A. Focal epilepsy associated with glioneuronal tumors. *ISRN Neurol 2011:867503 doi: 10 5402/2011/867503 Epub 2011 Jul 7.* 2011.

[113] Rossetti AO, Stupp R. Epilepsy in brain tumor patients. *Curr Opin Neurol.* 2010;23:603-609.

[114] White JC, Liu CT, Mixter WJ. Focal epilepsy; a statistical study of its causes and the results of surgical treatment; epilepsy secondary to intracranial tumors. *N Engl J Med.* 1948;238:891-899.

[115] Zaatreh MM, Firlik KS, Spencer DD, Spencer SS. Temporal lobe tumoral epilepsy: characteristics and predictors of surgical outcome. *Neurology.* 2003;61:636-641.

[116] Consales A, Striano P, Nozza P et al. Glioneuronal tumors and epilepsy inchildren:seizureoutcome related to lesionectomy. *Minerva Pediatr.* 2013;65:609-616.

[117] Kim SK, Wang KC, Hwang YS et al. Epilepsy surgery in children: outcomes and complications. *J Neurosurg Pediatr.* 2008;1:277-283.

[118] Hirsch JF, Sainte Rose C, Pierre-Kahn A, Pfister A, Hoppe-Hirsch E. Benign astrocytic and oligodendrocytic tumors of the cerebral hemispheres in children. *J Neurosurg.* 1989;70:568-572.

[119] Luat AF, Behen ME, Juhasz C, Sood S, Chugani HT. Secondary tics or tourettism associated with a brain tumor. *Pediatr Neurol.* 2009;41:457-460.

[120] Goh KY, Conway EJ, DaRosso RC, Muszynski CA, Epstein FJ. Sympathetic storms in a child with a midbrain glioma: a variant of diencephalic seizures. *Pediatr Neurol.* 1999;21:742-744.

[121] Hottinger AF, Khakoo Y. Neuro-oncology of Neurofibromatosis Type 1. *Curr Treat Options Neurol.* 2009;11:306-314.

[122] Lu-Emerson C, Plotkin SR. The neurofibromatoses. Part 2: NF2 and schwannomatosis. *Rev Neurol Dis.* 2009;6:E81-E86.

[123] Goh S, Butler W, Thiele EA. Subependymal giant cell tumors in tuberous sclerosis complex. *Neurology.* 2004;63:1457-1461.

[124] Ferner RE, Huson SM, Thomas N et al. Guidelines for the diagnosis and management of individuals with neurofibromatosis 1. *J Med Genet.* 2007;44:81-8.

[125] Hou JW, Wang PJ, Wang TR. Tuberous sclerosis in children. *Zhonghua Min Guo Xiao Er Ke Yi Xue Hui Za Zhi.* 1994;35:102-107.

[126] Roaches ES, Gomez MR, Northrup H. Tuberous sclerosis complex consensus conference: revised clinical diagnostic criteria. *J Child Neurol.* 1998;13:624-628.

[127] Guerrini R, Rosati A, Giordano F, Genitori L, Barba C. The medical and surgical treatment of tumoral seizures: current and future perspectives. *Epilepsia.* 2013;54:84-90.

[128] Jansky J, Kovacs N, Gyimesi C, Fogarasi A, Doczi T, Wiebe S. Epilepsy surgery, antiepileptic drug trials, and the role of evidence. *Epilepsia.* 2010;51:1004-1009.

[129] Kumar A, Juhasz C, Asano E, Sood S, Muzik O, Chugani HT. Objective detection of epileptic foci by 18F-FDG PET in children undergoing epilepsy surgery. *J Nucl Med.* 2010;51:1901-1907.

[130] Maytal J, Krauss JM, Novak G, Nagelberg J, Patel M. The role of brain computed tomography in evaluating children with new onset of seizures in the emergency department. *Epilepsia.* 2000;41:950-954.

[131] Prabhu VC, Khaldi A, Barton KP et al. Management of diffuse low-grade cerebral gliomas. *Neurol Clin.* 2010;28:1037-1059.

[132] Sandberg DI, Ragheb J, Dunoyer C, Bhatia S, Olavarria G, Morrison G. Surgical outcomes and seizure control rates after resection of dysembryoplastic neuroepithelial tumors. *Neurosurg Focus.* 2005;18:E5.

[133] Spooner CG, Berkovic SF, Mitchell LA, Wrennal JA, Harvey AS. New-onset temporal lobe epilepsy in children: lesion on MRI predicts poor seizure outcome. *Neurology.* 2006;67:2147-2153.

[134] Taheri MR, Krauthamer A, Otjen J, Khanna PC, Ishak GE. Neuroimaging of migrational disorders in pediatric epilepsy. *Curr Probl Diagn Radiol.* 2012;41:11-19.

[135] Hardasmalani MD, Saber M. Yield of diagnostic studies in children presenting with complex febrile seizures. *Pediatr Emerg Care.* 2012;28:789-791.

[136] Lote K, Egeland T, Hager B et al. Survival, prognostic factors, and therapeutic efficacy in low-grade glioma: a retrospective study in 379 patients. *J Clin Oncol.* 1997;15:3129-3140.

[137] Recinos PF, Sciubba DM, Jallo GI. Brainstem tumors: where are we today? *Pediatr Neurosurg.* 2007;43:192-201.

[138] Shuper A, Kornreich L, Loven D, Michowitz S, Schwartz S, Cohen IJ. Diffuse brain stem gliomas. Are we improving outcome? *Childs Nerv Syst.* 1998;14:578-581.

[139] Freeman CR, Farmer JP. Pediatric brain stem gliomas: a review. *Int J Radiat Oncol Biol Phys.* 1998;40:265-271.

[140] van Breeman MS, Vecht CJ. Optimal seizure management in brain tumor patients. *Curr Neurol Neurosci Rep.* 2005;5:207-213.

[141] Vecht CJ, Wilms EB. Seizures in low-and high-grade gliomas: current management and future outlook. *Expert Rev Anticancer Ther.* 2010;10:663-669.

[142] Kwan P, Brodie MJ. Early identification of refractory epilepsy. *N Engl J Med.* 2000;342:314-319.

[143] Kwan P, Arzimanoglou A, Berg AT et al. Definition of drug resistant epilepsy: consensus proposal by the ad hoc Task Force of the ILAE Commission on Therapeutic Strategies. *Epilepsia.* 2010;51:1069-1077.

[144] Wiebe S. Effectiveness and safety of epilepsy surgery: what is the evidence? *CNS Spectr.* 2004;9:120-122.

[145] Kim YH, Park CK, Kim TM et al. Seizures during the management of high-grade gliomas: clinical relevance to disease progression. *J Neurooncol.* 2013;113:101-109.

[146] Verla T, Babu R, Agarwal V, Halvorson KG, Adamson DC. Treatment outcomes and prognostic factors of pediatric glioblastoma multiforme. *Neurosurgery.* 2014;61:217-218.

[147] Napolitino M, Vaz G, Lawson TM et al. Glioblastoma surgery with and without intraoperative MRI at 3.0T. *Neurochirurgie 2014 Jun 26 pii: S0028-3770(14)00064-2 doi: 10 1016/j neuchi 2014 03 010 [Epub ahead of print].* 2014.

[148] Cataltepe O, Turanli G, Yalnizoglu D, Topcu M, Akalan N. Surgical management of temporal lobe tumor-related epilepsy in children. *J Neurosurg.* 2005;102:280-287.

[149] Uliel-Sibony S, Kramer U, Fried I, Fattal-Valevski A, Constantini S. Pediatric temporal low-grade glial tumors: epilepsy outcome following resection in 48 children. *Childs Nerv Syst.* 2011;27:1413-1418.

[150] Sherman JH, Moldovan K, Yeoh HK et al. Impact of temozolomide chemotherapy on seizure frequency in patients with low-grade gliomas. *J Neurosurg.* 2011;114:1617-1621.

[151] Cramer JA, Mintzer S, Wheless J, Mattson RH. Adverse effects of antiepileptic drugs: a brief overview of important issues. *Expert Rev Neurother.* 2010;10:885-891.

[152] Maschio M, Dinapoli L. Lecture: profile of risks and benefits of new antiepileptic drugs in brain tumor-related epilepsy. *Neurol Sci.* 2011;32:S259-S262.

[153] Taphoorm MJ. Neurocognitive sequelae in the treatment of low-grade gliomas. *Semin Oncol.* 2003;30:45-48.

[154] Chang EF, Quigg M, Oh DC et al. Predictors of efficacy after stereotactic radiosurgery for medial temporal lobe epilepsy. *Neurology.* 2010;74:165-172.

[155] Grenier Y, Tomita T, Marymont MH, Byrd S, Burrowes DM. Late postirradiation occlusive vasculopathy in childhood medulloblastoma. Report of two cases. *J Neurosurg.* 1998;89:460-464.

[156] Shuper A, Yaniv Y, Michowitz S et al. Epilepsy associated with pediatric brain tumors: the neuro-oncologic perspective. *Pediatr Neurol.* 2003;29:232-235.

[157] Jooma R, Yeh HS, Privitera MD, Gartner M. Lesionectomy versus electrophysiologically guided resection for temporal lobe tumors manifesting with complex partial seizures. *J Neurosurg.* 1995;83:231-236.

[158] Siegel AM. Presurgical evaluation and surgical treatment of medically refractory epilepsy. *Neurosurg Rev.* 2004;27:1-18.

[159] Pati S, Alexopoulos AV. Pharmacoresistant epilepsy: from pathogenesis to current and emerging therapies. *Cleve Clin J Med.* 2010;77:457-467.

[160] Riva M, Salmaggi A, Marchioni E et al. Tumour-associated epilepsy: clinical impact and the role of referring centres in a cohort of glioblastoma patients. A multicentre study from the Lombardia Neurooncology Group. *Neurol Sci.* 2006;27:345-351.

[161] Alexiou GA, Varela M, Sfakianos G, Prodromou N. Benign lesions accompanied by intractable epilepsy in children. *J Child Neurol.* 2009;24:697-700.

[162] Benifla M, Otsubo H, Ochi A et al. Temporal lobe surgery for intractable epilepsy in children: an analysis of outcomes in 126 children. *Neurosurgery.* 2006;59:1203-1213.

[163] Berger MS, Ghatan S, Haglund MM, Dobbins J, Ojemann GA. Low-grade gliomas associated with intractable epilepsy: seizure outcome utilizing electrocorticography during tumor resection. *J Neurosurg.* 1993;79:62-69.

[164] Chang EF, Christis C, Sullivan JE et al. Seizure control outcomes after resection of dysembryoplastic neuroepithelial tumor in 50 patients. *J Neurosurg Pediatr.* 2010;5:123-130.

[165] Duffau H, Capelle L, Lopes M, Bitar.A., Sichez JP, van Effenterre R. Medically intractable epilepsy from insular low-grade gliomas: improvement after an extended lesionectomy. *Acta Neurochir (Wien).* 2002;144:563-572.

[166] Fried I, Kim JH, Spencer DD. Limbic and neocortical gliomas associated with intractable seizures: a distinct clinicopathological group. *Neurosurgery.* 1994;34:815-823.

[167] Giuloni M, Rubboli G, Marucci G et al. Seizure outcome of epilepsy surgery in focal epilepsies associated with temporomesial glioneuronal tumors: lesionectomy compared with tailored resection. *J Neurosurg.* 2009;111:1275-1282.

[168] Packer RJ, Sutton LN, Patel KM et al. Seizure control following tumor surgery for childhood cortical low-grade gliomas. *J Neurosurg.* 1994;80:998-1003.

[169] Zentner J, Hufnagel A, Wolf HK et al. Surgical treatment of neoplasms associated with medically intractable epilepsy. *Neurosurgery.* 1997;41:378-386.

[170] Mehrotra N, Shamji MF, Vassilyada M, Ventureyra EC. Intracranial tumors in first year of life: the CHEO experience. *Childs Nerv Syst.* 2009;25:1563-1569.

[171] Steinbok P, Gan PY, Connolly MB et al. Epilepsy surgery in the first 3 years of life: a Canadian survey. *Epilepsia.* 2009;50:1442-1449.

[172] Stevens GH. Antiepileptic therapy in patients with central nervous system malignancies. *Curr Neurol Neurosci Rep.* 2006;6:311-318.

[173] Glantz MJ, Cole BF, Forsyth PA et al. Practice parameter: anticonvulsant prophylaxis in patients with newly diagnosed brain tumors. Report of the Quality Standards Subcommittee of the American Academy of Neurology. *Neurology.* 2000;54:1886-1893.

[174] Siomin V, Angelov L, Li L, Vogelbaum MA. Results of a survey of neurosurgical practice patterns regarding the prophylactic use of anti-epilepsy drugs in patients with brain tumors. *J Neurooncol.* 2005;74:211-215.

[175] van Breeman M, Wilms EB, Vecht CJ. Epilepsy in patients with brain tumours: epidemiology, mechanisms, and management. *Lancet Neurol.* 2007;6:421-430.

[176] Vecht CJ, van Breeman M. Optimizing therapy of seizures in patients with brain tumors. *Neurology.* 2006;67:S10-S13.

[177] Sirven JI, Wingerchuk DM, Drazkowski JF, Lyons MK, Zimmerman RS. Seizure prophylaxis in patients with brain tumors: a meta-analysis. *Mayo Clin Proc.* 2004;79:1489-1494.

[178] North JB, Penhall RK, Hanieh A, Frewin DB, Taylor WB. Phenytoin and postoperative epilepsy. A double-blind study. *J Neurosurg.* 1983;58:672-677.

[179] Hardesty DA, Sanborn MR, Parker WE, Storm PB. Perioperative seizure incidence and risk factors in 223 pediatric brain tumor patients without prior seizures. *J Neurosurg Pediatr.* 2011;7:609-615.

[180] Wu AS, Trinh VT, Suki D et al. A prospective randomized trial of perioperative seizure prophylaxis in patients with intraparenchymal brain tumors. *J Neurosurg.* 2013;118:873-883.

[181] Khan RB, Onar A. Seizure recurrence and risk factors after antiepilepsy drug withdrawal in children with brain tumors. *Epilepsia.* 2006;47:375-379.

[182] Bilginer B, Yalnizoglu D, Soylemezoglu F et al. Surgery for epilepsy in children with dysembryoplastic neuroepithelial tumor: clinical spectrum, seizure outcome, neuroradiology, and pathology. *Childs Nerv Syst.* 2009;25:485-491.

[183] Chan CH, Bittar RG, Davis GA, Kalnins RM, Fabinyi GC. Long-term seizure outcome following surgery for dysembryoplastic neuroepithelial tumor. *J Neurosurg.* 2006;104:62-69.

[184] Lee J, Lee BL, Joo EY et al. Dysembryoplastic neuroepithelial tumors in pediatric patients. *Brain Dev.* 2009;31:671-681.

[185] Ramantani G, Kadish NE, Anastasopoulos C et al. Epilepsy surgery for glioneuronal tumors in childhood: avoid loss of time. *Neurosurgery.* 2014;74:648-657.

[186] Chassoux F, Daumas-Duport C. Dysembryoplastic neuroepithelial tumors: where are we now?Chassoux F1, Daumas-Duport C. *Epilepsia.* 2013;54:129-134.

[187] Ruggiero A, Rizzo D, Mastrangelo S, Battaglia D, Attina G, Riccardi R. Interactions between antiepileptic and chemotherapeutic drugs in children with brain tumors: is it time to change treatment? *Pediatr Blood Cancer.* 2010;54:193-198.

[188] Baker SD, Wirth M, Statkevich P et al. Absorption, metabolism, and excretion of 14C-temozolomide following oral administration to patients with advanced cancer. *Clin Cancer Res.* 1999;5:309-317.

[189] Yang LJ, Zhou CF, Lin ZX. Temozolomide and radiotherapy for newly diagnosed glioblastoma multiforme: a systematic review. *Cancer Invest.* 2014;32:31-36.

[190] Pouratian N, Schiff D. Management of low-grade glioma. *Curr Neurol Neurosci Rep.* 2010;10:224-231.

[191] van den Bent MJ, Snijders TJ, Bromberg JE. Current treatment of low grade gliomas. *Memo.* 2012;5:223-227.

[192] Zhu W, Zhou L, Qian JQ, Qiu TZ, Shu YQ, Liu P. Temozolomide for treatment of brain metastases: A review of 21 clinical trials. *World J Clin Oncol.* 2014;5:19-27.

[193] Hummel TR, Chow LM, Fouladi M, Franz D. Pharmacotherapeutic management of pediatric gliomas : current and upcoming strategies. *Paediatr Drugs.* 2013;15:29-42.

[194] Packer RJ, Lange B, Ater J et al. Carboplatin and vincristine for recurrent and newly diagnosed low-grade gliomas of childhood. *J Clin Oncol.* 1993;11:850-856.

[195] Packer RJ, Ater J, Allen J et al. Carboplatin and vincristine chemotherapy for children with newly diagnosed progressive low-grade gliomas. *J Neurosurg.* 1997;86:747-754.

[196] Maschio M, Dinapoli L, Saveriano F et al. Efficacy and tolerability of zonisamide as add-on in brain tumor-related epilepsy: preliminary report. *Acta Neurol Scand.* 2009;120:210-212.

[197] Maschio M, Dinapoli L, Mingoia M et al. Lacosamide as add-on in brain tumor-related epilepsy: preliminary report on efficacy and tolerability. *J Neurol.* 2011;258:2100-2104.

[198] Maschio M, Dinapoli L, Sperati F et al. Levetiracetam monotherapy in patients with brain tumor-related epilepsy: seizure control, safety, and quality of life. *J Neurooncol.* 2011;104:205-214.

[199] Maschio M, Dinapoli L, Sperati F et al. Effect of pregabalin add-on treatment on seizure control, quality of life, and anxiety in patients with brain tumour-related epilepsy: a pilot study. *Epileptic Disord.* 2012;14:388-397.

[200] Maschio M, Dinapoli L, Sperati F et al. Oxcarbazepine monotherapy in patients with brain tumor-related epilepsy: open-label pilot study for assessing the efficacy, tolerability and impact on quality of life. *J Neurooncol.* 2012;106:651-656.

[201] Newton HB, Goldlust SA, Pearl D. Retrospective analysis of the efficacy and tolerability of levetiracetam in brain tumor patients. *J Neurooncol.* 2006;78:99-102.

[202] Newton HB, Dalton J, Goldlust SA, Pearl D. Retrospective analysis of the efficacy and tolerability of levetiracetam in patients with metastatic brain tumors. *J Neurooncol.* 2007;84:293-296.

[203] Novy.J., Stupp R, Rossetti AO. Pregabalin in patients with primary brain tumors and seizures: a preliminary observation. *Clin Neurol Neurosurg.* 2009;111:171-173.

[204] Rossetti AO, Jeckelmann S, Novy.J., Roth P, Weller M, Stupp R. Levetiracetam and pregabalin for antiepileptic monotherapy in patients with primary brain tumors. A phase II randomized study. *Neuro Oncol.* 2014;16:584-588.

[205] Cabanas R, Saurez G, Alert J et al. Prolonged use of nimotuzumab in children with central nervous system tumors: safety and feasibility. *Cancer Biother Radiopharm.* 2014;29:173-178.

[206] Narayana A, Kunnakkat S, Chacko-Mathew J et al. Bevacizumab in recurrent high-grade pediatric gliomas. *Neuro Oncol.* 2010;12:985-990.

[207] Boon P, Raedt R, de Herdt V, Wyckhuys T, Vonck K. Electrical stimulation for the treatment of epilepsy. *Neurotherapeutics.* 2009;6:218-227.

[208] Chalifoux R, Elisevich K. Effect of ionizing radiation on partial seizures attributable to malignant cerebral tumors. *Stereotact Funct Neurosurg.* 1996;67:169-182.

[209] Aronica E, Leenstra S, van Veelen CW et al. Glioneuronal tumors and medically intractable epilepsy: a clinical study with long-term follow-up of seizure outcome after surgery. *Epilepsy Res.* 2001;43:179-191.

[210] Chuang NA, Yoon JM, Newbury RO, Crawford JR. Glioblastoma Multiforme Arising From Dysembryoplastic Neuroepithelial Tumor in a Child in the Absence of Therapy. *J Pediatr Hematol Oncol 2013 Dec 4 [Epub ahead of print].* 2013.

[211] Moazzam AA, Wagle N, Shiroishi MS. Malignant transformation of DNETs: a case report and literature review. *Neuroreport.* 2014;25:894-899.

[212] Moreno A, de Felipe J, Garcia Sola R, Navarro A, Ramon y Cajal S. Neuronal and mixed neuronal glial tumors associated to epilepsy. A heterogeneous and related group of tumours. *Histol Histopathol.* 2001;16:613-622.

[213] Yang T, Pruthi S, Geyer JR, Ojemann JG. MRI changes associated with vigabatrin treatment mimicking tumor progression. *Pediatr Blood Cancer.* 2010;55:1221-1223.

[214] Gelinas JN, Battison AW, Smith S, Connolly MB, Steinbok P. Electrocorticography and seizure outcomes in children with lesional epilepsy. *Childs Nerv Syst.* 2011;27:381-390.

[215] Giulioni M, Galassi E, Zucchelli M, Volpi L. Seizure outcome of lesionectomy in glio-neuronal tumors associated with epilepsy in children. *J Neurosurg Ped.* 2005;102:288-293.

[216] Im SH, Chung CK, Cho BK, Lee SK. Supratentorial ganglioglioma and epilepsy: post-operative seizure outcome. *J Neurooncol.* 2002;57:59-66.

[217] Kan P, Van Orman C, Kestle JR. Outcomes after surgery for focal epilepsy in children. *Childs Nerv Syst.* 2008;24:587-591.

[218] Khajavi K, Comair YG, Wyllie E, Palmer J, Morris HH, Hahn JF. Surgical management of pediatric tumor-associated epilepsy. *J Child Neurol.* 1999;14:15-25.

[219] Kim SK, Wang KC, Cho BK. Intractable seizures associated with brain tumor in childhood: lesionectomy and seizure outcome. *Childs Nerv Syst.* 1995;11:634-638.

[220] Kim SK, Wang KC, Hwang YS, Kim KJ, Cho BK. Intractable epilepsy associated with brain tumors in children: surgical modality and outcome. *Childs Nerv Syst.* 2001;17:445-452.

[221] Consales A, Striano P, Nozza P et al. Glioneuronal tumors and epilepsy inchildren:seizureoutcome related to lesionectomy. *Minerva Pediatr.* 2013;65:609-616.

[222] Babini M, Giulioni M, Galassi E et al. Seizure outcome of surgical treatment of focal epilepsy associated with low-grade tumors in children. *J Neurosurg Pediatr.* 2013;11:214-223.

[223] Jo KI, Chung SB, Jo KW, Kong DS, Seol HJ, Shin HJ. Microsurgical resection of deep-seated lesions using transparent tubular retractor: pediatric case series. *Childs Nerv Syst.* 2011;27:1989-1994.

[224] Karnofsky DA, Burchenal JH. The Clinical Evaluation of Chemotherapeutic Agents in Cancer. In: MacLeod CM, ed. *Evaluation of Chemotherapeutic Agents*. New York, NY: Columbia University Press; 1949:196.

[225] Grajkowska W, Kotulska K, Jurkiewicz E, Matyja E. Brain lesions in tuberous sclerosis complex. Review. *Folia Neuropathol.* 2010;48:139-149.

[226] Orlova KA, Crino PB. The tuberous sclerosis complex. *Ann N Y Acad Sci.* 2010;1184:87-105.

[227] Bourgeois M, Sainte-Rose C, Lellouch-Tubiana A et al. Surgery of epilepsy associated with focal lesions in childhood. *J Neurosurg.* 1999;90:833-842.

[228] Sonderkaer S, Schmiegelow M, Carstensen H, Nielsen LB, Muller J, Schmiegelow K. Long-term neurological outcome of childhood brain tumors treated by surgery only. *J Clin Oncol.* 2003;21:1347-1351.

[229] Mekitarian Filho E, Brunow de Carvalho W, Cavalheiro S, Horigoshi NK, Freddi NA. Perioperative factors associated with prolonged intensive care unit and hospital length of stay after pediatric neurosurgery. *Pediatr Neurosurg.* 2011;47:423-429.

[230] Drake JM, Riva-Cambrin J, Jea A, Auguste K, Tamber M, Lamberti-Pasculli M. Prospective surveillance of complications in a pediatric neurosurgery unit. *J Neurosurg Pediatr.* 2010;5:544-548.

[231] Graham GR. Blood volume in children. *Ann R Coll Surg Engl.* 1963;33:149-158.

[232] Guidance: Blood Draw Guidelines. University of Michigan Medical School. 2013. Ref Type: Electronic Citation

[233] Lobel DA. Pediatric Intensive Care Unit Management of Neurosurgical Diseases. In: Lobel DA, Lee MR, Duhaime A-C, eds. *The Central Nervous System in Pediatric Critical Illness and Injury*. London: Springer; 2009:1-10.

[234] Hammer GB, Krane EJ. Perioperative care of the child with acute neurological disease. In: Hammer GB, Andrews BT, eds. *Pediatric Neurosurgical Intensive Care*. Park Ridge, IL: American Association of Neurological Surgeons (AANS); 1997:25-36.

[235] Segura Matute S, Balaguer Gargallo M, Cambra Lasaosa FJ, Zambudio Sert S, Martin Rodrigo JM, Palomeque Rico A. [Fluid and electrolyte disorders following surgery for brain tumors]. [Article in Spanish]. *An Pediatr (Barc).* 2007;67:225-230.

[236] Hiranrat P, Katavetin P, Supornsilchai V, Wacharasindhu S, Srivuthana S. Water and sodium disorders in children undergoing surgical treatment of brain tumors. *J Med Assoc Thai.* 2003;86:S152-S159.

[237] Spentzas T, Escue JE, Patters AB, Varelas PN. Brain tumor resection in children: neurointensive care unit course and resource utilization. *Pediatr Crit Care Med.* 2010;11:718-722.

[238] Pruitt AA. Treatment of Medical Complications in Patients with Brain Tumors. *Curr Treat Options Neurol.* 2005;7:323-336.

[239] Michelucci R. Optimizing therapy of seizures in neurosurgery. *Neurology.* 2006;67:S14-S18.

[240] Asano E, Benedek K, Shah A et al. Is intraoperative electrocorticography reliable in children with intractable neocortical epilepsy? *Epilepsia.* 2004;45:1091-1099.

[241] Wennberg R, Quesney LF, Lozano A, Olivier A, Rasmussen T. Role of electrocorticography at surgery for lesion-related frontal lobe epilepsy. *Can J Neurol Sci.* 1999;26:33-39.

[242] Lombardi D, Marsh R, de Tribolet N. Low grade glioma in intractable epilepsy: lesionectomy versus epilepsy surgery. *Acta Neurochir Suppl.* 1997;68:70-74.

[243] Terra-Bustamante VC, Inuzuka LM, Fernandes RM et al. Outcome of hemispheric surgeries for refractory epilepsy in pediatric patients. *Childs Nerv Syst.* 2007;23:321-326.

[244] Butman JA, Linehan WM, Lonser RR. Neurologic manifestations of von Hippel-Lindau disease. *JAMA.* 2008;300:1334-1342.

[245] Richard S, Campello C, Taillandier L, Parker F, Resche F. Haemangioblastoma of the central nervous system in von Hippel-Lindau disease. French VHL Study Group. *J Intern Med.* 1998;243:547-553.

[246] Shanley S, Ratcliffe J, Hockey A, et al. Nevoid basal cell carcinoma syndrome: review of 118 affected individuals. *Am J MedGenet.* 1994;50:282-290.

[247] Yang T, Temkin N, Barber J et al. Gross total resection correlates with long-term survival in pediatric patients with glioblastoma. *World Neurosurg.* 2013;79:537-544.

[248] Hart MG, Garside R, Rogers G, Stein K, Grant R. Temozolomide for high grade glioma. *Cochrane Database Syst Rev 2013 Apr 30;4:CD007415 doi: 10 1002/14651858 CD007415 pub2.* 2013.

[249] Ho RHVK, Reijneveld JC, Enting et al. Changing incidence and improved survival of gliomas. *Eur J Cancer 2014 Jun 24 pii: S0959-8049(14)00718-7 doi: 10 1016/j ejca 2014 05 019 [Epub ahead of print].* 2014.

[250] Weller M, Gorlia T, Cairncross JG et al. Prolonged survival with valproic acid use in the EORTC/NCIC temozolomide trial for glioblastoma. *Neurology.* 2011;77:1156-1164.

[251] Evans DG, Birch JM, Ramsden RT, Sharif S, Baser ME. Malignant transformation and new primary tumours after therapeutic radiation for benign disease: substantial risks in certain tumour prone syndromes. *J Med Genet.* 2006;43:289-294.

[252] Osipov V, Ho KC, Krouwer HG, Meyer G, Shidham VB. Post-radiation dedifferentiation of meningioma into osteosarcoma. *BMC Cancer.* 2002;2:34.

[253] Pereira EA, Dabbous B, Qureshi HU, Ansorge O, Bojanic S. Rapid development of glioblastoma at the site of atypical meningioma resection. *Br J* Neurosurg. 2010;24:471-473.

[254] Gonzalez-Martinez JA, Srikijvilaikul T, Nair D, Bingaman WE. Long-term seizure outcome in reoperation after failure of epilepsy surgery. Neurosurgery. 2007;60:873-880.

[255] Ojemann JG, Hersonskey TY, Abeshaus S et al. Epilepsy surgery after treatment of pediatric malignant brain tumors. Seizure. 2012;21:624-630.

[256] Tian AG, Edwards MS, Williams AJ, Olson DM. Epilepsy surgery following brain tumor resection in children. J Neurosurg Pediatr. 2011;7:229-234.

3

Diagnostic Testing in Epilepsy Genetics Clinical Practice

Birute Tumiene, Algirdas Utkus, Vaidutis Kučinskas,
Aleš Maver and Borut Peterlin

Abstract

Changing landscape of epilepsy genetic testing gives vast opportunities to both patients and clinicians. Significance of precise genetic diagnosis in patients affected by epilepsy cannot be overestimated: it not only gives the opportunities of personalized therapeutical approaches but is also associated with multiple additional benefits for patients, their families, and society. Although the burden of Mendelian and chromosomal diseases amenable to current diagnostic testing measures is unknown, recently, we have comprised a database of more than 880 human genes associated with monogenic diseases involving epilepsy or seizures, EpiGene database (http://www.kimg.eu/en/tools/epigene-database). Besides, more than 50 chromosomal syndromes are related to epilepsy or seizures. Currently, there are no recommendations or guidelines for genetic testing in epilepsy patients addressing specificities of next-generation sequencing technologies. However, as every genetic testing modality has its own characteristics of specificity/sensitivity, range of clinical indications, and possible bioethical and psychosocial implications, genetic testing in epilepsies must be properly selected and applied along with proper clinical genetics/genetic counseling services. In this chapter, an overview of genetic testing modalities and workflows taking into account genetic architecture of epilepsies is given, and practical aspects of genetic testing in epilepsies, including advantages/limitations and clinical utility of tests, are discussed.

Keywords: algorithm, diagnostic yield, clinical utility, next-generation sequencing, exome, molecular karyotyping

1. Introduction

Recent genetic revolution due to advancements in genomic testing technologies evolves into fundamental changes in clinical practice of not only clinical genetics but also other medical specialties. Changing landscape of epilepsy genetic testing gives vast opportunities to both patients and clinicians, however, not without additional challenges. Although the burden of Mendelian and chromosomal diseases, amenable to current diagnostic testing measures, among all patients with epilepsy or seizures is currently unknown, significance of precise genetic diagnosis in patients affected by epilepsy cannot be overestimated: it not only gives the opportunities of personalized therapeutical approaches but is also associated with multiple additional benefits for patients, their families, and society. However, as every genetic testing modality has its own characteristics of specificity/sensitivity, range of clinical indications, and possible bioethical and psychosocial implications, genetic testing in epilepsies must be properly selected and applied along with proper clinical genetics/genetic counseling services. In this chapter, an overview of genetic testing modalities and workflows taking into account genetic architecture of epilepsies is given, and practical aspects of genetic testing in epilepsies, including advantages/limitations and clinical utility of tests, are discussed.

2. Diagnostic testing in epilepsy genetics clinical practice[1]

2.1. Genetic and clinical heterogeneity of epilepsy

Both traditional and genomic heritability studies unequivocally show the importance of genetic factors in epilepsy [1, 2]. Genetic factors play a role in more than half of all epilepsies [3]. Although a part of these epilepsies may not be amenable for genetic testing in current clinical practice (e.g., multifactorial or those due to somatic mutations), many monogenic and chromosomal diseases related to epilepsy or seizures may and should be diagnosed. Most of these diagnosable diseases belong to a category of rare diseases (in the European Union defined as a disease affecting less than 1 in 2000). One of the main factors delaying diagnostics of any rare disease is a low index of suspicion [4]. Indeed, for a referral to medical genetic clinic, a neurologist must raise a possibility of a genetic disorder in a patient with epilepsy or seizures first.

In any human disorder with a substantial genetic background, the choice of genetic testing modalities and workflows depends crucially on the genetic and clinical heterogeneity of a given disorder. The overall genetic heterogeneity and number of genetic nosologies involving epilepsy or seizures are largely unknown; however, epilepsy or seizures may be a symptom of many diverse conditions including channelopathies, neurodevelopmental diseases, inborn errors of metabolism, and congenital malformation syndromes [5]. Recently, we have comprised the most extensive to our knowledge database of more than 880 human genes associated with human monogenic diseases involving epilepsy or seizures, EpiGene database (http://www.kimg.eu/en/tools/epigene-database). Besides, more than 50 chromosomal syndromes are related to epilepsy or seizures (see Section 2.5). These numbers give important insights into the huge genetic heterogeneity of human disorders involving epilepsy or seizures, comparable to that of intellectual disabilities [6].

[1]Discussions about usefulness of genetic testing in multifactorial epilepsies (including pharmacogenetic testing) go beyond the scope of this chapter.

For many years the prevailing "dogma" was that epilepsy is a channelopathy [7], and the first unveiled channelopathy due to mutations in nicotinic acetylcholine receptor gene CHRNA4 became one of long-standing prototypes of genetic epilepsies [8]. Multiple channelopathies presenting with variable phenotypes are currently known (e.g., epileptic encephalopathies (due to mutations in genes HCN1, KCNA2, KCNB1, SCN8A, SLC13A5, STXBP1, and SYN1), benign neonatal seizures (genes KCNQ2 and KCNQ3), a spectrum of generalized epilepsy plus to Dravet syndrome due to SCN1A gene mutations). One of the major targets of current epilepsy genetic research is a group of disorders defined as epileptic encephalopathies; more than 70 genes have been related to this phenotype, explaining 20–25% of epileptic encephalopathy cases [9]. Relatively, homogenous clinical presentation of this epilepsy phenotype may aid in the recruitment of patients for genetic testing in both clinical setting and research. Distinct group of inherited epilepsies comprises progressive myoclonic epilepsies—an umbrella term for childhood- or adolescence-onset conditions characterized by myoclonus and relentlessly progressive neurodegeneration [10], including Unverricht-Lundborg, Lafora disease, neuronal ceroid lipofuscinoses, type 1 sialidosis, GM2 gangliosidosis, Gaucher disease, MERRF, and some other mitochondrial diseases—and other progressive myoclonic epilepsies due to mutations in genes ASAH1, CERS1, GOSR2, KCNC1, PRICKLE1, PRICKLE2, and SERPINI1. Other epilepsy phenotypes are much more heterogeneous. Surprisingly, the most extensive group of monogenic epilepsies is inherited metabolic diseases, encompassing 373 genes (42% of all genes) in EpiGene database (discussed more extensively below). The most frequent genetic epilepsy-associated symptoms are psychomotor retardation and intellectual disability (419 and 386 EpiGene diseases, respectively). Indeed, epilepsy is a frequent comorbidity (20–30% of cases) of syndromic and non-syndromic intellectual disabilities and vice versa; 30% of patients with epilepsy have intellectual disabilities [11]. Epilepsy or seizure is an accompanying symptom of a vast range of inherited neuromuscular and neurologic diseases, sometimes preceding development of other neurologic symptoms such as spastic paraplegias (SPG6, SPG11, SPG18, SPG35, SPG47, SPG49, SPG50, SPG51, and SPG52), muscular dystrophies (dystroglycanopathies due to mutations in genes B4GAT1, DAG1, FKRP, FKTN, GMPPB, ISPD, LARGE, POMGNT1, POMK, POMT1, and POMT2, congenital megaconial dystrophy (CHKB), merosin-deficient muscular dystrophy (LAMA2)), hereditary ataxias (spastic ataxia 5, ataxia with oculomotor apraxia (APTX), and ataxia-telangiectasia (ATM), spinocerebellar ataxias (SCA) SCA10 (ATXN10), SCA13 (GRM1), SCA15 (KIAA0226), SCA20 (SNX14), SCA17 (TBP), SCA12 (WWOX)), demyelinating diseases (e.g., hypomyelinating leukodystrophy due to mutations in genes AIMP1, FAM126A, GJC2, HSPD1, POLR3A, TUBB4A, leukoencephalopathy with vanishing white matter, megalencephalic leukoencephalopathy with subcortical cysts (HEPACAM, MLC1), adrenoleukodystrophy, metachromatic leukodystrophy, Krabbe disease); and hereditary dystonias (dentatorubropallidoluysian atrophy, dystonia 24 (ANO3), juvenile onset Parkinson disease 19 (DNAJC6), infantile striatonigral degeneration (NUP62)). Paving embryonic neurodevelopmental processes, epilepsy or seizures are very frequent symptoms in syndromes with malformations of cortical development, including megalencephalies (AKT3, EZH2, FGFR3, and PIK3CA), lissencephalies (ARX, RELN, VLDLR, ACTB, ACTG1, DCX, DYNC1H1, KIF2A, LIS1, TUBA1A, TUBB2B, and TUBG1), polymicrogyrias (NDE1, WDR62, FH, KIAA1279, NSDHL, OCLN, GPSM2, RAB3GAP1, RAB3GAP2, RAB18,

CHD7, and SRPX2), periventricular nodular heterotopia (ARFGEF2) [12], and neurocutaneous syndromes (tuberous sclerosis (TSC1 and TSC2), Sturge-Weber syndrome (GNAQ), incontinentia pigmenti (IKBKG), neurofibromatosis (NF1 and NF2)). However, epilepsy or seizures may also be variably present in multiple other congenital malformation syndromes, including not only CNS malformations (e.g., holoprosencephaly spectrum, pontocerebellar hypoplasia, and corpus callosum agenesis) but also malformations in any other organ. More than 130 congenital malformation syndromes include epilepsy or seizures as phenotypic features (http://www.kimg.eu/en/tools/epigene-database). Five hundred thirty-seven (61%) of EpiGene disorders are autosomal recessive, 234 (27%) (autosomal dominant) and 79 (9%) (X-linked).

It is not credible that any physician would be able to recognize and differentiate about 1000 genetic nosologies involving epilepsy or seizures, especially so that most of them are very rare and/or have just recently been described. Indeed, 228 of 880 EpiGene diseases (26%) are ultrarare, described just in several patients or families. Moreover, nonspecific and overlapping symptoms are frequent characteristics of these disorders. For many genetic epilepsies, mutations in a single gene may lead to a broad range of possible phenotypes and vice versa; patients with different genetic etiologies may have the same phenotype. To complicate matters still further, characteristic MRI and/or EEG features are very rare pointers or even supporters for a specific genetic etiology [13, 14]. Therefore, in clinical practice, genetic evaluation of a patient with epilepsy or seizures is usually not an easy task.

2.2. Genetic diagnostics of epilepsies: from traditional approach

Conventional etiological evaluation of epilepsy patients was complex and traditionally included karyotype, molecular karyotyping, and individually tailored serial metabolic and molecular genetic tests [5]. Secondary invasive tests such as biopsies and cerebrospinal fluid examination, aid in diagnosis in a small percentage of additional cases [15]. The main performance characteristic of any genetic testing modality is a diagnostic yield [16]. Clinical utility of various modes of genetic testing was recently evaluated in a retrospective analysis of 110 patients with various epileptic encephalopathies [17]. Genetic causes were identified in 26% of these patients by applying biochemical genetic testing, array comparative genome hybridization (aCGH), single-gene testing, targeted next-generation sequencing (NGS) testing (gene panels of 38, 70, or 327 genes), and whole-exome sequencing (WES) in six patients. In two patients, diagnosis was made on clinical grounds and not confirmed by genetic testing (1.8%), three patients (2.7%) had microdeletions revealed by aCGH, eight patients (7.2%) had inherited metabolic disorders (IEM), and targeted NGS testing resulted in diagnosis in 14 cases (12.7%) of patients [17]. The whole diagnostic pathway leading to the final diagnosis is not analyzed in this publication; however, a comparable pathway in patients with developmental delay/intellectual disability, many of whom had epilepsy, was described by López-Pisón et al. [18]. In a total of 686 cases (69% of all cases) in whom etiological diagnosis was not established had 8 tests each on average, including 2887 biochemistry tests, 1582 metabolic tests, 516 karyotyping/subtelomeric deletion tests, and 525 single-gene testing. Indeed, with sequential targeted testing, despite considerable efforts to reach the diagnosis, final diagnosis is frequently not established leading to a long "diagnostic odyssey" arduous for both patients and healthcare systems. Moreover, in many clinical situations, traditional approach is not only lengthy but also costly. In a study by Soden et al. before WES or whole-genome sequencing (WGS), patients had an average of 13.3 prior tests for the cost of $19,100 per family (seizures were observed in 39 of 100 patients in this study) [19]. The entire traditional diagnostic trajectory average cost was $16,409 per patient, substantially higher than the $3972 trio-WES cost, in 17 patients investigated by Monroe et al. [20]. The first and the only to date prospective comparison of cost-effectiveness of clinical whole-exome sequencing with a usual testing shows even more cost savings: in a cohort of 40 infants with neurodevelopmental disorders and congenital malformations, standard traditional testing had an average cost per diagnosis of US$21,099 compared to US$3937 for singleton WES. The use of WES early in the diagnostic pathway resulted in more than three times bigger diagnostic yield, while the price of testing was three times smaller [21]. It must be also noted that although Sanger sequencing is frequently entitled as the gold standard in genetic diagnostic accuracy, there are several recent reports about missed variants. In 9/105 families diagnosed through WES, the causative variant has not been detected by previous Sanger testing of a gene [22]. Finally, all the main professional genetic organizations, including the European Society of Human Genetics (ESHG), American College of Medical Genetics and Genomics (ACMG), and Canadian College of Medical Geneticists (CCMG), recognize that NGS testing may be a more practical approach than traditional gene-by-gene testing in certain clinical situations [23–25].

Nevertheless, traditional approach of genetic diagnostics with thorough phenotyping followed by targeted genetic testing can still be of value even in the era of NGS testing. Recently, a retrospective data analysis of 500 unselected consecutive patients coming to a university medical genetic clinic revealed a diagnostic rate of traditional approach reaching 46%. In this study, however, the reason for referral of 31% of diagnosed (14% of all) patients was a suspected specific diagnosis or a family history of a definite or suspected genetic disorder (i.e., confirmation or ruling out by a targeted genetic testing was needed only). Importantly, 72% of the diagnoses were made during the first visits (presumably, due to a highly suggestive phenotype), and further targeted testing resulted in huge expenses [26]. However, in patients with early onset epilepsy and developmental delay, standard clinical evaluation suggested a diagnosis in only 15% of them (11/71) [27]. Therefore, besides confirmation of the known family mutation, targeted testing is most suitable in cases with distinctive clinical features and minimal locus heterogeneity, for example, MECP2 gene analysis in a girl with characteristic Rett syndrome symptoms and clinical course or 15q11q13 methylation analysis in a patient with presumable Angelman syndrome. Targeted testing may also be important in selected cases where diagnosis cannot be captured by NGS (see Section 2.6). Otherwise, sequential targeted testing is largely inefficient and highly time- and cost-consuming.

2.3. To genomic testing technologies

In contrast, next-generation sequencing (NGS) technologies allow for untargeted testing of almost all genomic sequence (whole-genome sequencing (WGS)), almost all coding part of the genome (whole-exome sequencing (WES)), or simultaneous testing of a predetermined set of genes (gene panels). The most comprehensive testing methods—WGS and WES—usually allow for the most extensive differential diagnostics; however, extraction of useful information from huge amounts of raw data is time- and resource-consuming. Besides, all the bioethical/psychosocial implications pertinent to exhaustive genomic testing technologies must be addressed properly (see Section 2.7). On the other hand, too restrictive diagnostic approach leads to missed diagnoses. In our current era of constant accumulation of knowledge in human genomic health and disease and continuous technological advances of NGS methods, creation of valid recommendations for diagnostic evaluation of human disorders with a considerable genetic background always lags behind scientific and technological achievements and is not an easy task in a constantly changing landscape. Currently, there are no recommendations or guidelines for genetic testing in epilepsy patients addressing specificities of NGS technologies [28].

Although sequencing of the first human genome took 15 years and costs approximately 3 billion US dollars, the new Illumina HiSeq X Ten System can sequence 40–50 genomes per day for approximately 1000 US dollars each [29]. However, amounts of obtained data are overwhelming. Human genome consists of roughly 3.2 billion bp and contains around 3–4 million variants (roughly, 1 out of every 1000 bases) [30]. Certainly, the vast majority of these variants are benign, determining personal particularities of any individual. Exome, the coding part of genome, comprises 1–2% of the whole-genome sequence (~65 Mb) and contains 30,000–60,000 variants [30, 31]. Human genomic variation is almost immeasurable: the most extensive to date human population exome database ExAC (http://exac.broadinstitute.org), encompassing more than 60,000 exomes, contains 7.4 million high-quality variants, a variant in one out of every eight bases on average. More than a half of these variants (54%) have been found just in one individual each [32].

Besides, extraction of useful information from the huge amounts of WGS/WES data is limited due to our limited knowledge about human genes. As of February 2015, of approximately ~19,000 protein-coding genes predicted to exist in the human genome, variants that cause Mendelian phenotypes have been identified in ~2937 (~15.5%), while the genes underlying about half of all known Mendelian phenotypes (i.e., 3152) have not yet been discovered, despite the fact that ~20% (i.e., 643) have been mapped. Moreover, ~16,063 other genes still remain candidates for Mendelian phenotypes [33]. Therefore, the major limiting factor of current genomic diagnostics is not data generation, but identification and proper interpretation of causative variants in the whole flood of "genomic noise." Multiple powerful bioinformatic approaches and tools are implemented in WGS/WES data mining; however, technologies cannot totally replace human workload. On the contrary, deep knowledge and extensive skills of multiple professionals are on a higher demand than ever in order to enable successful usage of the technological advances of NGS.

Nevertheless, hundreds of thousands of exomes and tens of thousands of genomes are already sequenced, and projects like 100K Genome Project in UK are well under way [30]. Data on diagnostic rates of WGS in epilepsy patients are limited: WGS revealed pathogenic and likely pathogenic mutations in all six (100% yield) patients with severe early onset epilepsy who had previously were refractory to molecular diagnosis by extensive genetic, biochemical, and imaging testing [34]. Other WGS studies mostly include patients with various neurodevelopmental phenotypes; however, considerable part of them have epilepsy or seizures: in 119 children WES resulted in a 33% and WGS achieved a remarkable 73% diagnostic rate, while cumulative rate of both WES and WGS was 45% [19]. WES gave a 27% diagnostic rate (27/100 patients), while WGS in patients with negative prior WES and aCGH testing resulted in 42% diagnostic yield (21/50 patients) [35]. Indeed, WGS is the most comprehensive genomic testing mode, encompassing the most extensive mutational spectrum and bypassing many of WES limitations in mutation detection (e.g., reliable identification of deep intronic/regulatory sequence variants or tandem repeats, see Section 2.6). In a recent study of 156 cases with variable phenotypes, an estimated ~15% of causal variants identified by clinical WGS would most likely have been missed by WES [36]. However, our limited knowledge and a huge interpretative workload currently limit the use of WGS, especially in a clinical setting. In the studies mentioned above, the vast majority of data obtained from WGS, especially variants beyond the coding part of human genome, did not have any diagnostic value and could not reliably be ascribed to either benign or pathogenic [35, 36].

Meanwhile, WES gets more and more applications in the diagnostic evaluation of patients with epilepsy or seizures. Recently, a study on WES in 314 consecutive patients with unselected epilepsies has shown a diagnostic yield of 38.2% [37]. WES in 10 sporadic cases of infantile spasms was diagnosed in 40% [38]. Diagnostic output of WES in neurodevelopmental disorders, including epilepsies, was 41% in a group of 78 pediatric patients (12% of them had epilepsy) [39]. In a cohort of 500 unselected patients coming to a university medical genetic clinic, diagnostic yield of WES was 30%, while that of patients with epilepsy was 35% [40]. The output of WES may also depend on when in a diagnostic process it is used: as a first-tier test when a genetically heterogeneous disorder is suspected, as a second-tier after the initial set of tests is normal, or at the end of the whole diagnostic odyssey. In a prospective study of 80 infants with mostly neurodevelopmental disorders and congenital malformations, first-tier singleton WES resulted in 57.5% diagnostic yield compared to 13.75% diagnostic yield of standard investigations (including gene panel testing) [41].

Despite the well-recognized benefits of WGS/WES approaches, they also carry with them a high burden of interpretative workload and an increased possibility of detecting incidental findings (see Section 2.6) [42]. According to the current European Society of Human Genetics (ESHG) recommendations, it is preferable to use a targeted approach of gene panels first in order to avoid unsolicited findings or findings that cannot be interpreted [23]. Indeed, about 80% of human genes are currently not associated with a disease. In the investigation of disorders with limited genetic and phenotypic heterogeneity, gene panels may outperform WES because of better coverage, time- and cost-efficiency, and a focused approach excluding incidental findings [29]. Multiple gene panels exist for the investigation of patients with epileptic encephalopathies, cortical malformations, groups of inborn errors of metabolism, various other clinical indications, and undifferentiated epilepsy phenotypes. However, due to a huge phenotypic and genetic heterogeneity characteristic of disorders involving epilepsy or seizures, as illustrated by EpiGene database (http://www.kimg.eu/en/tools/epigene-database), gene panels may lead to smaller diagnostic yields due to their restrictiveness. Testing of 500 epileptic encephalopathy patients with a gene panel containing 65 genes gave a diagnostic yield of 10% [43], 30 gene or 90 gene panels in 349 patients with treatment-resistant epilepsies gave a diagnostic yield of 20.3% [44], a gene panel of 46 genes in 216 patients with various epilepsies gave 23% diagnostic yield [45], a gene panel trio-testing of 412 genes in 63 probands with variable epilepsies gave 23.8% diagnostic yield [46], and a combined approach of 46 gene panel and targeted exon-level aCGH in 400 patients with early onset epilepsy and developmental delay gave 18% diagnostic yield [27]. Comparisons of gene panel testing studies are hindered by a huge phenotypic and gene panel variability in all these studies. Indeed, Genetic Testing Registry (http://www.ncbi.nlm.nih.gov/gtr/) database lists more than 60 epilepsy gene panels from several to 377 genes in size (as of 09/04/2016), and the most comprehensive commercially available epilepsy gene panels include from 100 to more than 400 genes, with a proportion of genes associated with epilepsy in animal or association studies only and up to 4% of included genes currently not related to epilepsy or seizures at all [47]. Moreover, there is a high inconsistency in both gene numbers and compositions of gene panels even though applied for similar groups of patients with epilepsy. In a clinical setting, selection of the most appropriate gene panel in a given patient may be challenging because of overlapping, not-full-blown, atypical clinical presentations [42]. Finally, gene panels rather quickly become outdated because of newly discovered genes [41]. A possible solution to these problems is the use of "virtual" gene panels applied to WES data. Such an approach gives a flexibility in "virtual" gene panel selection and, in cases of negative findings, further possibilities to eventually proceed to a much more untargeted analysis of the whole WES data. Besides, carefully selected and applied to WES sequencing data, "virtual" gene panels can act as a supplementary filtering system aiding in time-efficient and better variant calling in terms of exclusion of both false-positive (by filtering out non-epilepsy-related genes) and false-negative (by inclusion of epilepsy-related genes which could be missed in the whole flood of variants) findings. Recently, we have created a web tool for a customized gene panel creation according to the phenotype (http://www.kimg.eu/generator). Application of this tool to 405 patients with various phenotypes increased diagnostic sensitivity from 25.4 to 29.7% [42] comparing to the whole WES data analysis.

2.4. Diagnoses not to miss: treatable inborn errors of metabolism

Metabolic epilepsies represent an unquestionable area of precision medicine where timely diagnosis and specific treatments tailored to the inherited metabolic defect may markedly improve both the seizures and associated comorbidities as intellectual disability [48]. Regrettably, diagnosis of these and other potentially treatable epilepsy-related diseases is still often delayed [49]. The reasons for that may be insufficient testing due to a low index of suspicion, phenotypic variability and nonspecificity, complexity and limited availability of metabolic testing, and invasiveness of some of the diagnostic methods.

More than 370 inborn errors of metabolism (IEM) can present with epilepsy or seizures, and more than 90 of these disorders have disease-specific treatments leading to a much more better prognosis, improved control of both seizures and comorbid symptoms, and complete avoidance of antiepileptic drugs if diagnosed timely (**Table 1**; http://www.kimg.eu/en/tools/epigene-database). However, traditional diagnostics of IEM may be cumbersome as it involves a range of metabolic tests performed in specialized laboratories. Urine and/or plasma specimen are mostly used; however, in some IEM characteristic metabolites can mainly or only be investigated in cerebrospinal fluid (CSF). Histological and/or biochemical investigations of biopsies (e.g., skin, conjunctiva, or muscle) can aid in the diagnostics of certain other IEM. Selection of tests is usually based on a diagnostic hypothesis and requires specialized

Inherited metabolic disease		Diagnostic metabolites	Gene	OMIM number
1. Disorders of amino acid and peptide metabolism				
1.	Glycine encephalopathy (GCE)	Hyperglycinemia Hyperglycinuria Elevated CSF glycine Elevated CSF/plasma glycine ratio	*AMT* *GCSH* *GLDC*	#605899 #605899 #605899
2.	Argininemia	Hyperarginemia Diaminoaciduria (arginuria, lysinuria, cystinuria, ornithinuria) Orotic aciduria Pyrimidinuria Increased CSF amino acids (arginine, ornithine, aspartate, threonine, glycine, and methionine)	*ARG1*	#207800
3.	Argininosuccinic aciduria	Increased citrulline (P) Increased glutamine (P) Argininosuccinic aciduria Orotic aciduria	*ASL*	#207900
4.	Citrullinemia, classic	Increased citrulline (P) Increased glutamine (P) Decreased arginine (P) Orotic aciduria	*ASS1*	#215700
5.	3-Methylglutaconic aciduria, type I (MGCA1)	Metabolic acidosis Increased 3-methylglutaconic acid (U) Increased hydroxyisovaleric acid (U)	*AUH*	#250950
6.	Maple syrup urine disease (MSUD)	Increased branched chain amino acids (leucine, isoleucine, valine) (P) Branched chain ketoaciduria (alpha-keto isocaproate, alpha-keto-beta methylisovalerate, alpha-keto isovalerate) Increased alloisoleucine(P) Positive urine DNPH screening test	*BCKDHA* *BCKDHB* *DBT*	#248600 #248600 #248600
7.	Homocystinuria due to cystathionine beta-synthase deficiency	Homocystinuria Methioninuria	*CBS*	#236200
8.	Carbamoyl phosphate synthetase I deficiency, hyperammonemia due to	Decreased citrulline (P) Decreased arginine (P) Decreased orotic acid (U)	*CPS1*	#237300

Inherited metabolic disease		Diagnostic metabolites	Gene	OMIM number
9.	Glutaric acidemia I	Glutaric aciduria	*GCDH*	#231670
10.	Hyperinsulinemic hypoglycemia, familial, 6 (HHF6)	Hyperinsulinemic hypoglycemia Hyperammonemia	*GLUD1*	#606762
11.	17-Beta-hydroxysteroid dehydrogenase X deficiency	Increased 2-methyl-3 hydroxybutyrate (U) Increased tiglylglycine (U)	*HSD17B10*	#300438
12.	Isovaleric acidemia (IVA)	Isovaleric acidemia Isovaleric aciduria Isovaleryl glycinuria	*IVD*	#243500
13.	Homocystinuria-megaloblastic anemia, cblG complementation type (HMAG)	Homocystinuria Hyperhomocysteinemia Hypomethioninemia	*MTR*	#250940
14.	Homocystinuria-megaloblastic anemia, cblE complementation type (HMAE)	Homocystinuria Hyperhomocysteinemia Hypomethioninemia	*MTRR*	#236270
15.	N-Acetylglutamate synthase deficiency (NAGSD)	Increased glutamine (P) Decreased or absent citrulline (P) Normal orotic acid (U)	*NAGS*	#237310
16.	Ornithine transcarbamylase deficiency, hyperammonemia due to	Decreased citrulline (P) Decreased arginine (P) Increased glutamine (P) Increased asparagine (P) Increased orotic acid (U) Increased ornithine (P)	*OTC*	#311250
17.	Phenylketonuria (PKU)	Hyperphenylalaninemia Phenylpyruvic acidemia	*PAH*	#261600
18.	Propionic acidemia	Increased propionate Increased 3-hydroxypropionic acid Increased 3-methylcitric acid Hyperglycinemia Hyperglycinuria	*PCCA* *PCCB*	#606054 #606054

Inherited metabolic disease		Diagnostic metabolites	Gene	OMIM number
19.	Phosphoglycerate dehydrogenase deficiency (PHGDHD)	Decrease serine (fasting) (P) Decreased serine (C) Normal-to-decreased glycine (fasting) (P) Decreased glycine (C)	*PHGDH*	#601815
20.	Phosphoserine aminotransferase deficiency (PSATD)	Decreased serine (P, C) Decreased glycine (P, C)	*PSAT1*	#610992
21.	Phosphoserine phosphatase deficiency (PSPHD)	Decreased serine (P) Decreased glycine (P)	*PSPH*	#614023
22.	Citrullinemia, type II, adult-onset (CTLN2)	Citrullinemia	*SLC25A13*	#603471
23.	Hyperornithinemia-hyperammonemia-homocitrullinuria syndrome	Hyperornithinemia Hyperammonemia Homocitrullinuria	*SLC25A15*	#238970
24.	3-Hydroxy-3-methylglutaryl-CoA lyase deficiency (HMGCLD)	Hypoketotic hypoglycemia	*HMGCL*	#246450
2. *Disorders of carbohydrate metabolism*				
25.	Fructose intolerance (hereditary)	Hypoglycemia Fructosemia	*ALDOB*	#229600
26.	Glut1 deficiency syndrome	Decreased CSF/plasma glucose ratio	*SLC2A1*	#614847
27.	Hyperinsulinemic hypoglycemia, familial, 1 (HHF1)	Hypoglycemia Hyperinsulinemia	*ABCC8*	#256450
28.	Hyperinsulinemic hypoglycemia, familial, 5 (HHF5)	Hypoglycemia, postprandial Hyperinsulinemia, fasting Elevated serum insulin-to-C-peptide ratio	*INSR*	#609968
29.	Hyperinsulinemic hypoglycemia, familial, 2 (HHF2)	Hypoglycemia Hyperinsulinemia	*KCNJ11*	#601820
3. *Disorders of fatty acid and ketone body metabolism*				

Inherited metabolic disease		Diagnostic metabolites	Gene	OMIM number
30.	Multiple acyl-CoA dehydrogenase deficiency (MADD)	Neonatal acidosis Hypoglycemia Glutaric aciduria Glutaric acidemia Ethylmalonic aciduria	*ETFA* *ETFB* *ETFDH*	#231680 #231680 #231680
31.	Neurodegeneration due to cerebral folate transport deficiency	Decreased methyltetrahydrofolate (MTHF) (C)	*FOLR1*	#613068
32.	3-Hydroxy-3-methylglutaryl-CoA synthase-2 deficiency (HMGCS2D)	Hypoketotic hypoglycemia	*HMGCS2*	#605911
4. Disorders of energy metabolism				
33.	Coenzyme Q10 deficiency, primary, 4 (COQ10D4)	Increased lactate (P, C)	*ADCK3*	#612016
34.	Coenzyme Q10 deficiency, primary, 1 (COQ10D1)	Lactic acidosis	*COQ2*	#607426
35.	Coenzyme Q10 deficiency, primary, 5 (COQ10D5)	Lactic acidosis	*COQ9*	#614654
36.	Encephalopathy, ethylmalonic (EE)	Lactic acidosis Ethylmalonic aciduria Methylsuccinic aciduria Increased C4 and C5 acylcarnitine esters (P) Increased isobutyryl glycine (U) Increased 2-methylbutyryl glycine (U) Increased thiosulfate (U)	*ETHE1*	#602473
37.	Cerebral creatine deficiency syndrome 2 (CCDS2)	Low creatine (C) Low creatinine (C)	*GAMT*	#612736
38.	Cerebral creatine deficiency syndrome 3 (CCDS3)	Decreased guanidinoacetate (GAA) (P, U)	*GATM*	#612718
39.	Pyruvate dehydrogenase E1-alpha deficiency (PDHAD)	Lactic acidosis Increased pyruvate (P, C, U) Increased lactate (P, C, U)	*PDHA1*	#312170
40.	Pyruvate dehydrogenase E1-beta deficiency (PDHBD)	Lactic acidosis	*PDHB*	#614111

Inherited metabolic disease		Diagnostic metabolites	Gene	OMIM number
41.	Pyruvate dehydrogenase E3-binding protein deficiency (PDHXD)	Lactic acidosis Increased pyruvate (P) Increased alanine (P)	*PDHX*	#245349
42.	Coenzyme Q10 deficiency, primary, 3 (COQ10D3)	Increased lactate (P)	*PDSS2*	#614652
5. Disorders of the metabolism of sterols				
43.	Cerebrotendinous xanthomatosis (CTX)	Increased cholestanol (P) Increased 7 alpha-hydroxylated bile alcohols (U)	*CYP27A1*	#213700
44.	Smith-Lemli-Opitz syndrome (SLOS)	Decreased cholesterol (P) Increased 7-dehydrocholesterol (P)	*DHCR7*	#270400
45.	Bile acid synthesis defect, congenital, 1 (CBAS1)	Increased serum bilirubin Abnormal liver function tests Decreased serum cholesterol	*HSD3B7*	#607765
6. Disorders of porphyrin and heme metabolism				
46.	Porphyria, acute intermittent (AIP)	Increased delta-aminolevulinic acid (ALA) and porphobilinogen (PBG) during acute attacks (U)	*HMBS*	#176000
47.	Porphyria variegata	Increased fecal protoporphyrin and coproporphyrin Increased porphyrins (U) Increased porphobilinogen (PBG) and delta-aminolevulinic acid (ALA) during acute attacks (U)	*PPOX*	#176200
48.	Porphyria, acute hepatic	Hemolytic anemia Elevated urinary delta-aminolevulinic acid and porphyrins	*ALAD*	#612740
49.	Coproporphyria, hereditary (HCP)	Increased coproporphyrin isomer III:I ratio (HCP, feces) Increased harderoporphyrin excretion (feces, harderoporphyria)	*CPOX*	#121300
7. Disorders of lipid and lipoprotein metabolism				
50.	Sjogren-Larsson syndrome (SLS)	Fatty alcohol: NAD+ oxidoreductase deficiency in leukocytes and fibroblasts	*ALDH3A2*	#270200
8. Congenital disorders of glycosylation and other disorders of protein modification				

Inherited metabolic disease		Diagnostic metabolites	Gene	OMIM number
51.	Congenital disorder of glycosylation, type IIc (CDG2C)	Neutrophilia, both basal and during infections Isoelectric focusing of serum transferrin (type II)	*SLC35C1*	#266265
10. Lysosomal disorders				
52.	Aspartylglucosaminuria (AGU)	Aspartylglucosaminuria	*AGA*	#208400
53.	Metachromatic leukodystrophy	Increased protein (C) Increased sulfatide (U)	*ARSA*	#250100
54.	Krabbe disease	Increased protein (C)	*GALC*	#245200
55.	Gaucher disease, type III	Gaucher cells in bone marrow	*GBA*	#231000
56.	Fabry disease	Bone marrow contains lipid-laden macrophages Increased globotriaosylceramide (GB3) (P, U) Increased globotriaosylsphingosine (lyso-GB3) (P)	*GLA*	#301500
57.	Mucopolysaccharidosis, type IIID (MPS3D)	Heparan sulfate (U)	*GNS*	#252940
58.	Mucopolysaccharidosis, type IIIC (MPS3C)	Heparan sulfate (U)	*HGSNAT*	#252930
59.	Mucopolysaccharidosis, type II (MPS2)	Dermatan and heparan sulfate (U)	*IDS*	#309900
60.	Mucopolysaccharidosis, type IIIB (MPS3B)	Heparan sulfate (U)	*NAGLU*	#252920
61.	Niemann-Pick disease, type C1 (NPC1)	Foam cells on bone marrow biopsy "Sea-blue" histiocytes Foam cells in visceral organs and CNS Foam cells contain polymorphic cytoplasmic inclusions consisting of lamellar osmiophilic membranes on electron microscopy	*NPC1*	#257220
62.	Niemann-Pick disease, type C2 (NPC2)	Foam cells on bone marrow biopsy "Sea-blue" histiocytes Foam cells in visceral organs and CNS Foam cells contain polymorphic cytoplasmic inclusions consisting of lamellar osmiophilic membranes on electron microscopy	*NPC2*	#607625
63.	Mucopolysaccharidosis, type IIIA (MPS3A)	Heparan sulfate (U)	*SGSH*	#252900
10. Peroxisomal disorders				
64.	Adrenoleukodystrophy (ALD)	Very long-chain fatty acids (P, U, C)	*ABCD1*	#300100

	Inherited metabolic disease	Diagnostic metabolites	Gene	OMIM number
11. Disorders of neurotransmitter metabolism				
65.	Succinic semialdehyde dehydrogenase deficiency (SSADHD)	Increased 4-hydroxybutyric acid (U, P, C) Increased gamma-aminobutyric acid (U, P, C)	*ALDH5A1*	#271980
12. Disorders in the metabolism of vitamins and (nonprotein) cofactors				
66.	Epilepsy, pyridoxine-dependent (PDE)	Increased pipecolic acid (U, P, C) Increased alpha-aminoadipic semialdehyde (P, U, C)	*ALDH7A1*	#266100
67.	Hypophosphatasia, infantile	Phosphoethanolaminuria Increased inorganic pyrophosphate (P, U) Decreased alkaline phosphatase (P)	*ALPL*	#241500
68.	Biotinidase deficiency	Increased beta-hydroxyisovalerate, lactate, beta-methylcrotonylglycine, beta-hydroxypropionate, methylcitrate (U)	*BTD*	#253260
69.	Hyperphenylalaninemia, BH4-deficient, B (HPABH4B)	Hyperphenylalaninemia Decreased homovanillic acid and 5-hydroxyindoleacetic acid (C) Decreased neopterin and biopterin (U, C)	*GCH1*	#233910
70.	Holocarboxylase synthetase deficiency	Increased beta-hydroxyisovalerate, beta-methylcrotonylglycine, beta-hydroxypropionate, methylcitrate, lactate, tiglylglycine (U) Normal serum biotin concentration	*HLCS*	#253270
71.	Methylmalonic aciduria and homocystinuria, cblF type	Methylmalonic acid (U, P) Homocystine (P, U) Cystathionine (P, U) Decreased adenosylcobalamin Decreased methylcobalamin	*LMBRD1*	#277380
72.	Methylmalonic aciduria, cblA type	Methylmalonic acid (P, U) Long-chain ketonuria Hyperglycinemia Decreased adenosylcobalamin Normal serum cobalamin (vitamin B12)	*MMAA*	#251100

Inherited metabolic disease		Diagnostic metabolites	Gene	OMIM number
73.	Methylmalonic aciduria and homocystinuria, cblC type	Homocystine (P, U) Methylmalonic acid (P, U) Decreased methionine (P) Cystathionine (P, U) Decreased adenosylcobalamin Decreased methylcobalamin Normal serum cobalamin	*MMACHC*	#277400
74.	Methylmalonic aciduria and homocystinuria, cblD type	Megaloblastic anemia Homocystinuria Homocystinemia Methylmalonic acid (P, U) Decreased methionine (P) Decreased adenosylcobalamin Decreased methylcobalamin Normal or mildly reduced serum cobalamin	*MMADHC*	#277410
75.	Molybdenum cofactor deficiency	Increased xanthine (U) Increased hypoxanthine (U) Increased S-sulfocysteine (U) Increased taurine (U)	*MOCS1* *MOCS2*	#252150 #252160
76.	Homocystinuria due to deficiency of N(5,10)-methylenetetrahydrofolate reductase activity	Low to normal methionine (P) Homocystinemia Homocystinuria	*MTHFR*	#236250
77.	Pyridoxamine 5-prime-phosphate oxidase deficiency	Normal to increased glycine (P) Normal to increased threonine (P) Decreased arginine (P) Increased vanillactic acid (U) Decreased homovanillic acid (C) Decreased 5-hydroxyindoleacetic acid (C) Increased 3-methoxytyrosine (C) Increased glycine, threonine, taurine, histidine (C) Decreased arginine (C) Decreased pyridoxal (C) Decreased pyridoxal 5-prime-phosphate (C)	*PNPO*	#610090

Inherited metabolic disease		Diagnostic metabolites	Gene	OMIM number
78.	Hyperphenylalaninemia, BH4-deficient, A (HPABH4A)	Hyperphenylalaninemia Decreased homovanillic acid and 5-hydroxyindoleacetic acid (C) Increased neopterin (U, C)	*PTS*	#261640
79.	Hyperphenylalaninemia, BH4-deficient, C (HPABH4C)	Hyperphenylalaninemia Decreased homovanillic acid and 5-hydroxyindoleacetic acid (C) Increased biopterin (U, C)	*QDPR*	#261630
80.	Salla disease (SD)		*SLC19A2*	#249270
81.	Thiamine-responsive megaloblastic anemia syndrome (TRMA)	0	*SLC19A3*	#607483
82.	Folate malabsorption, hereditary	Megaloblastic anemia, folate-responsive Decreased folate (P, C) Decreased methionine (P) Increased formiminoglutamic acid (U)	*SLC46A1*	#229050
83.	Dystonia, dopa-responsive, due to sepiapterin reductase deficiency	Decreased 5-hydroxyindoleacetic acid (C) Decreased homovanillic acid (C) Increased sepiapterin (C) Increased biopterin (C) Increased dihydrobiopterin (C) Decreased HVA, 5-HIAA, and vanillylmandelic acid (U) Normal urinary pterins No hyperphenylalaninemia	*SPR*	#612716
13. Disorders in the metabolism of trace elements and metals				
84.	Menkes disease	Decreased copper and ceruloplasmin (P)	*ATP7A*	#309400
85.	Wilson disease	Decreased ceruloplasmin (P) Increased copper (U)	*ATP7B*	#277900

Table 1. Treatable inborn errors of metabolism (IEM) associated with epilepsy or seizures.

knowledge in IEM. Unfortunately, characteristics of seizure semiology, EEG, or head magnetic resonance imaging/spectroscopy (MRI/MRS) can only seldom guide differential diagnostics of these IEM [13, 48, 50–52]. Besides, there is a huge phenotypic diversity: epilepsy or seizures are usually accompanied by other signs and symptoms; multisystem involvement is common. Seizures can be the main and the first symptom (e.g., in pyridoxine-dependent epilepsy) or a late presentation (e.g., in some of lysosomal storage diseases). Intermediary metabolism defects can present with symptomatic seizures during acute crises only [48, 53]. Consequently, diagnostics of IEM is sophisticated, time-consuming, and sometimes invasive and requires a high degree of specialization, experience, and investments into the diagnostic laboratory equipment and human resources (**Table 1**).

Molecular genetic tests are usually performed for the confirmation of IEM diagnosis and/or genetic counseling purposes [52]. However, recent emergence of NGS technologies provides us entirely new diagnostic possibilities. Indeed, previously unsuspected IEM were frequently diagnosed in patients with epilepsy through NGS studies [19, 54], and, vice versa, other genetic diseases were diagnosed in patients with suspected IEM [55]. Noninvasiveness is a further advantage of NGS tests. Therefore, NGS testing might be considered as a primary test and as the most comprehensive screening test for these IEM.

Many IEM present with acute symptoms and metabolic testing in this setting can give the only opportunity for timely diagnosis. However, with ever progressing technological advancements, application of NGS methods can be comparably time-efficient and gives very high diagnostic yield rates. In a study by Soden et al. [19], accelerated whole-genome sequencing has been performed in 15 acutely ill patients in 50 hours (7 of them presented with seizures) with a remarkable diagnostic rate of 73%, while turnaround times of whole-exome sequencing (applied mostly for outpatients) were on average of 16 days. About 20% of all diagnosed patients (9 patients of 45 diagnosed) were diagnosed with IEM [19].

2.5. Chromosomal disorders with epilepsy or seizures

Several hundreds of chromosomal disorders are associated with epilepsy or seizures including aneuploidies (e.g., ~10% of Down syndrome patients have epilepsy), chromosomal rearrangements (e.g., balanced translocations and disrupting known epilepsy-associated genes), and structural variants (syndromic and non-syndromic deletions, duplications, and inversions) [56]. In most of these disorders, epilepsy or seizure is a variable feature, and most of these chromosomal disorders are associated with developmental delay/intellectual disability (DD/ID), autism, and/or congenital malformations (CM). Historically, G-banding karyotype was used for the detection of aneuploidies and large-scale chromosomal rearrangements with an average diagnostic yield in patients with DD/ID and/or CM not exceeding 3% (excluding Down syndrome; [57]). Fluorescent in situ hybridization (FISH) technique was mostly used for the diagnosis of known, recognizable microdeletion and microduplication syndromes (e.g., 4pdel (Wolf-Hirschhorn), 17pdel (Miller-Dieker), 15q11q13del maternal (Angelman), and 18qdel (de Grouchy), all including seizures), and subtelomeric FISH/subtelomeric MLPA allowed for identification of subtelomeric gains or losses with additional ~3–6% of diagnoses [58, 59]. The major breakthroughs came with the advent of microarrays that have evolved from rather crude bacterial artificial chromosome (BAC)-based platforms to the contemporary platforms allowing copy number variation (CNV) analysis down to an exon level. These methods increased diagnostic rates in patients with ID/DD and/or CM by ~15% [60] and allowed for elucidation of multiple other microdeletion/microduplication syndromes associated with epilepsy or seizures (**Table 2**). Besides, NGS approaches for CNV variant calling (e.g., by using depth-of-coverage analysis-based tool CoNIFER [61] have been developed. Importantly, these methods are restricted to unbalanced chromosomal rearrangements solely; therefore, they do not abolish completely the need for karyotyping. For example, a small part of patients with ring 14

1q21.1del/dup	14q23.3del
1q31.3q41dup	15q11.2del
1q41q42.12del	15q13.2q13.3del
1q43q44del	15q13.3del
2q23.1del/dup	15q26.1del
2q23.3q24.2del	15q26.3del
2q24.1del	16p11.2del/dup
2q24dup	16p13.11del
2q24.3del/dup	16p12del
3p25.3del	16p11.2dup
5p15.31p15.2del	16q22.1del/dup
5q11.2del	17p13.3del
5q14.3q15del	17p13.1del
6q22.1del	17p11.2del
6q25.3q27del	17q11.2del/dup
6q26q27del	17q21.31del/dup
7q11.23q21.12del	19p13.2del
7q11.23dup	20p13del
7q22.2q22.3del	20q13.33del
8p23.3p23.1del	21q22del
8q22.2del	22q11.2del
9p24.1del	Xp22.33del
9q22.3del	Xp11.4dup
9q34.3del	Xq11.11del
14q12q22.1del	Xq27q28dup

References: 1. Leu et al. [110]; 2. Nevado et al. [111].

Table 2. Microdeletion and microduplication syndromes, associated with epilepsy or seizures.

and ring 20 chromosomal syndromes do not have any chromosomal material loss [62, 63]. It was estimated that <1% of all diagnoses will be undetected by array-based investigations due to balanced chromosomal rearrangements [64]. Moreover, different ranges of CNV size are typically captured by array-based and NGS-based methods. Although WGS may capture the whole spectrum of CNVs (and other structural variations), costs and large amounts of data requiring analysis and interpretation currently limits its use [65, 66].

Currently, copy number variation is defined as a genomic segment of at least 50 bp that differs in copy number based on two or more genome comparisons (the smaller elements are known as insertions or deletions, indels) [65]. Copy number variation of human genome is even more extensive than single-nucleotide variation (a median of 8.9 Mb of sequence is affected by structural variants in comparison to 3.6 Mb of single-nucleotide polymorphisms [67]). As of 2014, the most extensive general population of CNV database of genomic variants (DGV) contains more than 2.3 million variants [68], and the bulk of structural variations identified in population controls are low-frequency variants (e.g., 65% of variants detected in 2504 individuals had VAF <0.2% [67]). Together with a limited knowledge on human pathological copy number variation and functional importance of these genome elements, it creates huge challenges in CNV data interpretation [69, 70]. Although the American College of Medical Genetics and Genomics provides some guidelines in CNV analysis [70], interpretation and reporting, multiple various workflows, and strategies exist [60, 69, 71], and diagnostic outputs may substantially differ even in the same cohort of patients investigated by the same professionals over just several years [72]. Currently, the most extensively investigated are heterozygous de novo or inherited dominant CNVs. However, autosomal recessive, imprinting, and X-linked disorders (as much as 10% of all identified causative CNVs in ID were X-linked in a study by Hehir-Kwa et al.) may also be uncovered [69, 73]. Although the pathogenic potential of 1–500 kb small CNVs has not been well elucidated and may not be reported in some laboratories performing aCGH (2010 consensus statement on diagnostic chromosomal microarray testing recommends a resolution of ≥400 kb as a balance of analytical and clinical sensitivity), small CNVs may account for a neurodevelopmental disease phenotype in at least 2% of patients, and this range of CNVs is of increasing importance due to spreading NGS-based CNV calling methods [74]. Although noncoding copy number variation is usually discarded as nonrelevant or uninterpretable, intergenic or intronic structural variation may affect gene regulation through position effect and disturbance of regulatory sequences or normal chromatin folding [75]. Moreover, somatically acquired structural variation may also play a role [76].

Since 2009, importance of CNVs in various epilepsy phenotypes has been shown in multiple studies. The biggest diagnostic yields have been achieved in patients with epilepsy and various brain malformations: pathogenic and likely pathogenic CNVs had 23.7% of 76 patients [77] and 22.5% of 169 patients [78]. Microarray testing has been informative in 3.4–8% of patients with epileptic encephalopathy [79, 80], 10.9% in 247 cases with epilepsy and associated ID/DD and/or CM [81], and 5% in 805 patients with unselected epilepsy phenotypes [82]. Both recurrent CNVs at 15q13.3, 15q11.2, 16p11.2, and 16p13.11 and rare CNVs may play a significant role as one of the major risk factors for common epilepsies, including genetic generalized epilepsy [83, 84], absence epilepsies [85, 86], and Rolandic epilepsy [87]; however, lack of knowledge on the whole phenotypic expression and penetrance of these CNVs present considerable challenges for genetic counseling.

2.6. Next-generation sequencing testing in epilepsies: current problems and limitations

There are two main groups of limitations and problems that must be taken into consideration while applying NGS technologies in a diagnostic testing: technological problems/limitations and psychosocial/bioethical implications (discussed in Section 2.7).

Although WGS interrogates almost the whole genome and WES—a coding part of the genome—diagnostic rate of WGS in patients with epilepsy and other phenotypically and genetically diverse neurodevelopmental disorders is seldom above 70%, while the rate of WES usually does not exceed 50%. Some types of mutations are reluctant to WGS (e.g., epigenetic mutations, structural chromosome rearrangements, tissue-restricted somatic mosaicism). Although our knowledge of WGS-reluctant human molecular pathology is very limited, there are several recent examples of such pathology discovered in patients with epilepsy. Postzygotic tissue-restricted somatic de novo mutations in *AKT3*, *MTOR*, and *PIK3CA* have been identified as the cause of cortical malformation syndromes associated with severe epilepsy [88], and somatic mutations in *DCX*, *LIS1*, *FLNA*, and *TUBB2B* genes as the cause of double cortex syndrome, periventricular nodular heterotopia, and pachygyria [89]. Recently found biallelic mutations in the box C/D snoRNA U8 gene *SNORD118* as a cause of the cerebral microangiopathy leukoencephalopathy with calcifications and cysts are an example of a pathogenic genomic variation, not amenable to current WES variant filtering practices restricted to coding regions and canonical splice sites [90].

Deep intronic, intergenic, regulatory sequence variants (noncoding parts of genome), tandem repeats, mtDNA variants, CNVs, variants in GC-rich, repetitive, and homologous regions of exome may not be detected in WES [91]. However, at least some of the technological limitations of WES technologies may be solved. Capturing of mtDNA variation (e.g., by using MitoSeek tool; [92]) and CNV variant calling (see Section 2.5) may be incorporated into the method and WES data analysis pipeline. Although detection of very large or small (one to two exons) deletions may be limited, sensitivity of identifying CNVs containing three or more exons has been estimated to be 76%, with a specificity of 94% [61]. As both CNVs and mtDNA variations [93] play a substantial role in the etiology of genetic epilepsies, these amendments are crucially important in this patient group. Unequal coverage of exome leading to missed variants (mostly in GC-rich, repetitive, and homologous regions) is a well-known problem [31, 91]. Therefore, when testing a limited number of genes in disorders with a limited genetic heterogeneity (~50–300 genes comprising about 0.5–2 Mb), gene panels, possibly supplemented with Sanger sequencing for poorly covered sequences, may be a better approach [29]. However, as it was recently shown in a retrospective study, 99.7% (1491/1533) of variants detected in gene panel testing had sufficient coverage for detection in WES [94]. Therefore, for disorders with extensive genetic and phenotypic heterogeneity, the minimal false-negative rate due to unequal coverage may be outweighed by a substantially larger diagnostic yield of WES due to a comprehensive nature of this technology. Sanger sequencing of potentially causative variants is also currently used for the confirmation of NGS testing. However, as it was shown by several groups, high-quality (≥500 Q) NGS variants do not require Sanger confirmation and restriction of Sanger confirmation to low-quality single-nucleotide variants, and all insertions/deletions <10 bp may reduce Sanger confirmation workload by 70–80% and enable cost savings [95].

Finally, the biggest part of false negatives in WES may be accounted for current variant filtration, annotation, and interpretation practices; therefore, rate of false negatives have a potential to diminish with accumulating information and bioinformatic/technological improvements [96, 97]. Although too stringent criteria can lead to false negatives, most likely they are unavoidable in a current setting of clinical practice. False-positive diagnoses can potentially have more devastating consequences for the family (e.g., through erroneous application of prenatal testing); therefore, all doubtful variants are usually ascribed to variants of unknown significance (VUS): it is easier to specify earlier suspected diagnosis than to refute previously established diagnosis [24].

There are some other non-laboratory-dependent problems potentially leading to missed or misinterpreted variants. One of the major steps in variant annotation process is assessing variant frequency in the general population. However, population databases cannot be assumed as containing data of healthy people only [24]. Besides, the prevalence of reported severe disease-causing variants in population controls points of the fact that incomplete penetrance and wider than appreciated expressivity are more inherent to genetic pathology than usually appreciated. One more problem potentially leading to a wrongful diagnosis is an erroneous annotation of variants and genes in databases and published data. Recently, several genes including *CACNA1H, SCN9A, EFHC1, CLCN2, GABRD,* and *SPRX2,* at first ascribed to various monogenic forms of epilepsy, have later been refuted as causative [9]. Finally, lots of very rare pathogenic variants are currently hiding in "private" databases of various laboratories. As both normal and pathogenic variation of human genome is almost endless (see Section 2.3), very large collaborative efforts for sharing both phenotypic and genotypic data of patients must be employed for the elucidation of these ultrarare variants and for ascribing them to certain phenotypes. Recently, the Epilepsy Genetics Initiative has created a database to house the clinically sequenced exomes (and, in due course, sequenced genomes) and phenotypic data of individuals with epilepsy; one unique purpose of which is to allow ongoing iterative reassessment of unsolved cases [49].

2.7. Building new healthcare practices in a responsible way

Incidental findings are not a new issue in clinical practice, for example, unanticipated findings in radiological imaging or even surgery, sometimes leading to dramatic changes in patient care, are well-known examples. However, all-inclusive nature of genomic testing, especially WES and WGS, means that the generation of a certain amount of unanticipated or incidental findings is unavoidable, currently confronted in 1–8% of all tested individuals [98]. Incidental findings in genetic testing have several definitions including more general "unexpected positive findings" [98] and deliberate search for pathogenic variants not related to the primary diagnostic question [99]. Some of these findings are "actionable," that is, measures may be implemented for preventing/alleviating the consequences of imminent genetic disorder. In other cases, no such measures exist. In any case, many psychosocial/bioethical issues may arise; therefore, all the main professional genetic organizations, including ESHG, ACMG, and CCMG, provide perspectives on how to handle unsolicited/incidental/secondary findings [23, 25, 98, 100].

Uncertainty of medical information, including pathogenicity assessments of laboratory or instrumental investigation results and prognostication, is also not a new issue in medicine. In genomic testing, a significant number of variants of unknown clinical significance (VUS) that cannot reliably be ascribed to either benign or pathogenic are generated. It is presumable that over time due to accumulating knowledge of benign and pathogenic human genome variation a considerable proportion of these VUS will receive their proper meaning. However, as a normal mutation rate will continue to generate a nearly infinite spectrum of variants, the challenge of VUS is going to persist; therefore, in clinical genetic practice, professionals must prepare their patients for the possibility of uncertainty due to VUS [23].

2.8. Clinical utility of genetic and genomic testing in epilepsies

Establishment of exact etiological diagnosis, where it is possible, is a standard of care in nowadays clinical practice. Precise genetic diagnosis has a huge impact on the individuals tested, their families, and community, as it allows timely medical interventions, informed reproductive choices, and avoidance of additional testing. In some cases it enables avoidance of inappropriate or detrimental treatments as illustrated by epilepsy due to *POLG1* gene mutations where valproates are contraindicated due to a threat of fatal hepatic failure [101]. Precise diagnosis can also determine the eligibility for clinical trials or enable engagement into appropriate patient support groups [102]. Psychosocial benefits of ending the diagnostic odyssey may also be substantial [103]. Finally, accurate prognostic information can be used by families for obtaining appropriate social and educational services and making personal and financial plans.

Undoubtedly, the most important benefits that may be enabled by exact genetic diagnosis are disease course-changing specific treatments. With timely diagnosis, there is an opportunity to provide life-saving and disability-preventing specific treatments to some epilepsy patients. Specific therapies have been initiated or adjusted in 6–8% of diagnosed patients in some studies [19, 22]. A significant group of treatable metabolic epilepsies provide one of the most veritable examples of precision medicine applications (see Section 2.4). Recent examples of specific treatments also include individuals with *KCNT1* mutations treated with quinidine, children with *KCNQ2* mutations treated with ezogabine (retigabine), individuals with *GRIN2A* mutations treated with memantine, and patients with mTORopathies treated with everolimus [49]. Fueled by novel epilepsy of genetic discoveries leading to further elucidation of pathogenetic disease mechanisms, the list of precision medicine applications in monogenic epilepsies will likely expand in the future. However, the first prerequisite to specific treatment applications in all these cases is an exact genetic diagnosis. Moreover, as currently up to one-third of all epilepsy cases are refractory to current treatments, new discoveries in monogenic forms of epilepsy may also fuel research and novel treatment target discoveries in common epilepsies.

In reaching diagnosis, comprehensiveness and untargeted approach of NGS technologies, especially WES, may be of special importance. It allows for elucidation of diagnoses in atypical, unusual, and not-full-blown (e.g., in young patients) phenotypes where phenotype-driven diagnostic hypothesis and targeted testing are impossible [19, 104]. Indeed, compatibility of a phenotype to that described in literature (the "first case bias") is one of the main factors in diagnostic hypothesis both raising and ascribing of pathogenicity to a novel variant. However, as of February 2015, 706 genes or ~24% of all genes associated with a Mendelian phenotype in OMIM database were responsible for at least two "clinically discrete" phenotypes [33]. Comprehensiveness of WES is also important for diagnostics of more than one genetic disease in a patient; such cases comprised four of 105 diagnosed patients in a study by Sawyer et al. [22]

and 4.6% of patients in a study by Yang et al. [105]. NGS testing may be the only opportunity for diagnosis in life-limiting disorders or in postmortem setting when DNA samples can be limited [41]. Finally, novel disease genes are also not an unusual finding in a clinical practice with WES or WGS testing and were found in 3.3–8.1% of patients in various studies [37, 40, 102, 104] and 23% of patients in FORGE study [22]. Importantly, each successful discovery opens horizons for diagnostic, preventive, and therapeutic opportunities for the corresponding disease [33]. The most common reasons for patients not to receive a diagnosis prior to WES in FORGE study were a significant genetic heterogeneity of the interrogated disorder, atypical presentation, missed diagnosis by other methods, and novel and ultrarare disorders [22].

2.9. The role of a clinical geneticist

Given all the complexities of genetic diseases' clinical presentation and phenotype evaluation, choice of the right genetic testing strategies, interpretation of genetic testing results and their communication to patients and families, genetic counseling regarding further risks and possibilities for prenatal diagnostics, and finally, sensitive and respectful consideration of all the psychosocial/bioethical aspects related to genetic diseases and genetic/genomic testing, the role of a clinical geneticist in the whole pathway of genetic diagnostics of a patient with epilepsy or seizures is undisputed. In the contemporary clinical genetic practice, geneticists must possess not only proper clinical skills but also abilities to use a vast range of bioinformatic tools and databases and have a deep knowledge of not only clinical genetics but also multiple genetic and genomic testing specificities.

Success of both targeted genetic testing and untargeted NGS approach is crucially dependent on the completeness and accuracy of phenotype evaluation [24, 26, 106]. Given the vast phenotypic variability of human monogenic and chromosomal disorders involving epilepsy or seizures, illustrated by EpiGene database (http://www.kimg.eu/en/tools/epigene-database), phenotyping of patient may include not only neurological examinations and tests but also thorough assessment of dysmorphic features, cutaneous signs, congenital malformations, variable symptoms of any other organ or organ system impairment, results of prior laboratory/radiological and other testings, information on cognitive functioning, etc. Family history/genealogy data may be helpful. Contrary to expectations of some people, with the advent of NGS testing, importance of thorough phenotyping did not diminish [106]. On the contrary, the final stages of variant annotation (gene level) and accurate variant interpretation are crucially dependent on the full phenotypic picture of a patient. Besides, as in many cases, phenotype-driven diagnostic hypothesis is not raised; a constant contact between laboratory and clinics with possibilities to perform a "reverse phenotyping" or "genotype to phenotype" correlation of identified variants is very important. Indeed, diagnostic yields were lower in studies where exome sequencing and interpretation of results were done in laboratories separate from clinical units (e.g., gene panel of 447 genes in 148 patients with a suspicion of mitochondrial diseases gave a diagnostic yield of only 9.4% in a separate laboratory [107] in comparison to 39% yield in a group of 109 patients tested with a gene panel of 238 genes in a laboratory connected to clinical unit [55]). In a recently published study, discordance rate in the initial interpretation of causal variants between laboratory and clinical geneticists was approximately 10% [108]. Finally, standardization and automation of phenotyping may be facilitated by tools like PhenoTips [109].

3. Diagnostic testing in epilepsy genetic clinical practice: proposed workflow

Currently, there are no recommendations or guidelines for genetic testing in epilepsy patients addressing specificities of NGS technologies [28]. We propose a simplified diagnostic workflow based on expected diagnostic yields and cost-effectiveness in various clinical situations encountered in epilepsy genetic clinical practice (**Figure 1**). The choice of a diagnostic route that is the most appropriate in a given clinical situation requires not only deep knowledge of

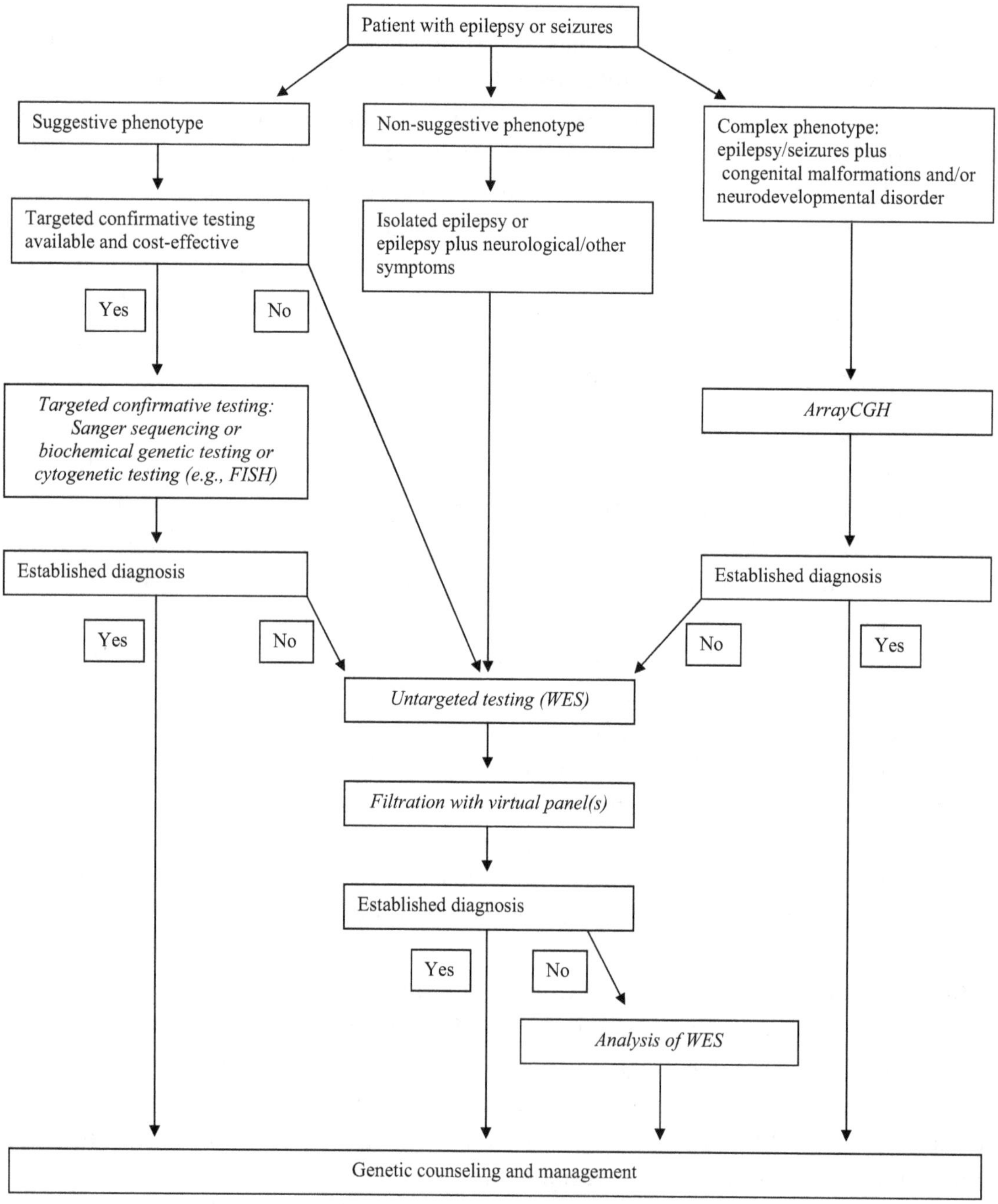

Figure 1. Provisional diagnostic workflow in patients with epilepsy or seizures.

a genetic architecture and a molecular pathology of a disorder; multiple technical specificities and limitations/disadvantages of diagnostic methods must be taken into consideration.

Author details

Birute Tumiene[1*], Algirdas Utkus[1], Vaidutis Kučinskas[2], Aleš Maver[3] and Borut Peterlin[3]

*Address all correspondence to: birute.tumiene@santa.lt

1 Department of Human and Medical Genetics, Centre for Medical Genetics, Vilnius University, Vilnius, Lithuania

2 Department of Human and Medical Genetics, Centre for Human Genomics, Vilnius University, Vilnius, Lithuania

3 Clinical Institute for Medical Genetics, Division of Gynecology, University of Ljubljana Medical Centre, Ljubljana, Slovenia

References

[1] Peljto AL, Barker-Cummings C, Vasoli VM, Leibson CL, Hauser WA, Buchhalter JR, Ottman R. Familial risk of epilepsy: A population-based study. Brain. 2014 Mar;**137**(Pt 3):795-805. DOI: 10.1093/brain/awt368

[2] Speed D, O'Brien TJ, Palotie A, Shkura K, Marson AG, Balding DJ, Johnson MR. Describing the genetic architecture of epilepsy through heritability analysis. Brain. 2014 Oct;**137**(Pt 10):2680-2689. DOI: 10.1093/brain/awu206

[3] Pal DK, Pong AW, Chung WK. Genetic evaluation and counseling for epilepsy. Nature Reviews Neurology. 2010 Aug;**6**(8):445-453. DOI: 10.1038/nrneurol.2010.92

[4] Kliegman RM, Bordini BJ, Basel D, Nocton JJ. How doctors think: Common diagnostic errors in clinical judgment-lessons from an undiagnosed and rare disease program. Pediatrics Clinics of North America. 2017 Feb;**64**(1):1-15. DOI: 10.1016/j.pcl.2016.08.002

[5] Sisodiya SM. Genetic screening and diagnosis in epilepsy? Current Opinion in Neurology. 2015 Apr;**28**(2):136-142. DOI: 10.1097/WCO.0000000000000180

[6] van Bokhoven H. Genetic and epigenetic networks in intellectual disabilities. Annual Review of Genetics. 2011;**45**:81-104. DOI: 10.1146/annurev-genet-110410-132512

[7] Greenberg DA, Subaran R. Blinders, phenotype, and fashionable genetic analysis: A critical examination of the current state of epilepsy genetic studies. Epilepsia. 2011 Jan;**52**(1):1-9. DOI: 10.1111/j.1528-1167.2010.02734.x

[8] Beck C, Moulard B, Steinlein O, Guipponi M, Vallee L, Montpied P, et al. A nonsense mutation in the alpha4 subunit of the nicotinic acetylcholine receptor (CHRNA4) cosegregates with 20q-linked benign neonatal familial convulsions (EBNI). Neurobiology of Disease. 1994 Nov;**1**(1-2):95-99

[9] Helbig I, Tayoun AA. Understanding genotypes and phenotypes in epileptic encephalopathies. Molecular Syndromology. 2016 Sep;**7**(4):172-181

[10] Malek N, Stewart W, Greene J. The progressive myoclonic epilepsies. Practical Neurology. 2015 Jun;**15**(3):164-171. DOI: 10.1136/practneurol-2014-000994

[11] Busch RM, Najm I, Hermann BP, Eng C. Genetics of cognition in epilepsy. Epilepsy Behaviour. 2014 Dec;**41**:297-306. DOI: 10.1016/j.yebeh.2014.05.026

[12] Guerrini R, Dobyns WB. Malformations of cortical development: Clinical features and genetic causes. Lancet Neurology. 2014 Jul;**13**(7):710-726. DOI: 10.1016/S1474-4422(14)70040-7

[13] Longo MG, Vairo F, Souza CF, Giugliani R, Vedolin LM. Brain imaging and genetic risk in the pediatric population, part 1: Inherited metabolic diseases. Neuroimaging Clinics of North America. 2015 Feb;**25**(1):31-51. DOI: 10.1016/j.nic.2014.09.004

[14] Longo MG, Félix TM, Ashton-Prolla P, Vedolin LM. Brain imaging and genetic risk in the pediatric population, part 2: Congenital malformations of the central nervous system. Neuroimaging Clinics of North America. 2015 Feb;**25**(1):53-67. DOI: 10.1016/j.nic.2014.09.003

[15] Patel J, Mercimek-Mahmutoglu S. Epileptic encephalopathy in childhood: A stepwise approach for identification of underlying genetic causes. Indian Journal of Pediatrics. 2016 Oct;**83**(10):1164-1174. DOI: 10.1007/s12098-015-1979-9

[16] Weiss MM, Van der Zwaag B, Jongbloed JD, Vogel MJ, Brüggenwirth HT, Lekanne Deprez RH, et al. Best practice guidelines for the use of next-generation sequencing applications in genome diagnostics: A national collaborative study of Dutch genome diagnostic laboratories. Human Mutation. 2013 Oct;**34**(10):1313-1321. DOI: 10.1002/humu.22368

[17] Mercimek-Mahmutoglu S, Patel J, Cordeiro D, Hewson S, Callen D, Donner EJ, et al. Diagnostic yield of genetic testing in epileptic encephalopathy in childhood. Epilepsia. 2015 May;**56**(5):707-716. DOI: 10.1111/epi.12954

[18] López-Pisón J, García-Jiménez MC, Monge-Galindo L, Lafuente-Hidalgo M, Pérez-Delgado R, García-Oguiza A, Peña-Segura JL. Our experience with the aetiological diagnosis of global developmental delay and intellectual disability: 2006-2010. Neurologia. 2014 Sep;**29**(7):402-407. DOI: 10.1016/j.nrl.2013.10.006

[19] Soden SE, Saunders CJ, Willig LK, Farrow EG, Smith LD, Petrikin JE, et al. Effectiveness of exome and genome sequencing guided by acuity of illness for diagnosis of neurodevelopmental disorders. Science Translational Medicine. 2014 Dec 3;**6**(265):265ra168. DOI: 10.1126/scitranslmed.3010076

[20] Monroe GR, Frederix GW, Savelberg SM, de Vries TI, Duran KJ, van der Smagt JJ, et al. Effectiveness of whole-exome sequencing and costs of the traditional diagnostic trajectory in children with intellectual disability. Genetics in Medicine. 2016 Sep;**18**(9):949-956. DOI: 10.1038/gim.2015.200

[21] Stark Z, Schofield D, Alam K, Wilson W, Mupfeki N, Macciocca I, et al. Prospective comparison of the cost-effectiveness of clinical whole-exome sequencing with that of usual care overwhelmingly supports early use and reimbursement. Genetics in Medicine. 2017 Jan 26. DOI: 10.1038/gim.2016.221

[22] Sawyer SL, Hartley T, Dyment DA, Beaulieu CL, Schwartzentruber J, Smith A, et al. Utility of whole-exome sequencing for those near the end of the diagnostic odyssey: Time to address gaps in care. Clinical Genetics. 2016 Mar;**89**(3):275-284. DOI: 10.1111/cge.12654

[23] van El CG, Cornel MC, Borry P, Hastings RJ, Fellmann F, Hodgson SV, et al. Whole-genome sequencing in health care. Recommendations of the European society of human genetics. European Journal of Human Genetics. 2013 Jun;**21**(Suppl 1):S1-S5

[24] Richards S, Aziz N, Bale S, Bick D, Das S, Gastier-Foster J, et al. Standards and guidelines for the interpretation of sequence variants: A joint consensus recommendation of the American College of Medical Genetics and Genomics and the Association for Molecular Pathology. Genetics in Medicine. 2015 May;**17**(5):405-424. DOI: 10.1038/gim.2015.30

[25] Boycott K, Hartley T, Adam S, Bernier F, Chong K, Fernandez BA, et al. The clinical application of genome-wide sequencing for monogenic diseases in Canada: Position statement of the Canadian College of Medical Geneticists. Journal of Medical Genetics. 2015 Jul;**52**(7):431-437. DOI: 10.1136/jmedgenet-2015-103144

[26] Shashi V, McConkie-Rosell A, Rosell B, Schoch K, Vellore K, McDonald M, et al. The utility of the traditional medical genetics diagnostic evaluation in the context of next-generation sequencing for undiagnosed genetic disorders. Genetics in Medicine. 2014 Feb;**16**(2):176-182. DOI: 10.1038/gim.2013.99

[27] Trump N, McTague A, Brittain H, Papandreou A, Meyer E, Ngoh A, et al. Improving diagnosis and broadening the phenotypes in early-onset seizure and severe developmental delay disorders through gene panel analysis. Journal of Medical Genetics. 2016 May;**53**(5):310-317. DOI: 10.1136/jmedgenet-2015-103263

[28] Ottman R, Hirose S, Jain S, Lerche H, Lopes-Cendes I, Noebels JL, et al. Genetic testing in the epilepsies--report of the ILAE Genetics Commission. Epilepsia. 2010 Apr;**51**(4):655-670. DOI: 10.1111/j.1528-1167.2009.02429.x

[29] Klein CJ, Foroud TM. Neurology individualized medicine: When to use next-generation sequencing panels. Mayo Clinic Proceedings. 2017 Feb;**92**(2):292-305. DOI: 10.1016/j.mayocp.2016.09.008

[30] Wright CF, Middleton A, Burton H, Cunningham F, Humphries SE, Hurst J, et al. Policy challenges of clinical genome sequencing. BMJ. 2013 Nov 22;**347**:f6845. DOI: 10.1136/bmj.f6845

[31] Xue Y, Ankala A, Wilcox WR, Hegde MR. Solving the molecular diagnostic testing conundrum for Mendelian disorders in the era of next-generation sequencing: Single-gene, gene panel, or exome/genome sequencing. Genetics in Medicine. 2015 Jun;**17**(6):444-451. DOI: 10.1038/gim.2014.122

[32] Lek M, Karczewski KJ, Minikel EV, Samocha KE, Banks E, Fennell T, et al. Analysis of protein-coding genetic variation in 60,706 humans. Nature. 2016 Aug 18;**536**(7616):285-291. DOI: 10.1038/nature19057

[33] Chong JX, Buckingham KJ, Jhangiani SN, Boehm C, Sobreira N, Smith JD, et al. The genetic basis of Mendelian phenotypes: Discoveries, challenges, and opportunities. American Journal of Human Genetics. 2015 Aug 6;**97**(2):199-215. DOI: 10.1016/j.ajhg.2015.06.009

[34] Martin HC, Kim GE, Pagnamenta AT, Murakami Y, Carvill GL, Meyer E, et al. Clinical whole-genome sequencing in severe early-onset epilepsy reveals new genes and improves molecular diagnosis. Human Molecular Genetics. 2014 Jun 15;**23**(12):3200-3211. DOI: 10.1093/hmg/ddu030

[35] Gilissen C, Hehir-Kwa JY, Thung DT, van de Vorst M, van Bon BW, Willemsen MH, et al. Genome sequencing identifies major causes of severe intellectual disability. Nature. 2014 Jul 17;**511**(7509):344-347. DOI: 10.1038/nature13394

[36] Taylor JC, Martin HC, Lise S, Broxholme J, Cazier JB, Rimmer A, et al. Factors influencing success of clinical genome sequencing across a broad spectrum of disorders. Natural Genetics. 2015 Jul;**47**(7):717-726. DOI: 10.1038/ng.3304

[37] Helbig KL, Farwell Hagman KD, Shinde DN, Mroske C, Powis Z, Li S, et al. Diagnostic exome sequencing provides a molecular diagnosis for a significant proportion of patients with epilepsy. Genetics in Medicine. 2016 Sep;**18**(9):898-905. DOI: 10.1038/gim.2015.186

[38] Dimassi S, Labalme A, Ville D, Calender A, Mignot C, Boutry-Kryza N, et al. Whole-exome sequencing improves the diagnosis yield in sporadic infantile spasm syndrome. Clinical Genetics. 2016 Feb;**89**(2):198-204. DOI: 10.1111/cge.12636

[39] Srivastava S, Cohen JS, Vernon H, Barañano K, McClellan R, Jamal L, et al. Clinical whole exome sequencing in child neurology practice. Annals of Neurology. 2014 Oct;**76**(4):473-483. DOI: 10.1002/ana.24251

[40] Farwell KD, Shahmirzadi L, El-Khechen D, Powis Z, Chao EC, Tippin Davis B, et al. Enhanced utility of family-centered diagnostic exome sequencing with inheritance model-based analysis: Results from 500 unselected families with undiagnosed genetic conditions. Genetics in Medicine. 2015 Jul;**17**(7):578-586. DOI: 10.1038/gim.2014.154

[41] Stark Z, Tan TY, Chong B, Brett GR, Yap P, Walsh M, et al. A prospective evaluation of whole-exome sequencing as a first-tier molecular test in infants with suspected monogenic disorders. Genetics in Medicine. 2016 Nov;**18**(11):1090-1096. DOI: 10.1038/gim.2016.1

[42] Ales M, Luca L, Marija V, Gorazd R, Karin W, Ana B, et al. Phenotype-driven gene target definition in clinical genome-wide sequencing data interpretation. Genetics in Medicine. 2016 Nov;**18**(11):1102-1110. DOI: 10.1038/gim.2016.22

[43] Carvill GL, Heavin SB, Yendle SC, McMahon JM, O'Roak BJ, Cook J, et al. Targeted resequencing in epileptic encephalopathies identifies denovo mutations in CHD2 and SYNGAP1. Nature Genetics. 2013 Jul;**45**(7):825-830. DOI: 10.1038/ng.2646

[44] Parrini E, Marini C, Mei D, Galuppi A, Cellini E, Pucatti D, et al. Diagnostic targeted resequencing in 349 patients with drug-resistant pediatric epilepsies identifies causative mutations in 30 different genes. Human Mutation. 2017 Feb;**38**(2):216-225. DOI: 10.1002/humu.23149

[45] Møller RS, Larsen LH, Johannesen KM, Talvik I, Talvik T, Vaher U, et al. Gene panel testing in epileptic encephalopathies and familial epilepsies. Molecular Syndromology. 2016 Sep;**7**(4):210-219

[46] Wang Y, Du X, Bin R, Yu S, Xia Z, Zheng G, et al. Genetic variants identified from epilepsy of unknown etiology in Chinese children by targeted exome sequencing. Scientific Reports. 2017 Jan 11;**7**:40319. DOI: 10.1038/srep40319

[47] Chambers C, Jansen LA, Dhamija R. Review of commercially available epilepsy genetic panels. Journal of Genetic Counseling. 2016 Apr;**25**(2):213-217. DOI: 10.1007/s10897-015-9906-9

[48] Pearl PL. Amenable treatable severe pediatric epilepsies. Seminars in Pediatrics Neurology. 2016 May;**23**(2):158-166. DOI: 10.1016/j.spen.2016.06.004

[49] EpiPM Consortium. A roadmap for precision medicine in the epilepsies. Lancet Neurology. 2015 Dec;**14**(12):1219-1228. DOI: 10.1016/S1474-4422(15)00199-4

[50] Oz G, Alger JR, Barker PB, Bartha R, Bizzi A, Boesch C, et al. Clinical proton MR spectroscopy in central nervous system disorders. Radiology. 2014 Mar;**270**(3):658-679. DOI: 10.1148/radiol.13130531

[51] Ibrahim M, Parmar HA, Hoefling N, Srinivasan A. Inborn errors of metabolism: combining clinical and radiologic clues to solve the mystery. AJR American Journal of Roentgenology. 2014 Sep;**203**(3):W315-W327. DOI: 10.2214/AJR.13.11154

[52] Dulac O, Plecko B, Gataullina S, Wolf NI. Occasional seizures, epilepsy, and inborn errors of metabolism. Lancet Neurology. 2014 Jul;**13**(7):727-739. DOI: 10.1016/S1474-4422(14)70110-3

[53] Kölker S, Garcia-Cazorla A, Valayannopoulos V, Lund AM, Burlina AB, Sykut-Cegielska J, et al. The phenotypic spectrum of organic acidurias and urea cycle disorders. Part 1: The initial presentation. Journal of Inherited Metabolic Disease. 2015 Nov;**38**(6):1041-1057. DOI: 10.1007/s10545-015-9839-3

[54] Lemke JR, Riesch E, Scheurenbrand T, Schubach M, Wilhelm C, Steiner I, et al. Targeted next generation sequencing as a diagnostic tool in epileptic disorders. Epilepsia. 2012 Aug;**53**(8):1387-1398. DOI: 10.1111/j.1528-1167.2012.03516.x

[55] Wortmann SB, Koolen DA, Smeitink JA, van den Heuvel L, Rodenburg RJ. Whole exome sequencing of suspected mitochondrial patients in clinical practice. Journal of Inherited Metabolic Disease. 2015 May;**38**(3):437-443. DOI: 10.1007/s10545-015-9823-y

[56] Zuberi SM. Chromosome disorders associated with epilepsy. Handbook of Clinical Neurology. 2013;**111**:543-548. DOI: 10.1016/B978-0-444-52891-9.00057-9

[57] Miller DT, Adam MP, Aradhya S, Biesecker LG, Brothman AR, Carter NP, et al. Consensus statement: Chromosomal microarray is a first-tier clinical diagnostic test for individuals with developmental disabilities or congenital anomalies. American Journal of Human Genetics. 2010 May 14;**86**(5):749-764. DOI: 10.1016/j.ajhg.2010.04.006

[58] Charalsawadi C, Khayman J, Praphanphoj V, Limprasert P. Screening for subtelomeric rearrangements in Thai patients with intellectual disabilities using FISH and review of literature on subtelomeric FISH in 15,591 cases with intellectual disabilities. Genetic Reseach International. 2016;**2016**:9153740

[59] Koolen DA, Nillesen WM, Versteeg MH, Merkx GF, Knoers NV, Kets M, et al. Screening for subtelomeric rearrangements in 210 patients with unexplained mental retardation using multiplex ligation dependent probe amplification (MLPA). Journal of Medical Genetics. 2004 Dec;**41**(12):892-899

[60] Hanemaaijer NM, Sikkema-Raddatz B, van der Vries G, Dijkhuizen T, Hordijk R, van Essen AJ, et al. Practical guidelines for interpreting copy number gains detected by high-resolution array in routine diagnostics. European Journal of Human Genetics. 2012 Feb;**20**(2):161-165. DOI: 10.1038/ejhg.2011.174

[61] Krumm N, Sudmant PH, Ko A, O'Roak BJ, Malig M, Coe BP, et al. Copy number variation detection and genotyping from exome sequence data. Genome Research. 2012 Aug;**22**(8):1525-1532. DOI: 10.1101/gr.138115.112

[62] Zollino M, Ponzi E, Gobbi G, Neri G. The ring 14 syndrome. European Journal of Medical Genetics. 2012 May;**55**(5):374-380. DOI: 10.1016/j.ejmg.2012.03.009

[63] Daber RD, Conlin LK, Leonard LD, Canevini MP, Vignoli A, Hosain S, et al. Ring chromosome 20. European Journal of Medical Genetics. 2012 May;**55**(5):381-387. DOI: 10.1016/j.ejmg.2012.02.004

[64] Hochstenbach R, van Binsbergen E, Engelen J, Nieuwint A, Polstra A, Poddighe P, et al. Array analysis and karyotyping: Workflow consequences based on a retrospective study of 36,325patients with idiopathic developmental delay in the Netherlands. European Journal of Medical Genetics. 2009 Jul–Aug;**52**(4):161-169. DOI: 10.1016/j.ejmg.2009.03.015

[65] Zarrei M, MacDonald JR, Merico D, Scherer SW. A copy number variation map of the human genome. Nature Reviews Genetics. 2015 Mar;**16**(3):172-183. DOI: 10.1038/nrg3871

[66] Ruderfer DM, Hamamsy T, Lek M, Karczewski KJ, Kavanagh D, Samocha KE, et al. Patterns of genic intolerance of rare copy number variation in 59,898 human exomes. Nature Genetics. 2016 Oct;**48**(10):1107-1111. DOI: 10.1038/ng.3638

[67] Sudmant PH, Rausch T, Gardner EJ, Handsaker RE, Abyzov A, Huddleston J, et al. An integrated map of structural variation in 2,504 human genomes. Nature. 2015 Oct 1;**526**(7571):75-81. DOI: 10.1038/nature15394

[68] MacDonald JR, Ziman R, Yuen RK, Feuk L, Scherer SW. The database of genomic variants: A curated collection of structural variation in the human genome. Nucleic Acids Researcch. 2014 Jan;**42**(Database issue):D986-D992. DOI: 10.1093/nar/gkt958

[69] Hehir-Kwa JY, Pfundt R, Veltman JA, de Leeuw N. Pathogenic or not? Assessing the clinical relevance of copy number variants. Clinical Genetics. 2013 Nov;**84**(5):415-421. DOI: 10.1111/cge.12242

[70] Kearney HM, Thorland EC, Brown KK, Quintero-Rivera F, South ST, Working Group of the American College of Medical Genetics Laboratory Quality Assurance Committee. American College of Medical Genetics standards and guidelines for interpretation and reporting of postnatal constitutional copy number variants. Genetics in Medicine. 2011 Jul;**13**(7):680-685. DOI: 10.1097/GIM.0b013e3182217a3a

[71] Carreira IM, Ferreira SI, Matoso E, Pires LM, Ferrão J, Jardim A, et al. Copy number variants prioritization after array-CGH analysis—a cohort of 1000 patients. Molecular Cytogenetics. 2015 Dec 30;**8**:103. DOI: 10.1186/s13039-015-0202-z

[72] Palmer E, Speirs H, Taylor PJ, Mullan G, Turner G, Einfeld S, et al. Changing interpretation of chromosomal microarray over time in a community cohort with intellectual disability. American Journal of Medical Genetics A. 2014 Feb;**164A**(2):377-385. DOI: 10.1002/ajmg.a.36279

[73] Paciorkowski AR, Keppler-Noreuil K, Robinson L, Sullivan C, Sajan S, Christian SL, et al. Deletion 16p13.11 uncovers NDE1 mutations on the non-deleted homolog and extends the spectrum of severe microcephaly to include fetal brain disruption. American Journal of Medical Genetics A. 2013 Jul;**161A**(7):1523-1530. DOI: 10.1002/ajmg.a.35969

[74] Asadollahi R, Oneda B, Joset P, Azzarello-Burri S, Bartholdi D, Steindl K, et al. The clinical significance of small copy number variants in neurodevelopmental disorders. Journal of Medical Genetics. 2014 Oct;**51**(10):677-688. DOI: 10.1136/jmedgenet-2014-102588

[75] Spielmann M, Mundlos S. Looking beyond the genes: The role of non-coding variants in human disease. Human Molecular Genetics. 2016 Oct 1;**25**(R2):R157-R165

[76] Magaard Koldby K, Nygaard M, Christensen K, Christiansen L. Somatically acquired structural genetic differences: A longitudinal study of elderly Danish twins. European Journla of Human Genetics. 2016 Oct;**24**(10):1506-1510. DOI: 10.1038/ejhg.2016.34

[77] Wincent J, Kolbjer S, Martin D, Luthman A, Åmark P, Dahlin M, Anderlid BM. Copy number variations in children with brain malformations and refractory epilepsy. American Journal of Human Genetics. 2015 Mar;**167A**(3):512-523. DOI: 10.1002/ajmg.a.36886

[78] Kariminejad R, Lind-Thomsen A, Tümer Z, Erdogan F, Ropers HH, Tommerup N, et al. High frequency of rare copy number variants affecting functionally related genes in patients with structural brain malformations. Human Mutation. 2011 Dec;**32**(12):1427-1435. DOI: 10.1002/humu.21585

[79] Mefford HC, Yendle SC, Hsu C, Cook J, Geraghty E, McMahon JM, et al. Rare copy number variants are an important cause of epileptic encephalopathies. Annals of Neurology. 2011 Dec;**70**(6):974-985. DOI: 10.1002/ana.22645

[80] Ma Y, Chen C, Wang Y, Wu L, He F, Chen C, et al. Analysis copy number variation of Chinese children in early-onset epileptic encephalopathies with unknown cause. Clinical Genetics. 2016 Nov;**90**(5):428-436. DOI: 10.1111/cge.12768

[81] Nicholl J, Waters W, Suwalski S, Brown S, Hull Y, Harbord MG, et al. Epilepsy with cognitive deficit and autism spectrum disorders: prospective diagnosis by array CGH. American Journal of Medical Genetics B Neuropsychiatry Genetics. 2013 Jan;**162B**(1):24-35. DOI: 10.1002/ajmg.b.32114

[82] Olson H, Shen Y, Avallone J, Sheidley BR, Pinsky R, Bergin AM, et al. Copy number variation plays an important role in clinical epilepsy. Annals of Neurology. 2014 Jun;**75**(6):943-958. DOI: 10.1002/ana.24178

[83] Mullen SA, Carvill GL, Bellows S, Bayly MA, Trucks H, Lal D, et al. Copy number variants are frequent in genetic generalized epilepsy with intellectual disability. Neurology. 2013 Oct 22;**81**(17):1507-1514. DOI: 10.1212/WNL.0b013e3182a95829

[84] Lal D, Ruppert AK, Trucks H, Schulz H, de Kovel CG, Kasteleijn-Nolst Trenité D, et al. Burden analysis of rare microdeletions suggests a strong impact of neurodevelopmental genes in genetic generalised epilepsies. PLoS Genetics. 2015 May 7;**11**(5):e1005226. DOI: 10.1371/journal.pgen.1005226

[85] Addis L, Rosch RE, Valentin A, Makoff A, Robinson R, Everett KV, Nashef L, Pal DK. Analysis of rare copy number variation in absence epilepsies. Neurology Genetics. 2016 Mar 22;**2**(2):e56. DOI: 10.1212/NXG.0000000000000056

[86] Depondt C. Copy number variants in absence epilepsy: Further complications of the picture. Neurology Genetics. 2016 Mar 22;**2**(2):e67. DOI: 10.1212/NXG.0000000000000067

[87] Reinthaler EM, Lal D, Lebon S, Hildebrand MS, Dahl HH, Regan BM, et al. 16p11.2 600 kb Duplications confer risk for typical and atypical Rolandic epilepsy. Human Molecular Genetics. 2014 Nov 15;**23**(22):6069-6080. DOI: 10.1093/hmg/ddu306

[88] Poduri A, Evrony GD, Cai X, Walsh CA. Somatic mutation, genomic variation, and neurological disease. Science. 2013 Jul 5;**341**(6141):1237758. DOI: 10.1126/science.1237758

[89] Jamuar SS, Walsh CA. Somatic mutations in cerebral cortical malformations. New England Journal of Medicine. 2014 Nov 20;**371**(21):2038. DOI: 10.1056/NEJMc1411784

[90] Jenkinson EM, Rodero MP, Kasher PR, Uggenti C, Oojageer A, Goosey LC, et al. Mutations in SNORD118 cause the cerebral microangiopathy leukoencephalopathy with calcifications and cysts. Nature Genetics. 2016 Oct;**48**(10):1185-1192. DOI: 10.1038/ng.3661

[91] Sun Y, Ruivenkamp CA, Hoffer MJ, Vrijenhoek T, Kriek M, van Asperen CJ, et al. Next-generation diagnostics: gene panel, exome, or whole genome? Human Mutation. 2015 Jun;**36**(6):648-655. DOI: 10.1002/humu.22783

[92] Guo Y, Li J, Li CI, Shyr Y, Samuels DC. MitoSeek: Extracting mitochondria information and performing high-throughput mitochondria sequencing analysis. Bioinformatics. 2013 May 1;**29**(9):1210-1211. DOI: 10.1093/bioinformatics/btt118

[93] Finsterer J, Zarrouk MS. Epilepsy in mitochondrial disorders. Seizure. 2012 Jun;**21**(5):316-321. DOI: 10.1016/j.seizure.2012.03.003

[94] LaDuca H, Farwell KD, Vuong H, Lu HM, Mu W, Shahmirzadi L, et al. Exome sequencing covers >98% of mutations identified on targeted next generation sequencing panels. PLoS One. 2017 Feb 2;**12**(2):e0170843. DOI: 10.1371/journal.pone.0170843

[95] Strom SP, Lee H, Das K, Vilain E, Nelson SF, Grody WW, Deignan JL. Assessing the necessity of confirmatory testing for exome-sequencing results in a clinical molecular diagnostic laboratory. Genetics in Medicine. 2014 Jul;**16**(7):510-515. DOI: 10.1038/gim.2013.183

[96] Shamseldin HE, Maddirevula S, Faqeih E, Ibrahim N, Hashem M, Shaheen R, Alkuraya FS. Increasing the sensitivity of clinical exome sequencing through improved filtration strategy. Genetics in Medicine. 2016 Oct 6. DOI: 10.1038/gim.2016.155

[97] Salgado D, Bellgard MI, Desvignes JP, Béroud C. How to identify pathogenic mutations among all those variations: Variant annotation and filtration in the genome sequencing era. Human Mutation. 2016 Dec;**37**(12):1272-1282. DOI: 10.1002/humu.23110

[98] Hehir-Kwa JY, Claustres M, Hastings RJ, van Ravenswaaij-Arts C, Christenhusz G, Genuardi M, et al. Towards a European consensus for reporting incidental findings during clinical NGS testing. European Journal of Human Genetics. 2015 Dec;**23**(12):1601-1606. DOI: 10.1038/ejhg.2015.111

[99] Green RC, Berg JS, Grody WW, Kalia SS, Korf BR, Martin CL, et al. ACMG recommendations for reporting of incidental findings in clinical exome and genome sequencing. Genetics in Medicine. 2013 Jul;**15**(7):565-574. DOI: 10.1038/gim.2013.73

[100] Kalia SS, Adelman K, Bale SJ, Chung WK, Eng C, Evans JP, et al. Recommendations for reporting of secondary findings in clinical exome and genome sequencing, 2016 update (ACMG SF v2.0): A policy statement of the American College of Medical Genetics and Genomics. Genetics in Medicine. 2017 Feb;**19**(2):249-255. DOI: 10.1038/gim.2016.190

[101] Hynynen J, Komulainen T, Tukiainen E, Nordin A, Arola J, Kälviäinen R, et al. Acute liver failure after valproate exposure in patients with POLG1 mutations and the prognosis after liver transplantation. Liver Transplantation. 2014 Nov;**20**(11):1402-1412. DOI: 10.1002/lt.23965

[102] Iglesias A, Anyane-Yeboa K, Wynn J, et al. The usefulness of whole-exome sequencing in routine clinical practice. Genetics in Medicine 2014;**16**(12):922-931

[103] Beaulieu CL, Majewski J, Schwartzentruber J, Samuels ME, Fernandez BA, Bernier FP, et al. FORGE Canada Consortium: Outcomes of a 2-year national rare-disease gene-discovery project. American Journal of Human Genetics. 2014 Jun 5;**94**(6):809-817. DOI: 10.1016/j.ajhg.2014.05.003

[104] Zhu X, Petrovski S, Xie P, Ruzzo EK, Lu YF, McSweeney KM, et al. Whole-exome sequencing in undiagnosed genetic diseases: Interpreting 119 trios. Genetics in Medicine. 2015 Oct;**17**(10):774-81. DOI: 10.1038/gim.2014.191

[105] Yang Y, Muzny DM, Xia F, Niu Z, Person R, Ding Y, et al. Molecular findings among patients referred for clinical whole-exome sequencing. JAMA. 2014 Nov 12;**312**(18):1870-1879. DOI: 10.1001/jama.2014.14601

[106] Hennekam RC, Biesecker LG. Next-generation sequencing demands next-generation phenotyping. Human Mutation. 2012 May;**33**(5):884-886. DOI: 10.1002/humu.22048

[107] DaRe JT, Vasta V, Penn J, Tran NT, Hahn SH. Targeted exome sequencing for mitochondrial disorders reveals high genetic heterogeneity. BMC Medical Genetics. 2013 Nov 11;**14**:118. DOI: 10.1186/1471-2350-14-118

[108] Shashi V, McConkie-Rosell A, Schoch K, Kasturi V, Rehder C, Jiang YH, et al. Practical considerations in the clinical application of whole-exome sequencing. Clinical Genetics. 2016 Feb;**89**(2):173-181. DOI: 10.1111/cge.12569

[109] Girdea M, Dumitriu S, Fiume M, Bowdin S, Boycott KM, Chénier S, et al. PhenoTips: Patient phenotyping software for clinical and research use. Human Mutation. 2013 Aug;**34**(8):1057-1065. DOI: 10.1002/humu.22347

[110] Leu C, Coppola A, Sisodiya SM. Progress from genome-wide association studies and copy number variant studies in epilepsy. Current Opinion in Neurology. 2016 Apr;**29**(2):158-167. DOI: 10.1097/WCO.0000000000000296

[111] Nevado J, Mergener R, Palomares-Bralo M, Souza KR, Vallespín E, Mena R, et al. New microdeletion and microduplication syndromes: A comprehensive review. Genetics in Molecular Biology. 2014 Mar;**37**(1 Suppl):210-219

4

Psychiatric Comorbidities and Quality of Life in Epilepsy

Ayşe Kutlu and Serap Mülayim

Abstract

Epilepsy is a chronic disorder characterized by a spontaneous tendency to recurrent seizures which affects patients' cognitive, behavioral, psychological, and social functioning. Epileptic patients face various problems that result in a lower quality of life. Seizure frequency, drug side effects, psychological comorbidity, and stigma are the major factors affecting the quality of lives of patients with epilepsy. Depression, anxiety, psychosis, and cognitive impairment are some of the comorbid psychiatric problems accompanying the clinical picture in epilepsy. Also the role of antiepileptic drugs (AEDs) in psychopathology of epilepsy should not be underestimated. One of the most important reasons why health-related quality of life (HRQOL) has become important for epileptic patients is related with well-known characteristics of this disorder. Its chronic nature, presence of unexpected, intractable and frequent seizures, and stigma are some of these characteristics among others. With the review of the current literature, it can be concluded that there is still a need for further scientific research to find out more clear relation between epilepsy, comorbidities, and HRQOL.

Keywords: epilepsy, psychiatric comorbidities, quality of life

1. Introduction

Epilepsy is a chronic disorder characterized by recurrent seizures which impairs patient's quality of life through cognitive, behavioral, psychological, and social functioning [1]. It has been reported that the total lifetime risk for epilepsy and for any unprovoked seizure are 3.1 and 4.1%, respectively in industrialized countries. The estimation of annual incidence of epilepsy is reported as high as 43 cases per 100,000 of the population in so-called developed countries, and is almost double this figure in the developing world [2]. Another estimation points out that there are 50 million people who have epilepsy in the world [3, 4]. It was suggested that more than 80% of people with epilepsy live in developing countries, where the condition remains largely untreated [5, 6].

The science of health-related quality of life (HRQOL) measurements rapidly evolved during the 1980s and 1990s within general health and in all medicine disciplines [7]. HRQOL has become so important for patients with epilepsy (PWE) because of well-known characteristics of this disorder. Among these characteristics, chronic nature, unexpectability, intractable and/ or frequent seizures, stigma, and side effects of the antiepileptic drugs are acknowledged. Also, neurobiological, cognitive, psychological, and social consequences of epilepsy are very important [8].

Patients with epilepsy (PWE) encounter various problems due to this disorder which conduce a lower quality of life (QOL). Seizure frequency, side effects of the antiepileptic drugs, psychological problems, and stigma are the major factors determining severity of the disease and these factors may cause an important impact on life quality of PWE. Therefore, identifying the factors which mostly affect are important for improving epileptic patients' quality of lives [9].

2. Psychiatric comorbidities

2.1. Depression

Psychiatric disorders are frequent in epilepsy and they have a marked effect in QOL, morbidity, and mortality. Mood and anxiety disorders are the most frequent problems [10]. Depression is the most frequent psychiatric comorbidity in epilepsy, affecting one of every three patients with epilepsy in clinical studies [11] and lifetime prevalence rates of depression range between 30 and 35% in patients with epilepsy [10].

The International League Against Epilepsy (ILAE) has recognized the importance of comorbidities in the management of PWE. But, these comorbidities are usually ignored, unless they lead to a major disability. This may be related to several factors, such as patients not giving enough information about their psychiatric state or neurologists may not be specifically trained for these comorbidities [12]. In a recent study reported by Kanner et al., it was demonstrated that comorbid psychiatric problems affect the quality of life, so patients with subsyndromic depressive episodes (SSDEs), major depressive episodes (MDEs), anxiety disorders, and mixed MDEs (or SSDEs) with anxiety disorders have a significantly worse QOL than asymptomatic patients [13]. Authors also demonstrated that occurrence of mixed disorders resulted with unfavorable HRQOL than the occurrence of anxiety disorders alone. Another important finding of this study was that the comorbid occurrence of depression and anxiety disorders accompanied to epilepsy cause to important clinical results beyond their impact on HRQOL which include:

1. An increased suicidal risk.

2. A worse course and poorer response to treatment of a depressive disorder.

3. An increased risk of MDE recurrence; types of anxiety increased the probability of a new depressive episode.
4. Pharmacoresistant temporal lobe epilepsy patients encountered unsatisfied results including increased risk of failure to achieve seizure-free state after anterotemporal lobectomy [13].

Literature survey reveals enough evidence regarding the negative impact of mood disorders and anxiety symptoms on the quality of life of PWEs [14–20]. Symptoms of depression and anxiety are independently associated with reduced HRQOL; psychiatric comorbidity explains more variance in HRQOL than the combined groups of clinical seizure or demographic variables [18]. A study with a large sample included 435 PWEs aiming to investigate the relative impact of mood and anxiety symptoms as well as social- and seizure-related variables on HRQOL [21]; the presence of depressive symptoms was the strongest predictor of the composite and subscales of the Quality of Life in Epilepsy instrument used (QOLIE-31). In other studies conducted on patients with pharmacoresistant temporal lobe epilepsy (TLE), symptoms of depression were found to be the strongest independent predictors of poor QOL but (unexpectedly) not the seizure frequency or severity [14, 15, 17].

Kim et al. studied impact of depression and anxiety on adverse event profiles in Korean people with epilepsy. Consecutively, 453 patients who took antiepileptic drugs for at least 1 year completed self-reported questionnaires. They used Liverpool adverse events profile (LAEP), Beck Depression Inventory (BDI), and Beck Anxiety Inventory (BAI). In this study, it was reported that BAI, BDI scores, and the duration of antiepileptic drug treatment were significant predictors [22].

Another important point is the women with epilepsy of childbearing age. Increased risk of depression is a considerable problem for these patients. Lack of occupation, the presence of an underlying disabling condition (with treatment), and the severity of epilepsy are the significant properties accompanied to depression. Compared with the general population depressed women with epilepsy display greater impairment of HRQOL with epilepsy also images the physical, social, and emotional aspects of the disease [23].

Depressive disorders are associated with a worse response of seizures to antiepileptic drug treatment [24]. Hitiris et al. [25] retrospectively searched 780 patients with new onset epilepsy. Epileptic patients with a history of depression had two times more risk in developing refractory epilepsy.

Endocrine, neurotransmitter, and immunologic disturbances were found to be related with depression in patients with epilepsy. Especially, serotonin, glutamate, and GABA have an important role in epileptic seizures. Fluoxetine, a selective serotonin reuptake inhibitor (SSRI), has been shown to be effective in seizure prevention in a focal epilepsy model in rats [26]. Mazarati et al. studied an animal model of status epilepticus demonstrated abnormal 5-HT secretion in the raphe-hippocampal serotonergic pathway, lower serotonin concentrations in the hippocampus, and decreased serotonin release from the hippocampus following raphe stimulation [27]. Also, fluoxetine administration reversed the cortical hyperexcitability following status epilepticus. In animal models of depression, dysfunction of glutamate transporter proteins was shown, causing neuronal hyperexcitability and neuronal death [28]. In humans with depression, reduced expression of several glutamate transporter proteins was found in the frontal cortex and striatum in postmortem brain tissue that resulted in elevated synaptic glutamate concentrations [29]. By depression decreased cerebrospinal fluid concentration of GABA [30] and intracortical GABA signal on MR spectroscopy (MRS) [21, 28, 31–34] arises as a result of decreased GABAergic activity. For example, Rajkowska et al. [35] determined a significant decrease in GABAergic interneurons in the dorsolateral prefrontal cortex of the brains of the major depressive disorder patients (MDD) in a postmortem study which included 14 MDD patients (nine of whom died because of suicide) and nine controls [36]. Studies designed with transcranial magnetic stimulation (TMS), as a treatment modality for resistant MDD, also display decreased GABAergic activity in patients with depression [24].

2.2. Anxiety

Clinical studies found that 11–25% of PWE suffered from anxiety, which are higher proportions than healthy people [37]. These rates of depression and anxiety were close to that of drug-refractory epilepsy in a long-term population-based study [38]. The prevalence of depression or anxiety is higher in refractory epilepsy, and especially temporal lobe epilepsy (TLE), than in the general population of PWE [39–41]. The amygdala is important for the fear sensation. The avoidance behavior associated with fear is related to the output of the amygdala to the peri-aqueductal gray matter. Symptoms of anxiety disorders image the activation of the fear circuit involving structures of the hippocampus which is related with re-experiencing fear [42, 43]. Both in anxiety and epilepsy neurons discharging excitatory currents are associated with similar mechanisms [44]. Therefore, the amygdala and hippocampus play a critical pathophysiological role in both anxiety and epilepsy. The orbitofrontal cortex, insula, and cingulate gyrus are also essential in the central mediation of anxiety [45]. Inhibition of γ-aminobutyric acid (GABA)is an important factor in the pathogenesis of anxiety [44]. The $GABA_A$ receptor has an important role in controlling fear. Drugs affecting on $GABA_A$ receptors (like benzodiazepines and barbiturates) may increase the seizure threshold and also control anxiety symptoms by reducing neuronal excitability [46].

Tellez-Zentano et al. studied anxiety disorders in PWE; they found that people without epilepsy reported a lifetime incidence of 11.2% for any anxiety disorder compared with 22.8% in the group with epilepsy [10]. Rai et al. reported increased prevalence of depressive and anxiety disorders in people with epilepsy [47, 48].

We may think that the prevalence of anxiety disorders should be higher in refractory patients than in well-controlled patients. Brandt and Mula displayed a prevalence of 19.6% in patients with refractory epilepsy which is not different than the ratios reported in general epilepsy population [47]. Another important point stated was that the people with shorter epilepsy duration and younger age were more likely to have an anxiety disorder. This could show that the PWE can learn how to cope with the disease as getting older or with increasing duration of the disease. Also, it has been shown that patients in younger age and shorter duration of epilepsy are more likely to have anxiety disorders. This may be explained by patients acquiring coping strategies as years go by Brandt and Mula [47].

Depression and anxiety increase suicide risk, suicidal ideation, and stigmatization in PWE [37, 39]. Recent studies performed with newly diagnosed epileptic patients, identified depression, and anxiety as risk factors of drug-refractory epilepsy [13, 25]. These risk factors have also been associated with worse outcomes of epileptic surgery [49, 50]. In addition, depression and anxiety have been associated with increased adverse events in response to antiepileptic drugs (AEDs)in PWE [51]. Ultimately, the psychiatric and clinical effects of depression and anxiety can impair the quality of life (QOL)of PWE. Therefore, early detection and management of depression and anxiety are critical for the management of PWE.

2.3. Psychosis

There is a higher incidence of psychosis (9%) in PWE, when compared to the general population (1%) [52]. Psychoses in epilepsy have a complex psychopathology that is similar to the positive symptoms of schizophrenia and usually without negative symptoms [53]. Psychoses with seizure disorders can be classified as ictal, postictal, and interictal, depending on the onset of symptoms. Postictal psychosis most commonly appears within a week of the last seizure, whereas psychosis in forced normalization continues to manifest after normalization and with a clear state of consciousness [54]. Forced normalization can be defined by the emergence of psychosis after the control of seizures. The mechanism is unknown, but it can occur whether convulsions are controlled by medication, surgery, or neurostimulation [55]. Hilger et al. retrospectively analyzed 1434 patients with epilepsy, evaluated with prolonged EEG monitoring in order to estimate the prevalence of postictal psychosis (PP) and interictal psychosis (IP) [56]. They found that the overall prevalence of psychosis was 5.9%; prevalence of PP; and IP was 3.7 and 2.2%, respectively. They showed that the 97.6% of the patients with psychosis had localization-related epilepsy. Prevalence of psychosis was highest (9.3%) in patients with temporal lobe epilepsy [56].

2.4. Cognitive impairment

Cognitive impairment is a very important problem for PWE and their families. Memory impairment in epilepsy has been shown in neuropsychological studies and temporal lobe epilepsy (TLE) is an important risk factor. Brain training exercises in the form of activities such as reading, doing crosswords, and sudoku have been shown to improve memory function. Thompson et al. studied patients with temporal lobe epilepsy who had memory impairments. They showed that the traditional memory rehabilitation techniques can help to reduce the burden of memory impairment in temporal lobe epilepsy [57, 58].

Regarding the psychiatric comorbidities of epilepsy, Kanner highlighted some important points. First, he stated that the psychiatric disorders and epilepsy had a bidirectional relationship. The PWE have an increased risk of developing psychiatric comorbidities, but also patients with a primary psychiatric disorder have a greater risk of developing epilepsy. Second, he reported that the PWE with psychiatric comorbidities are less likely to become seizure-free with antiepileptic drugs (AEDs) and with epilepsy surgery. In addition, they are more likely to develop adverse events to AEDs. Finally, Kanner pointed out the importance of psychiatric evaluation of the patients with epilepsy especially who are being considered for surgery.

Because after epilepsy surgery, presurgical comorbid disorders may remit, recur, or be exacerbated [59].

2.5. Stigma

Stigma is associated with feared or perceived discrimination and an important psychosocial burden in people with epilepsy. Stigma among people with epilepsy brings out impairment in quality of life. Also, stigma is associated with aggravation of psychosocial burden like anxiety and depression for people with epilepsy [60]. Generally, prevention of seizures is not adequate in order to relieve the burden of epilepsy, also attenuating of perception of stigma matters for quality of life of individual with epilepsy [61]. Beside impact of stigma on quality of life of individual with epilepsy is frequently underestimated whereas stigma affects quality of life more than frequency of seizure and adverse effects of antiepileptic drugs.

Fisher demonstrated psychosocial symptoms like depression were quite important as initial reaction to the diagnosis of epilepsy and perceived stigma was associated with psychosocial symptoms [62]. A study which was intended to obtain certain demographic, clinical, and psychosocial traits associated with perceived stigma indicated that; being single, having poor quality of life, having difficulty in understanding the written information, and use of behavioral disengagement as a coping mechanism were enhancing factors for perceived stigma [63]. Previous studies demonstrated that low socioeconomic status compared with high socioeconomic status worsens the perception of stigma among PWE [61, 64]. Baker et al. published the largest population-based study to evaluate the stigma of epilepsy in 15 European countries [65]. Stigma data were collected from over 5000 PWE. Perception of stigma was correlated with anxiety, long-term health problems, injuries, and adverse effect of antiepileptic drugs [65]. Another study performed which the epilepsy-related stigma percentages were obtained from the previous largest population-based study. Results of the study suggested overall quality of health system, the health expenditure per capita, and the perceived quality of life have little effect on perceived stigma among individuals with epilepsy. Mentioned trail indicated the role of the public health system invests on awareness programs to increase public knowledge and reduce stigma [60]. Increasing the level of contact between PWE and people without epilepsy may lead changing negative public attitudes [66]. A trial aimed to investigate the relation between the level of knowledge about epilepsy and perception of stigma in adolescents and their mothers was performed. This trial demonstrated that the level of knowledge about epilepsy among adolescents with epilepsy was significantly related to their perception of stigma. As a result, knowledge of epilepsy can minimize the impact of perceived stigma, depressive feelings, and anxiety. This trial indicated also that correlation between the level of the maternal concealment behavior and adolescent with epilepsy's perception of stigma was more significant than maternal knowledge of epilepsy or maternal perception of stigma [67].

Stigma can be categorized into enacted stigma and perceived stigma [63]. Actual disapprobation and discrimination determined against individual with epilepsy is accepted as enacted stigma. However, perceived stigma is characterized as fear of encountering enacted stigma, feeling guilty, and shame about epilepsy. Epilepsy is not the only highly stigmatized illness but one of the most important of them like tuberculosis, leprosy, or HIV/AIDS [61].

In conclusion, epilepsy is a disease with many complications which lowers quality of life of PWE. Stigma, seizure frequency, drugs' adverse reactions, and neuropsychiatric issues are the major factors which are associated with the quality of lives of PWE.

2.6. Self-esteem

Self-esteem has been shown as the most important part of the ego and a major factor effecting psychosocial well-being [68]. The most important determinants of self-esteem are what we think of ourselves, how we assess ourselves when compared to others [68]. Literature analysis shows different results in the correlation between epilepsy and self-esteem [69–70]. Gauffin et al. studied self-esteem in young PWE and compared it with the earlier results [71]. They found that there was a decline in both sense of coherence and self-esteem overtime in young adults with epilepsy. On the other hand, Lee et al. reported that epilepsy in general has little impact on overall self-esteem in adolescents [71].

3. Antiepileptic drugs and suicidality

The pathogenesis of AED induced depressive symptoms is probably multifactorial. In which some of the factors are associated with the drug and other factors may be related to the patient. GABAergic properties, rapid titration of the drug, interaction with folate metabolism may be the drug-related factors. Whereas, poorly controlled seizures, structural abnormalities in the limbic system like small hippocampal volumes may be the patient-related factors [72].

May be the result of effects on the function of two types of receptor GABAergic and antiglutamatergic receptors are considered to be the two main receptors responsible from the psychotropic effects of AEDs but there may also be other possible mechanisms. Presumably, other neurochemical pathways especially a serotonergic mechanism should be considered in psychotropic effects of AEDs [73].

People with epilepsy seemed to have an increased risk for suicide. The risk increases with a history of a psychiatric illness. The AEDs may increase the risk of suicide in PWE, but it is not certain. Some AEDs shown to have negative effects on mood. Especially, barbiturates, vigabatrin, tiagabine, and topiramate were associated with depressive symptoms. In 2008, the Food and Drug Administration (FDA) drew attention on an increased risk of suicidality in people taking AEDs [74] and pharmaceutical companies had been asked to submit data from placebo-controlled trials of AEDs. Suicide-related adverse events occurring during double-blind treatment with an AED (concerning 11 AEDs) were searched. In this study, nearly 28,000 people taking AEDs and more than 16,000 people taking placebo were analyzed. In this analysis, the odds ratios for suicidality were increased for topiramate, but neither barbiturates nor vigabatrin were included in the analysis, and there were few suicidality events reported in the tiagabine trials. Carbamazepine, lamotrigine, and valproate are used as mood stabilizers. In the FDA analysis, carbamazepine and valproate were shown to have a nonsignificant protective effect against suicidality, whereas odds ratios of lamotrigine were significantly increased.

Further clinical prospective studies are needed to evaluate the relation between AEDs and suicidality because FDA analysis may have methodological concerns [72, 74].

Mood disorders, family history of a psychiatric illness, and risk of suicide must be carefully monitored in PWE. Psychiatry consultation must be organized for patients with such symptoms and it is very important to choose the AEDs according to both seizure type and the risk of possible drug induced depressive symptoms [72].

4. Quality of life in PWE

Previous researches regarding quality of life (QOL) in epilepsy showed many different results [75, 76]. Although most studies highlighted the negative effects of epilepsy on patients' quality of lives, there are still some other reports which showed minor or no effect [75, 76]. Some authors suggested that the impact of epilepsy might be minimal if the disease is stabile [75, 76]. On the other hand, epileptic patients living in Europe and North America were reported to have important impairment in HRQOL [77, 78]. The different results reported may be associated with the methodological and/or cultural factors. However, it can be easily noticed that especially in studies with larger samples, HRQOL is decreased in PWE [79, 80].

Baker et al. reported that epilepsy has the potential to negatively affect different aspects of quality of life [79]. They collected data from 3889 PWE from 10 different countries. In this multicenter study, it was shown that nervousness, headaches, and tiredness were the most frequent factors affecting the daily activities.

Short Form-36 (SF-36) was used in Baker et al.'s study and patients scored significantly lower in domains such as physical and social functioning, energy, and vitality [76]. In another multicenter study conducted by Baker et al., data from more than 5000 patients were analyzed and reported that epilepsy had a negative effect on patients' social and psychological well-being [80].

Kutlu et al. investigated the HRQOL, anxiety, and depression states of patients with epilepsy (PWE) [81]. The SF-36 scores were significantly lower in all subscales in PWE compared with the control group. Total scores for Beck Depression Inventory (BDI) were significantly higher in epilepsy patients. Hamilton anxiety scale was also significantly increased in PWE. It was concluded that epilepsy significantly effects with QOL of patients. In the patient group relationship between the seizure frequency and vitality was found to be statistically significant [81]. Birbeck et al. in their study evaluating ability of HRQOL measures to detect change overtime in people with epilepsy, suggested that SF-36 yielded responsiveness indices comparable to those of the epilepsy targeted measures [82].

Recently, Chen et al. studied factors affecting QOL in 260 PWE in Taiwan in a cross-sectional, correlational study. They used the Quality of Life in Epilepsy-31 (QOLIE-31) questionnaire for evaluating HRQOL [9]. In this study, scores for the QOLIE-31 were correlated with the demographic characteristics, sleep quality, symptoms of anxiety and depression, epilepsy-specific variables such as, seizure frequency; types, number, and frequency of AEDs; and adverse events of AED and social support. They reported that seven factors were predictive for quality of life: anxiety, depression, adverse events of AEDs, social support, seizure frequency of at least once in 3 months, household income of male gender. Another recent study was conducted by Mutluay et al., which they investigated the HRQOL in 124 PWE in Turkey [83]. This study measured the QOL in epilepsy and determined associated demographic and clinical factors by means of the Short Form-36 health survey. They found that patients with epilepsy do not perceive impaired physical health status. However, their mental health appears vulnerable, especially in women. In this study, the major burden was in the mental health category. They also reported that a positive treatment response is an important determinant of the HRQOL in PWE. Temporal lobe epilepsy (TLE) is the most common type of medically intractable epilepsy and is accepted as a prototype for a surgically remediable epilepsy when hippocampal sclerosis is the pathological substrate [84]. A reduction in seizure frequency and an improvement in the HRQOL are expected for patients with intractable epilepsy after epilepsy surgery [85]. Several studies indicate that complete seizure freedom is a strongly associated with psychosocial adjustment [86]. However, others show a poor correlation with postoperative seizure freedom. After surgery even if the seizures are completely lost, patients may still suffer from comorbidities such as depression, anxiety, and stigma. This can be explained by the "burden of normality" concept [84]. Patients' status changes from chronically ill to cured state in which the patient has to face the responsibilities of a normal life like finding a job and learn to continue and adjust life without the "advantages" of a chronic illness. Aydemir et al. studied 20 patients with intractable temporal lobe epilepsy who were waiting for surgery and 21 patients who had surgery. They used SF-36, Beck Depression Inventory, State Trait Anxiety Inventory, stigma and impact of epilepsy inventories, and a form asking their own perspectives about epilepsy and surgery. They found that QOL of patients after surgery was found to be better than before surgery. They also reported that seizure frequency, comorbidity, and AEDs affected HRQOL negatively. Impact of epilepsy levels was found to be higher among the preoperative patients [84]. A very important study was conducted by Taft et al. [87]. In this prospective study, HRQOL, mood, and patient satisfaction in epilepsy surgery candidates before and 2 years after epilepsy surgery was studied. They used Short Form Health Survey (SF-36), the Hospital Anxiety and Depression scale (HAD) at baseline and after 2-year follow-ups and also operated patients answered patient satisfaction questions. In patients who were seizure-free after epilepsy surgery HRQOL improved and anxiety decreased. Operated patients found surgery beneficial. But a very important point noticed in this study was that only about half of the seizure-free patients showed HRQOL improvements, in which that seizure freedom does not always improve patients' quality of lives.

5. Conclusion

Psychologically, PWE may have feelings of worthlessness, fear, stigma, anger, and hopelessness, and may exhibit passive behavior [88]. Stigmatization leads to discrimination, and PWE have been the target of prejudicial behavior in many aspects of life, over many centuries and in many cultures [89]. These factors decrease their psychosocial function, self-efficacy, and quality of life [90, 91] and even increase the suicide rate [90–92].

Recognition of the past and current comorbid psychiatric disorders needs to be incorporated into the evaluation of every PWE, including those with a newly diagnosed seizure disorder. Future research will need to determine whether an early remission of psychiatric disorders reverses the worse course of the seizure disorder. Finally, presurgical psychiatric evaluations must be conducted in all patients undergoing a presurgical evaluation.

Epilepsy, with its rich clinical features, is particularly important for HRQOL research. Epileptic patients may experience various problems which will result in a lower quality of life. Seizure frequency, side effects of the antiepileptic drugs, psychological comorbidity, and stigma are important factors associated with the severity of the disease and these factors may cause an important impact on life quality of epileptic patients. Stemming from a thorough review of the current literature, we can conclude that there is still a need for further scientific research with further validated instruments to find out more clear relation between epilepsy and HRQOL.

Author details

Ayşe Kutlu* and Serap Mülayim

*Address all correspondence to: draysekutlu@yahoo.com

Department of Neurology, Faculty of Medicine, Kocaeli University, Kocaeli, Turkey

References

[1] Foldwary N, Wyllie E. Epilepsy. In: Goetz GC, Pappert EJ, eds. Textbook of Clinical Neurology. Philedelphia: W.B. Saunders Company; 1999:1059–1088.

[2] McHugh JC, Delanty N. Epidemiology and classification of epilepsy. Int Rev Neurobiol. 2008;83:11–26.

[3] World Health Organization. International Classification of Functioning Disability and Health: ICF. Geneva: WHO; 2001.

[4] Leonardi M, Ustun TB. The global burden of epilepsy. Epilepsia. 2002;43(Suppl. 6):21–5.

[5] ILAE/IBE/WHO. "Out of the shadows": global campaign against epilepsy. ILAE/IBE/WHO Annual Report. Geneva: WHO; 1999.

[6] Meinardi H, Scott RA, Reis R, Sander JW. The treatment gap in epilepsy: the current situation and ways forward. Epilepsia. 2001;42:136–49.

[7] Tulsky DS, Rosenthal M. Quality of life measurement in rehabilitation medicine: building an agenda for the future. Arch Phys Med Rehabil. 2002;83(Suppl. 2):1–3.

[8] Mula M, Cock HR. More than seizures: improving the lives of people with refractory epilepsy. Eur J Neurol. 2015;22:24–30.

[9] Chen HF, Tsai YF, Mo-Song Hsi MS, Chen J. Factors affecting quality of life in adults with epilepsy in Taiwan: a cross-sectional, correlational study. Epilepsy Behav. 2016;58(26–32).

[10] Tellez-Zenteno JF, Patten SB, Jette N, Williams J, Wiebe S. Psychiatric comorbidity in epilepsy: a population-based analysis. Epilepsia. 2007;48:2336–2344.

[11] Kanner AM, Schachter SC, Barry JJ, Hersdorffer DC, Mula M, Trimble M, et al. Depression and epilepsy: epidemiologic and neurobiologic perspectives that may explain their high comorbid occurrence. Epilepsy Behav. 2012;24(156–168).

[12] Mula M, Kanner AM. Introduction—treatment of psychiatric disorders in adults with epilepsy: what every epileptologist should know. Epilepsia. 2013;54(Suppl. 1):1–2.

[13] Kanner AM, Barry JJ, Gilliam F, Hermann B, Meador KJ. Anxiety disorders, subsyndromic depressive episodes, and major depressive episodes: do they differ on their impact on the quality of life of patients with epilepsy? Epilepsia. 2010;51(7):1152–1158.

[14] Perrine K, Hermann BP, Meador KJ, Vickrey BG, Cramer JA, Hays RD, Devinsky O. The relationship of neuropsychological functioning to quality of life in epilepsy. Arch Neurol. 1995;52:997–1003.

[15] Gilliam FG. Optimizing health outcomes in active epilepsy. Neurology. 2002;58(Suppl. 5):9–19.

[16] Cramer JA, Blum M, Reed M, Fanning K, Epilepsy Impact Project. The influence of comorbid depression on quality of life for people with epilepsy. Epilepsy Behav. 2003;4:515–521.

[17] Boylan LS, Flint LA, Labovitz DL, Jackson SC, Starner K, Devinsky O. Depression but not seizure frequency predicts quality of life in treatment-resistant epilepsy. Neurology. 2004;62:258–261.

[18] Johnson EK, Jones JE, Seidenberg M, Hermann BP. The relative impact of anxiety, depression, and clinical seizure features on health related quality of life in epilepsy. Epilepsia. 2004;45:544–550.

[19] Loring DW, Meador KJ, Lee GP. Determinants of quality of life in epilepsy. Epilepsy Behav. 2004;5:976–980.

[20] Tracy JI, Dechant V, Sperling MR, Cho R, Glosser D. The association of mood with quality of life ratings in epilepsy. Neurology. 2007;68:1101–1107.

[21] Tracy JI, Dechant V, Sperling MR, Cho R, Glosser D. The association of mood with quality of life ratings in epilepsy. Neurology 2007; 68:1101–1107.

[22] Kim SK, Park SP, Kwon O. Impact of depression and anxiety on adverse event profiles in Korean people with epilepsy. Epilepsy Behav. 2015;46:185–191.

[23] Beghi E, Roncolato M, and Visona G. Depression and altered quality of life in women with epilepsy of childbearing age. Epilepsia. 2004;45(1):64–70.

[24] Kanner AM. Is depression associated with an increased risk of treatment-resistant epilepsy? Research strategies to investigate this question. Epilepsy Behav. 2014;38:3–7.

[25] Hitiris N, Mohanraj R, Norrie J, et al. Predictors of pharmacoresistant epilepsy. Epilepsy Res. 2007;75:192–6.

[26] Prendiville S, Gale K. Anticonvulsant effect of fluoxetine on focally evoked limbic motor seizures in rats. Epilepsia. 1993;34(2):381–4.

[27] Mazarati AM, Siddarth P, Baldwin RA, Sankar R. Depression after status epilepticus: behavioural and biochemical deficits and effects of fluoxetine. Brain. 2008;131:2071–83.

[28] Sanacora G, Mason GF, Rothman DL, Krystal JH. Increased occipital cortex GABA concentrations in depressed patients after therapy with selective serotonin reuptake inhibitors. Am J Psychiatry 2002;159:663–5.

[29] Zink M, Vollmayr B, Gebicke-Haerter PJ, Henn FA. Reduced expression of glutamate transporters vGluT1, EAAT2 and EAAT4 in learned helpless rats, an animal model of depression. Neuropharmacology. 2010;58:465–73.

[30] Bonanno G, Giambelli R, Raiteri L, et al. Chronic antidepressants reduce depolarization-evoked glutamate release and protein interactions favoring formation of SNARE complex in hippocampus. J Neurosci. 2005;25:3270–9.

[31] Gerner RH, Hare TA. CSF GABA in normal subjects and patients with depression, schizophrenia, mania, and anorexia nervosa. Am J Psychiatry. 1981;138:1098–101.

[32] Sanacora G, Gueorguieva R, Epperson, et al. Subtype-specific alterations of gamma-aminobutyric acid and glutamate in patients with major depression. Arch Gen Psychiatry. 2004;61:705–13.

[33] Bhagwagar Z, Wylezinska M, Jezzard, et al. Reduction in occipital cortex gamma-aminobutyric acid concentrations in medication-free recovered unipolar depressed and bipolar subjects. Biol Psychiatry. 2007;61:806–12.

[34] Sanacora G, Mason GF, Rothman DL, et al. Increased cortical GABA concentrations in depressed patients receiving ECT. Am J Psychiatry. 2003;160:577–9.

[35] Rajkowska G, O'Dwyer G Zsofia Teleki Z, Stockmeier CA, Miguel-Hidalgo JJ. GABAergic Neurons Immunoreactive for Calcium Binding Proteins are Reduced in the Prefrontal Cortex in Major Depression. Neuropsychopharmacology 2007 ;32(2):471–82.

[36] Price RB, Shungu DC, Mao X, Nestadt P, Kelly C, Collins KA, et al. Amino acid neurotransmitters assessed by proton magnetic resonance spectroscopy: relationship to treatment resistance in major depressive disorder. Biol Psychiatry. 2009;65:792–800.

[37] Kwon O, Park S-P. Depression and anxiety in people with epilepsy. J Clin Neurol 2014;10(3):175–88.

[38] Sillanpää M, Schmidt D. Natural history of treated childhood-onset epilepsy: prospective, long-term population-based study. Brain. 2006;129(Pt 3):617–24.

[39] Jacoby A, Baker GA, Steen N, Potts P, Chadwick DW. The clinical course of epilepsy and its psychosocial correlates: findings from a U.K. Community study. Epilepsia. 1996;37:148–161.

[40] Gaitatzis A, Trimble MR, Sander JW. The psychiatric comorbidity of epilepsy. Acta Neurol Scand. 2004;110:207–220.

[41] Perini GI, Tosin C, Carraro C, Bernasconi G, Canevini MP, Canger R, et al. Interictal mood and personality disorders in temporal lobe epilepsy and juvenile myoclonic epilepsy. J Neurol Neurosurg Psychiatry. 1996;61:601–5.

[42] Stahl SM. Brainstorms: symptoms and circuits, part 2: anxiety disorders. J Clin Psychiatry. 2003;64:1408–9.

[43] Rogawski MA, Löscher W. The neurobiology of antiepileptic drugs for the treatment of nonepileptic conditions. Nat Med. 2004;10:685–692.

[44] Mula M, Pini S, Cassano GB. The role of anticonvulsant drugs in anxiety disorders: a critical review of the evidence. J Clin Psychopharmacol. 2007;27:263–72.

[45] Rauch SL, Savage CR, Alpert NM, Miguel EC, Baer L, Breiter HC, et al. A positron emission tomographic study of simple phobic symptom provocation. Arch Gen Psychiatry. 1995;52:20–28.

[46] Mula M, Monaco F. Antiepileptic drugs and psychopathology of epilepsy: an update. Epileptic Disord. 2009;11:1–9.

[47] Brandt C, Mula M. Anxiety disorders in people with epilepsy. Epilepsy Behav. 2016;59:87–91.

[48] Rai D, Kerr MP, McManus S, Jordanova V, Lewis G, Brugha TS. Epilepsy and psychiatric comorbidity: a nationally representative population-based study. Epilepsia. 2012;53:1095–103.

[49] Cleary RA, Thompson PJ, Fox Z, Foong J. Predictors of psychiatric and seizure outcome following temporal lobe epilepsy surgery. Epilepsia. 2012;53:1705–12.

[50] de Araújo Filho GM, Gomes FL, Mazetto L, Marinho MM, Tavares IM, Caboclo LO, et al. Major depressive disorder as a predictor of a worse seizure outcome one year after

surgery in patients with temporal lobe epilepsy and mesial temporal sclerosis. Seizure. 2012;21:619–23.

[51] Liik M, Vahter L, Gross-Paju K, Haldre S. Subjective complaints compared to the results of neuropsychological assessment in patients with epilepsy: The influence of comorbid depression. Epilepsy Res. 2009;84:194–200.

[52] Kanner AM, Palac S. Neuropsychiatric complications of epilepsy. Curr Neurol Neurosci Rep. 2002;2(4):365–72.

[53] Hasija D, Jadapalle SLK, Badr A. Status epilepticus and psychosis of epilepsy. Psychiatr Ann. 2012;42(1):11–13.

[54] Schachter SC, Holmes GL, Trenité DK. Behavioral Aspects of Epilepsy: Principles and Practice. New York: Demos Medical Publishing; 2008:489–495.

[55] Loganathan MA, Enja M, Steven Lippmann S. Epilepsy and psychosis interaction. Innov Clin Neurosci. 2015;12(5–6):38–41.

[56] Hilger E, Zimprich F, Pataraia E, Aull-Watschinger S, Jung R, Baumgartner C, Bonelli S. Psychoses in epilepsy: a comparison of postictal and interictal psychoses. Epilepsy Behav. 2016;60:58–62.

[57] Thompson PJ, Duncan JS. Cognitive decline in severe intractable epilepsy. Epilepsia. 2005;46(11):1780–7.

[58] Thompson PJ, Baxendale SA, McEvoy AW, Duncan JS. Cognitive outcomes of temporal lobe epilepsysurgery in older patients. Seizure. 2015;29:41–5.

[59] Andres M. Kanner AM. Do psychiatric comorbidities have a negative impact on the course and treatment of seizure disorders? Curr Opin Neurol. 2013;26:2.

[60] Brigo F, Igwe SC, Ausserer H, Tezzon F, Nardone R, Otte WM. Epilepsy-related stigma in European people with epilepsy: correlations with health system performance and overall quality of life. Epilepsy Behav. 2015;42:18–21.

[61] Leaffer EB, Hesdorffer DC, Begley C. Psychosocial and sociodemographic associates of felt stigma in epilepsy. Epilepsy Behav. 2014;37:104–9.

[62] Fisher RS. Epilepsy from the patient's perspective: review of results of a community-based survey. Epilepsy Behav. 2000;1(4):9–14.

[63] Bautista RED, Shapovalov D, Shoraka AR. Factors associated with increased felt stigma among individuals with epilepsy. Seizure. 2015;30:106–112.

[64] Begley CE, Shegog R, Iyagba B, Chen V, Talluri K, Dubinsky S, et al. Socioeconomic status and self-management in epilepsy: comparison of diverse clinical populations in Houston, Texas. Epilepsy Behav. 2010;19:232–8.

[65] Baker GA, Brooks J, Buck D, Jacoby A. The stigma of epilepsy: a European perspective. Epilepsia. 2000;41:98–104.

[66] De Boer HM, Mula M, Sander JW. The global burden and stigma of epilepsy. Epilepsy Behav. 2008;12:240–6.

[67] Ryu HU, Lee SA, Eom S, Kim HD. Perceived stigma in Korean adolescents with epilepsy: effects of knowledge about epilepsy and maternal perception of stigma. Seizure. 2015;24:38–43.

[68] Winter DG. Personality, Analysis and Interpretations of Lives. New York: McGraw-Hill; 1996.

[69] Baker GA, Spector S, McGrath Y, Soteriou H. Impact of epilepsy in adolescence: a UK controlled study. Epilepsy Behav. 2005;6:556–62.

[70] Reeve DK, Lincoln NB. Coping with the challenge of transition in older adolescents with epilepsy. Seizure. 2002;11:33–9.

[71] Gauffin H, Landtblom AM, Räty L. Self-esteem and sense of coherence in young people with uncomplicated epilepsy: A 5-year follow-up. Epilepsy & Behavior 2010;17:520–524.

[72] Marco Mula M, Gail S. Bell GS, Sander JW. Suicidality in epilepsy and possible effects of antiepileptic drugs. Curr Neurol Neurosci Rep. 2010;10:327–32.

[73] Kalinin VV. Suicidality and antiepileptic drugs: is there a link? Drug Saf. 2007;30(2): 123–42.

[74] US Food and Drug Administration. Antiepileptic drugs and suicidality; 2008 May 23. Available at http://www.fda.gov/ohrms/dockets/ac/08/briefing/2008-4372b1-01-FDA.pdf. Accessed June 2008.

[75] Jacoby A. Felt versus inacted stigma: a concept revisited. Soc Sci Med. 1994;38:269–74.

[76] Leidy NK, Elizhauser A, Vickrey B, et al. Seizure frequency and health-related quality of life in adults with epilepsy. Neurology. 1999;53:162–6.

[77] Stavem K, Loge JH, Kaasa S. Health status of people with epilepsy compared with a general reference population. Epilepsia. 2000;41:85–90.

[78] Buck D, Jacoby A, Baker GA, et al. Cross-cultural differences in health-related quality of life of people with epilepsy: findings from a European study. Quality Life Res 1999;8:675–85.

[79] Baker GA, Jacoby A, Gorry J, Doughty J, Ellina V; on Behalf of the SIGN Group. Quality of life of people with epilepsy in Iran, the Gulf, and Near East. Epilepsia. 2005;46(1): 132–40.

[80] Baker GA, Jacoby A, Buck D, Stalgis C, Monnet D. Quality of life in people with epilepsy: a European study. Epilepsia. 1997;38(3):353–62.

[81] Kutlu A, Başaran S, Altun NS, Unalan H, Komsuoğlu SS. Quality of life, depression and anxiety in patients with epilepsy: controlled study with Short Form 36 Question-

naire, Beck Depression Inventory and Hamilton Anxiety Scale. Neurosurg Q. 2010;20(2):95–99.

[82] Birbeck GL, Kim S, Hays RD, Wickrey BG. Quality of life measures in epilepsy: how well can they detect change overtime? Neurology. 2000;54:1822–7.

[83] Mutluay FK, Gunduz A, Tekeoglu A, Oguz S, Yeni SN. Health related quality of life in patients with epilepsy in Turkey. J Phys Ther Sci. 2016 Jan;28(1):240–5.

[84] Aydemir N, Ozkara C, Canbeyli R, Tekcan A. Changes in quality of life and self-perspective related to surgery in patients with temporal lobe epilepsy. Epilepsy Behav. 2004;5(5):735–42.

[85] Kellett MW, Smith DF, Chadwick DW. Quality of life after epilepsy surgery. J Neurol Neurosurg Psychiatry. 1997;63:52–8.

[86] Selai CE, Elstner K, Trimble MR. Quality of life pre and post epilepsy surgery. Epilepsy Res. 1999;38:67–74.

[87] Taft C, Magnusson ES, Ekstedt G, and Malmgren K. Health-related quality of life, mood, and patient satisfaction after epilepsy surgery in Sweden—a prospective controlled observational study. Epilepsia. 2014;55(6):878–85.

[88] Chen HF, Tsai YF, Lin YP, Mo-Song Shih MS, Chen JC . The relationships among medicine symptom distress, self-efficacy, patient–provider relationship, and medication compliance in patients with epilepsy. Epilepsy Behav. 2010;19:43–9.

[89] Pahl K, de Boer HM. Epilepsy and rights. In: Atlas: epilepsy care in the world. Geneva: WHO; 2005. p. 72–3.

[90] Pramuka M, Hendrickson R, Zinski A, Van Cott AC. A psychosocial self-management program for epilepsy: a randomized pilot study in adults. Epilepsy Behav. 2007;11:533–45.

[91] Bell GS, Gaitatzis A, Bell CL, Johnson AL, Sander JW. Suicide in people with epilepsy: how great is the risk? Epilepsia. 2009;50:1933–42.

[92] Chen HF, Tsai YF. The psychosocial responses and coping strategies in the epilepsy. Chang Gung Nursing 2003;14:21–30.

5

Autoimmune Epilepsy: New Development and Future Directions

Sandra Orozco-Suarez, Angélica Vega-Garcia, Iris Feria-Romero, Lourdes Arriaga-Pizano, Emmanuel Rodriguez-Chavez and Israel Grijalva

Abstract

In recent years, there has been accumulating evidence to support an autoimmune etiology for some patients with drug-resistant seizures, typically in the context of an antibody-mediated encephalopathy; any seizure disorder that may be caused by pathogenic autoantibodies, are an example of autoimmune epilepsy. Autoimmunity is characterized by loss of immune tolerance that causes the destruction of cells and tissues. The largest complex histocompatibility system has had a strong association with autoimmune disease, although certain genes encoding cytokines and co-stimulatory molecules increase genetic susceptibility. In spite of having scientific advances in this research area, the conditions underlying mechanisms are unknown. **Goal**: this chapter aims to present in synthesized form, the genetic, immunological, and environmental factors role in the autoimmunity to epilepsy, as well as the therapeutic approach that has been used to control seizures, mainly where there is a suspected anti-neuronal-antibodies circulation. **Methods**: a review of the work achieved during the last years in patients with this condition provides information and experience in the diagnosis and treatment of this epilepsy type. For this, a systematic search of PUBMED is conducted using the search terms "autoimmune and epilepsy, auto antibodies and epilepsy, NMDA and epilepsy, AMPA and epilepsy, and GAD and epilepsy." The list of identified articles was complemented by additional searches for relevant articles in the reference section of the publications captured by the initial search.

Keywords: epilepsy, autoimmune encephalitis, NMDAr, immunotherapy

1. Introduction

Epilepsy is considered, as one disease with the highest prevalence of 1% population suffering from it. This pathology is defined as a cerebral disorder that is characterized by the predisposition to generate epileptic seizures, as well as the neurobiological, cognitive, psychological and social factors associated with this condition [1]. There is evidence that specific neuronal auto antibodies with pathogenic potential may be present in a subset of patients with epilepsy. Importantly, it has recently been shown that some patients with these serum auto antibodies and mainly in CSF are often refractory to treatment with standard antiepileptic drugs (AEDs) and, on the other hand, may respond well to immunomodulatory therapies. In this way, it has been possible to make a therapeutic approach. The autoimmune basis led to the introduction of immunotherapy (IT) in some drug-resistant syndromes [2], prompted by an intensive search for self-antibodies (Abs) in epilepsy. The findings of limbic encephalitis associated with self-Abs against neuronal plasma membrane (receptors, ion channels) and intracellular proteins have further fueled this search. As seizures are key to the infestation manifest, this disorder serves as a model for understanding epilepsy-immune system interaction [3], evoking the possibility that said antibodies could cause patients with epilepsy alone, and leading to the search for self-Acs in patients with pharmacoresistant epilepsy (PE). Recent prospective study found neuronal auto-Acs in about 10% of pediatric patients with seizures, a rate twice as high as in controls with other systemic diseases; this creates a quandary for clinicians as to when treatment should be chosen in pharmaco-resistant epilepsy patients [4].

2. Genetic and clinical heterogeneity of epilepsy

Autoimmune conditions are the result of multifactorial processes involving dysregulation of both the innate and adaptive immune system, and the possession of predisposing gene alleles, which ultimately at a certain moment in time "trigger" a sustained loss of self-tolerance resulting in an immune-mediated damage of autologous tissues [5]. The innate immune response is the host's first line of defense against invading microorganisms, while the adaptive immune responds to the infection in a time-delayed but antigen-specific manner. Adaptive immune responses are driven by specific components of bacteria or antigen, require several days to develop, and exhibit immunological memory for a lifetime, such that a second exposure to the same antigen results in an accelerated and specific response. Cell populations of the innate immune system, such as dendritic cells (DCs), which are antigen-presenting cells, promote primary T cells and B cell responses and therefore relate innate and adaptive immunity [6]. T cells that are reactive to self- antigens are largely deleted in the thymus in an active process termed thymic or central tolerance induction. Central tolerance induction occurs in both the immature thymus T cells and bone marrow for B cells. During the ontogeny of lymphocytes, T lymphocytes receptors (TCRs) that recognize high affinity, self-peptides exposed in The HLA molecules are deleted by clonal deletion, in order to avoid self-reactive clones. Only the clones whose TCRs recognize their own peptides with medium affinity, mature in secondary lymphoid organs. This shows that the HLA molecules themselves determine the TCR repertoire. Peripheral tolerance mechanisms include clonal anergy (absence of co-stimulatory molecules), unawareness and suppression by the activation of CD4 + CD25 + FOXP3 + regulatory T cells. In the antigen recognition, the segments $\alpha 1$ and $\beta 1$ of the HLA molecules (both polymorphic), the processed peptide and the TCR are involved [7]. In fact, some processed peptides are only exposed in certain HLA molecules. So the molecules of the HLA itself also determine which peptide can be recognized by the mature T lymphocytes TCR. The HLA molecules of an individual, determine their immune response at two levels: during negative selection in the thymus and in the selection of peptides at the periphery [7, 8]. By the other way, the new lines of AEs research focused on the genes coding for molecules involved in the central tolerance and peripheral induction. These genes found on any chromosome encode for proteins involved in the lymphocytes and molecules selection, acting as death receptors or co-stimulatory molecules. Most AEs caused the difficulty in knowing the triggering agents. The AEs caused by a mutation in a single gene (monogenic), which are small, provide clinical and experimental evidence of the contribution of different control mechanisms of self-reactivity [9].

2.1. Genetic diagnostics of epilepsies

In epilepsy, there are no studies associating autoimmunity with genetic factors; however, studies have focused on other autoimmune diseases and focuses are mainly associated with major histocompatibility system. Several alleles of classical human leukocyte antigen (HLA) genes in the MHC locus have been linked to autoimmune diseases. The genes coding for HLA molecules are located on the short arm of chromosome 6 in the region of the major histocompatibility complex (MHC). The HLA-I genes encoded by the HLAA, B, C, E, F, and G genes are expressed in all the genes encoding the class I, II, and III molecules. The nucleated cells and the platelets and HLA-II molecules are products of the HLA-DP, DQ, DR, DM, DO genes and are constitutively expressed in B lymphocytes, monocytes, macrophages, dendritic cells, endothelial cells, intestinal epithelial cells, cells early hematopoietic and activated T lymphocytes. The class III region called HLA non-classical contains a collection of approximately 20 genes. This region includes those encoding complement proteins, components involved in the intracellular processing of peptides (TAP1, TAP2) and epithelial cell surface molecules (MICA-MICB) [10, 11]. The fundamental function of molecules HLA-I and HLA-II is to bind their own and foreign peptides in order to transport them to the cell membrane. Once exposed, they are recognized by the TCR, so they have a central role in the execution of the immune response. HLA-I molecules primarily present cytosolic (such as a viral or tumor) peptides to CD8+ cytotoxic T cells, whereas HLA class II molecules generally have extracellular peptides (such as bacterial) to CD4+ helper T lymphocytes. This functional division of peptide presentation ensures the activation of T cells (CD8+ and CD4+) and therefore the appropriate immune response for each type of antigen [10]. The HLA system has two fundamental properties that make it difficult to understand, the genes involved in the predisposition to AEs: polymorphism and linkage disequilibrium (LD) [12]. I-II molecules are the most polymorphic of the whole genome. This property determines that for each loci, there are multiple alleles whose DNA sequences only differ by a few nucleotides. These local mutations are known as single nucleotide polymorphism (NSP). Genes located in the MHC region have a high genetic association. This property is known as linkage disequilibrium (LD) and describes the tendency of certain genes to inherit together given their closeness. The above determines that the frequency of these genes (in a single haplotype) in the population is greater than their individual inheritance [13, 14]. Inside the AEs gene, the greatest association is with the molecules of the HLA. The siblings concordance with identical HLA is 15% compared to 1% for siblings with a non-identical HLA. This figure is indicative of the strong association between HLA molecules and a risk to develop an autoimmune disease. In some diseases, this association is stronger as in ankylosing spondylitis (AS), while in others, it is weaker than in the myasthenia gravis (MG) [15].

Genetic study with a cohort of 24 cases of Rasmussen (RE) autoimmune encephalitis, the human leukocyte antigen (HLA) class I and class II genes were sequenced; they got the association of three C*07 alleles: 02:01:01, DQA1*04:01:01, and DQB1*04:02:01, that increased the relative risk of RE. It has been shown that HLA-B*07:02 is a risk factor for Graves' disease. In addition, 33% of patients in that study had HLA-A*03:01:01:01, which is considered a risk factor to multiple sclerosis. 17% of patients had a combination of three HLA class II alleles that were associated with type 1 diabetes; DQA1*, 05*01:01:01, DQB1*02:01:01 and 20% patients showed a combination of HLA alleles (DQA1*01:02:01:01, DQB1*06:02:01, DRB1*15:01:01:01), that have been linked to the risk of developing multiple sclerosis [15].

The same way, anti-leucine-rich glioma-inactivated (LGI1) encephalitis was associated [16] with the DRB1*07:01-DQB1*02:02 haplotype (10 patients, 91%) in HLA class II genes, as well as with B*44:03 (8 patients, 73%) and C*07:06 (7 patients, 64%) in the HLA class I region. The prevalence of these alleles in anti-LGI1 encephalitis was significantly higher than that in the epilepsy controls or healthy controls. By contrast, anti-NMDAR encephalitis was not associated with HLA genotypes. Additional analysis using HLA-peptide binding prediction algorithms and computational docking underpinned the close relationship; this finding suggests that most anti-LGI1 encephalitis develop in a population with specific HLA subtypes [17].

2.2. Influence of environmental factors

The concordance values between monozygotic twins are indicative of the role of environmental factors in the development of autoimmunity. Within this group are infections (viruses, parasites, bacteria, and fungi), hormones and immune system regulation loss. The action mechanism proposed for these factors is based on the release of pro-inflammatory substances inducing the danger signals expression and the consequent activation of auto-reactive T lymphocyte clones.

T cell TCRs recognize different peptides in the groove of the HLA molecule as long as they maintain the same charge distribution and spatial orientation. Hence, own and foreign molecules that have this similarity are recognized by lymphocytes and produce an immune response [18]. The creation of an inflammatory microenvironment increases the presence of antigens due to tissue damage and the expression of co-stimulatory molecules. In this medium, the anergized T lymphocytes may activate and stimulate the immune response against antigens themselves [19].

Nevertheless, infections can also modify the clinical manifestations associated with autoimmune epilepsy (AE) in such a way that infections are involved in the induction and protection of AEs in genetically predisposed individuals. This dual role underlying mechanism compression offers new ways of controlling and treating these diseases [20].

3. Conventional etiological mechanisms of neural proteins as antibodies

The target antigens that play a critical role in neuronal transmission and in plasticity include the N-methyl-D-aspartate (NMDA) receptor, alpha-amino-3-hydroxy-5-methyl-4-isoxazole-propionic acid (AMPA), the gamma-aminobutyric acid receptor (GABA), the glioma-inactivating leucine-rich protein (LGI1) and the contacting-associated protein 2 (CASPR2), a protein that plays a key role in the normal function of voltage-dependent potassium channels [21].

The structure of NMDA receptors (R-NMDA) are formed by combinations of different subunits: NMDAR1 (NR1), NMDAR2 (NR2), and NMDAR3 (NR3); which form a Ca++ permeable ion channel. A single gene encodes the NR1 subunit; however, transcription can generate at least eight isoforms, whereas for NR2-type subunits there are four different genes encoding NR2A, NR2B, NR2C, and NR2D7 subunits. Functional NMDA receptors are composed of heterotetramers, and formed by two dimers twisted by the subunits NR1-NR2, where in the NR1 subunit it possesses a glycine binding site and each in the NR2 subunit, a glutamate binding site, with two binding sites for glycine (S1) and two for glutamate (S2) in each receptor. The NR1-NR2 dimmer is considered the basic functional structure at each receptor, where different physiological and pharmacological binding sites are found for different ligands [22, 23]. Each ionotropic receptor subunit has similar molecular structure, which is organized into four functional domains, which are: an extracellular domain with the amino (N) terminal (DNT), a ligand binding domain (DBL), a region (M1–M4), where the M2 segment that partially enters the membrane forms the ion channel, and finally, a carboxyl domain (C) in the intracellular region (DCT) (**Figure 1(A)**) [24, 25].

In NMDARAS, IgG antibodies are directed to the N-terminal extracellular domain of the GluN1 subunit of the NMDA receptor (**Figure 1**), specifically an epitope region at GluN1 aa369 [26–28]; the cultures of dissociated rat hippocampal neurons and antibody-containing cerebrospinal fluid (CSF) from patients with NMDARAS have been used to study the molecular mechanism by which IgG antibodies cause hypo function of the NMDAR [29]; antibodies decrease the levels of synaptic NMDA receptor and disrupt NMDA receptor currents in cultured neurons. In addition, antibodies disrupt the interaction between NMDAR and the ephrin B2 receptor (EphB2R), a major stabilizer of NMDARs at postsynaptic sites, facilitating the displacement of NMDARs from the synapse [29]. The antibody does not act as a receptor antagonist, by modulating the physiological receptor binding domain, but causes capping and internalization of the receptor [30]. Antibody-mediated internalization is independent of NMDAR activity and does not occur as a compensatory response to the agonism of the receptor, suggesting that the mechanism of internalization is primarily NMDAR cross-linking by patient antibodies [29].

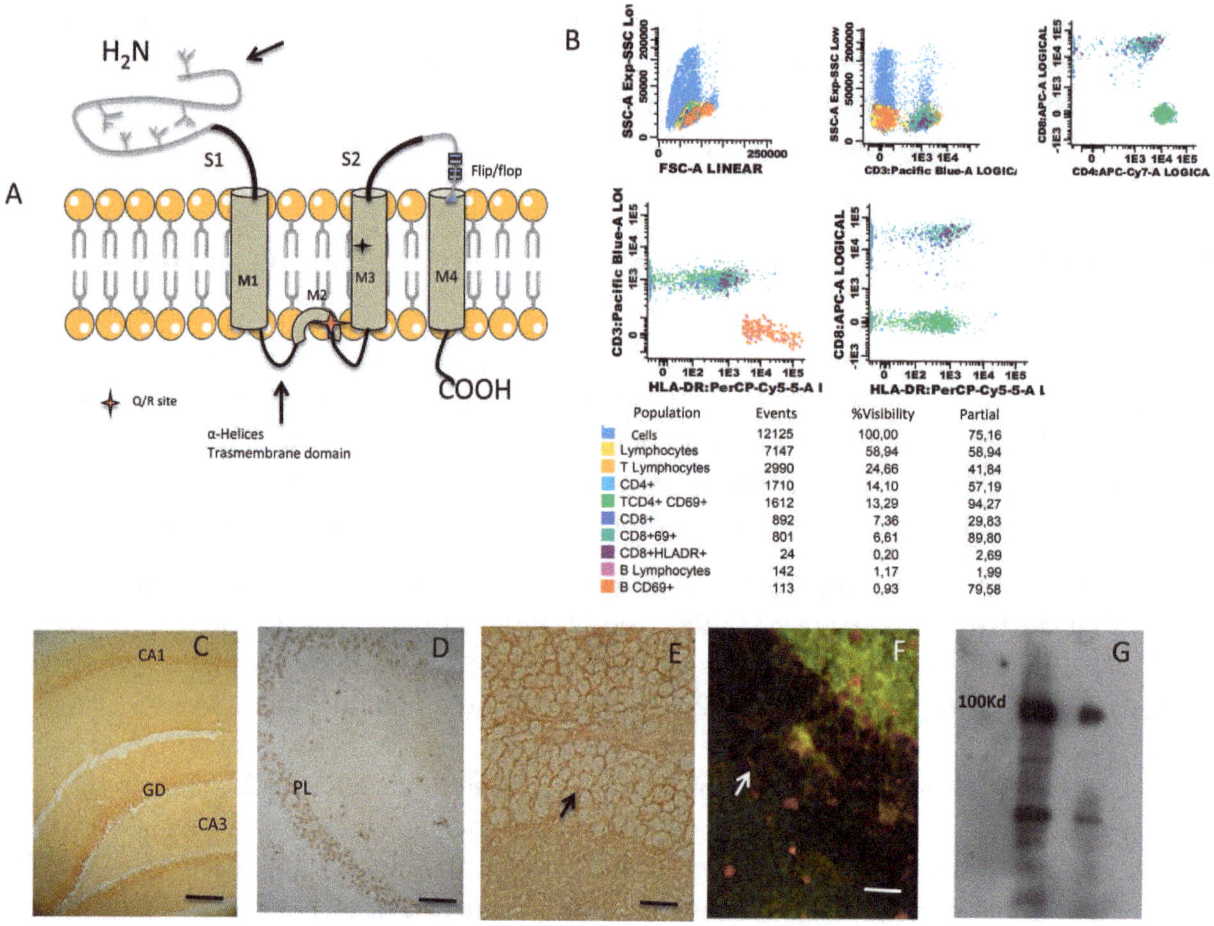

Figure 1. (A) Structure of AMPA receptor subunits. The transmembrane topology is shown, along with the flip/flop alternatively spliced exon, and the two ligand-binding domains (S1 and S2). Glycosylation sites are shown as trees in the N-terminal region; this region is associated with immune response. (B) Flow cytometry demonstrates the presence of T lymphocytes of the CD8+ class with greater activation, as well as B lymphocytes; here it can be known that the immune process has extravasated to the cerebral parenchyma, (C) and (D) the tissue based assay. Mouse brain tissue sections, such as hippocampus are stained with the patient's serum or CSF by indirect immunoperoxidase technique. (C) Shows CSF immunoreaction at the hippocampus level of the cytoplasmic and a neuronal surface in D (anti-human IgG-Px, Abcam-ab97225). (E) TBA in F, shown a reaction at neuronal surface level that colocalizes with GAD65 / 67 (Alexafluor 546, Invitrogen Molecular probes). (G) Immunoblot, CSF recognizes 100 and 50 Kd proteins(Anti-human IgG-Px, Abcam- ab97225).

Encephalitis associated with antibodies against GABAB1 receptor is generally presented as limbic encephalitis, as well as drug-refractory seizures. In a series of 15 patients, the mean age of presentation was 62 years (range 24–75) and both sexes were similarly affected. About half of the patients had an associated tumor, either a small cell lung carcinoma or a neuroendocrine lung tumor. These patients usually have antibodies to various non-neuronal proteins of uncertain significance, which suggests a susceptibility to autoimmunity [30].

In the knockout mice to the GABAB1 receptor, a variety of neurological and behavioral alterations are found, including spontaneous seizures, increased anxiety, hyperactivity, hyperalgesia and memory impairment, suggesting a dysfunction of the limbic system [31, 32].

In contrast, patients present with limbic encephalitis in conjunction with antibodies to the AMPAR were not present with seizures as frequently: only 3/10 had seizures as presenting feature with one other patient having seizures after a relapse [33].

Besides, anti-AMPA-GluR3B antibodies have been associated with many pathological effects: they activate glutamate, AMPA receptors, and are involved in the processes of "excitotoxicity." The phenomenon is associated with various pathological states of the CNS including: epilepsy, hypoxia/ischemia, and trauma. In animal and *in vitro* models, anti-NMDA-NR1 antibodies may be highly pathogenic, as they may cause a decrease in surface NMDA receptors expressed in hippocampal neurons, and also decrease the density and synaptic localization of receptors NMDA. The expression of these NR1a subunits correlates with the distribution of high-affinity NMDA receptors by agonists. Anti-NMDA-NR1 antibodies induces reduction in expression through cross-linking and internalization of NMDA receptors. Such changes may impair glutamate signaling through NMDA receptors and lead to various abnormal neuronal /behavioral/cognitive/psychiatric disorders.

Nevertheless, anti-AMPA-GluR3B antibodies induce many pathological effects that activate glutamate/AMPA receptors,which are involved in excitotoxic damage, the complement activation is modulated by regulatory proteins in which the activation plays a central role in the pathogenesis of brain damage and induces behavior and motor impairments. It has been observed in animal and *in vitro* models that anti-NMDA-NR1 antibodies can be highly pathogenic, as they may cause a decrease in surface NMDA receptors expressed in hippocampal neurons, and the density and synaptic localization of NMDA, probably by the internalization of receptors, which can impair glutamate signaling through NMDA receptors and lead to various neuronal/behavior/cognitive and psychiatric alterations. Knock-out mice to the GluR2 gene show reduced scanning and motor coordination. In these animals, the AMPA receptor-mediated synaptic transmission is reduced, but the long-term potentiation is better [34]. Knock-out mice to the GluR2 gene also exhibit increased cell death, possibly due to the excitotoxicity related to the greater insertion of the compensating homomeric GluR1 protein in AMPA receptors [35, 36].

4. Clinical features of epilepsy-associated autoimmune encephalitis

Each of the currently known neuronal cell surface or synaptic autoantibody associates with a specific syndrome or limited set off symptoms (**Table 1**). NMDAR antibody-associated encephalitis is a recently described disorder in which infrequent seizures are associated with the presence of autoantibodies directed against the extracellular domain of the NR1 subunit of the NMDAR. This disorder was first described as a clinical entity in 2005, in one in four young women who developed acute psychiatric symptoms, seizures, memory deficit, in association with the presence of an ovarian teratoma. In a study of 100 patients, it was shown that although the majority are young women (mean age 23 years), the disorder could occur in men and in children. This fact has allowed the number of pediatric cases to grow steadily and appears to represent approximately 40% of all cases [27, 37, 38].

4.1. NMDA receptor

Symptoms of anti-NMDA receptor encephalitis develop and resolve in a multi-stage process; most patients experience a prodromal similar to a viral picture, which is followed by a pattern

Epilepsy-associated antibody	Anti-LGI1 vs. LGI1 (*Channels Kv+*)	Anti-CASPR2 vs. CASPR2	LGI1 > CASPR2 (VGKC-complex) vs. LGI1 > CASPR2	NMDAR vs. Subunit NR1	GAD vs. GAD-65	$GABA_BR$ vs. $GABA_BR$	AMPA vs. GluR1/2
Gender/Age of involvement	M > F	M > F	M > F >50 years	F > M 70% childhood	F > M >20 years	M > F >40 years	F > M >40 years
Clinical manifestations	Hyponatremia. Cognitive impairment. It is associated with the presence of a thymoma or SCLC	Morvan syndrome Complication with Myasthenia gravis Not associated with neoplasias	TLE Hyponatremia and Synchronus dystonic arm posturing and grimacing facial ipsilateral associated with paraneoplasias (thymomas and lung cancer (SCLC)).	Viral pathway: fever, headache and fatigue of infectious etiology, delirium and disorientation. 10–20 days of evolution: orofacial dyskinesias, choreoatetotic movements, nystagmus, decreased consciousness and dysautonomia	Diabetes mellitus type 1, Stiff-person syndrome, cerebellar ataxia, non-paraneoplastic LE Severe cognitive impairment	LE It is associated with the presence of SCLC	LE It is associated with the presence of SCLC, thymus and breast cancer tumors
Psychiatric comorbidity	Confusion and behavior and REM sleep disorders	Cognitive impairment, memory loss and hallucinations	Sub-acute amnesia, confusion, sleep disorders, psychosis, anxiety, personality changes and depression	Personality changes, hallucinations (visual and auditory), difficulty speaking	Depression and anxiety.	Cognitive impairment, behavioral disorders such as psychosis and hallucinations	Confusion, amnesia, disorientation and psychosis
Seizure activity	GTC	GTC	FBDS GTC CPS	GTC CPS SE refractory to treatment	CPS. CTsG	CPS GTC SE	GTC CPS
Electrographic activity (EEG)	Slow focal or generalized activity	Slow focal or generalized activity	Slow focal or generalized activity	Focal or diffuse delta/theta activity and delta brush activity	Slow focal or generalized activity	Slow focal or generalized activity	Focal activity

Epilepsy-associated antibody	**Anti-LGI1 vs. LGI1 (*Channels Kv+*)**	**Anti-CASPR2 vs. CASPR2**	**LGI1 > CASPR2 (VGKC-complex) vs. LGI1 > CASPR2**	**NMDAR vs. Subunit NR1**	**GAD vs. GAD-65**	**$GABA_BR$ vs. $GABA_BR$**	**AMPA vs. GluR1/2**
Treatment and prognosis	Good response to immunotherapy	Good response to immunotherapy	Good response to immunotherapy	Slow response to Immunotherapy with recurrence	Refractory to treatment with AED's and immunotherapy	Good response to immunotherapy	Good response to immunotherapy with recurrence
References	[49, 54–56]	[31]	[31, 63]	[31, 55, 58, 65, 67]	[59–61]	[31, 41, 51, 57, 62, 64]	[34, 57, 61, 66]

NMDAR, N-methyl-D-aspartate receptor; LGI1, leucine-rich glioma-inactivated 1; CASPR2, contactin-associated protein-like 2; AMPAR, amino-3-hydroxy-5-hydroxy-5-methyl-4-isoxazolepropionic acid receptor; GABA a/B R, gamma-aminobutyric acid A/B receptor; mGluR1/2, metabotropic glutamate receptor type 1/2; LE, limbic encephalitis; SPS, stiff-person syndrome; CPS, complex partial seizure; EEG, electroencephalogram; FBDS , faciobrachial dystonic seizures; GTC, generalized tonic-clonic.

Table 1. Neuronal cell surface autoantibodies, associated epilepsy, and the clinical symptoms.

of memory alterations, behavior, cognition, developing psychotic pictures, convulsions, dyskinesia (orofacial, trunk, and limb), and autonomic respiratory instability. Most adults are initially seen by psychiatric services and may be confused with acute psychotic disturbance or drug abuse. Most children are taken to medical care due to changes in mood, behavior and/or personality, seizures, or language impairment [38–40]. Autonomic instability is a common manifestation in adults. Some patients develop severe cardiac arrhythmias that require the use of pacemakers. Signs of more frequent autonomic dysfunction in children include urinary incontinence and sleep disturbances [38]. Nuclear magnetic resonance (MRI) findings in these patients may be hyperintensities in FLAIR or T2 sequences in the cerebral cortex, cerebellar or temporal medial lobes, as well as in the corpus callosum and brainstem. In some cases, a transient increase in contrast, of the cerebral cortex, cerebellum, basal ganglia and meninges is observed.

Movement disorders are common and can be misinterpreted as a convulsive activity, the most common being dyskinesia, usually orofacial, choreoatetoid limb movements, rigidity, opisthotonos, or a combination of these. In most patients, EEG shows a slow generalized activity, disorganized without ictal discharges. These findings may overlap with ictal discharges in the EEG [41]. Niehusmann and colleagues [42] reported presence of NMDAR-antibodies in women (age range, 15–45 years), which had extra-temporal epilepsy, a reduction in level of consciousness and altered speech, as well as nystagmus, dyskinesia, dystonia, and hypoventilation. Clinical improvements in seizure frequency were seen in treatment of three patients treated with an immunomodulator such as corticosteroids and IVIg.

4.2. GABAb

GABA receptors are essential to inhibition. The presence of autoantibodies against these receptors has been associated with seizures and changes in memory and behavior. In a study with 15 patients with GABABR and LE antibodies (median age of 62 years, range 24–75 years), the clinical features where the presence of seizures, confusion and altering memory. Seizures were the predominant characteristic in 87%, and were mainly onset of temporal lobe with secondary generalization. 13% of patients presented epileptic status. CSF findings showed lymphocytic pleocytosis (n = 4) and MRI showed an increased signal, typical of LE. Clinical improvement was observed in 40% of patients who received IT alone and 20% who had IT, and 46% of patients were taken for a surgery to remove tumors. On the other hand, in a series of 15 patients, the mean age of presentation was 62 years (range 24–75) and both sexes were equally affected. About half of the patients had an associated tumor, either a small cell lung carcinoma or a neuroendocrine lung tumor. These patients often have additional antibodies to glutamic acid decarboxylase (anti-GAD) and several non-neuronal proteins of uncertain significance, suggesting a susceptibility to autoimmunity [32, 43].

4.3. AMPA receptor

Antibodies to the AMPAR have recently been described in patients with limbic encephalitis (LE). The AMPAR antibodies are the least frequent of these antibodies, however, also these patients develop a limbic dysfunction that may be associated with significant psychiatric symptoms. The most common disorder effects were in the middle-aged women. Most patients present with a sub-acute appearance of confusion, disorientation and memory loss, and seizures may also be part of the clinical describe. About 70% of patients have an underlying tumor in the lung, breast, or thymus. AMPAR is the predominant receptor subtype in the hippocampus, and it has been found that these antibodies in patients caused a decrease in the pre- and postsynaptic GluR1/2 receptor groups in cultures of rat hippocampal neurons. Since the receptor levels have been more affected at synapses than along dendrites, the findings suggested a mechanism by which patients' antibodies disrupted the receptor traffic, moving them from synaptic sites to extra-cellular sites and intracellular pool. These effects are similar to neuronal plasticity models that decrease synaptic strength, also called long-term depression. The effects of the antibodies were shown to be reversible [42, 45].

4.4. GAD

Glutamic acid decarboxylase (GAD) is a cytoplasmic enzyme that catalyzes the conversion of L-glutamic acid to gamma-aminobutyric acid (GABA), considered the main inhibitory neurotransmitter of the central nervous system. GAD is expressed primarily in GABAergic neurons and in pancreatic β cells, and has two isoforms with different molecular weight; GAD65 and GAD67. GAD antibodies act as a marker of the underlying autoimmune disease, although it is not known how antibodies against an intracellular enzyme can directly initiate pathological events; however, it is known that anti-GAD Abs inhibit the activity of GAD, and the synthesis of GABA antibodies to GAD is associated with several autoimmune disorders, including limbic encephalitis [44, 45], type 1 diabetes mellitus [46]. Stiff Person Syndrome (SPS) [47], and cerebellar ataxia [48], as well as overlapping syndromes. Recent work highlighting the response of these patients to immunotherapy and association with forms of epilepsy related to localization suggest that antibodies may also be present with specific cell surface. This is supported by a functional study of magnetic resonance spectroscopy in patients with TLE and elevated levels of serum GAD antibodies that demonstrated significantly lower GABA levels within their cortex compared to paired control patients [44]. On the other hand, in one study with 138 patients over 18 years old, investigated with recent onset epilepsy, were prospectively studied to determine the clinical and radiological characteristics of LE, and response to treatment. Fifty-three adult patients fulfilled the criteria for LE; nine had high-titer GAD antibodies and ten had voltage-controlled potassium channel (VGKC) antibodies. Patients with GAD antibodies were younger's (range, 17–66 years) and had seizures only, whereas polymorphic limbic features were more frequent in the VGKC positive group. Patients with anti-GAD antibodies had more frequently oligoclonal bands of cerebrospinal fluid and intrathecal secretion of the specific antibody. Which after monthly, patients were treated with intravenous methylprednisolone pulses, however GAD antibodies remained elevated in 6/6 patients, however VGKC antibodies normalized in 6/9 patients ($p < 0.03$). Despite the more intense anticonvulsant treatment in the group with anti-GAD antibodies ($p < 0.01$), none of these patients were seizure free, unlike all patients with VGKC antibodies ($p < 0.001$). High-titer GAD antibodies define a form of non-paraneoplasic LE. It is a chronic non-persistent disorder, and should be included in the differential diagnosis of patients with LE and mediotemporal encephalitis [49].

4.5. LGI

Studies describing treatment of LGI1-antibody associated encephalopathy, LGI1 is a protein secreted by neurons that interact with pre- and postsynaptic receptors. LGI1 mutations have been associated with autosomal dominant temporal lobe epilepsy syndrome [50, 51]. Patients with antibodies against LGI1 develop alterations of memory, confusion, and seizures. The MRI results are typical of limbic encephalitis. Memory and cognitive deficits can be preceded by brief tonic seizures that can be confused for mimic myoclonic movements. Observational studies have provided evidence of a marked improvement with for high-dose steroids, IVIG and PLEX for patients with auto-antibodies to LGI1 and CASPR [37, 50–52]. In a retrospective study of 10 patients with high titers of VGKC-complex antibodies that had seizures and memory disorders, who received IVIG 2 g/kg/day, 100 mg prednisolone on alternate days and PLEX for 5 days, improvement was observed in frequency of seizures and cognition in six patients within 2 weeks to 12 months, correlating with reductions in antibody titers [37]. Earlier treatment, and possibly corticosteroids, appeared to provide greater benefits than before. This disorder had been included previously within the spectrum of antibodies against voltage-dependent potassium channels. Some patients develop hyponatremia and behavior or REM sleep disorders. Only 20% of cases are associated with a neoplasm, usually thymoma or small cell lung carcinoma.

5. Diagnostic approach

The laboratory diagnosis of AD depends on the identification of the clinical symptoms of the patient, their association with each disease and their correspondence with the detection of AA. For this reason, laboratory tests are of great importance for the evaluation of patients when an AE is suspected. The results can confirm the diagnosis, estimate the severity of the disease, and are useful to follow up its evolution and establish a prognosis. The presence of autoantibodies (AA) alone in a patient does not mean the diagnosis of an AD, the associated signs and symptoms help to achieve the definitive diagnosis and are of crucial importance. Analysis of CSF plays a central part in all diagnostic criteria for encephalitis, including infectious encephalitis, relevant antibodies might be found only in the CSF, because the repertoire of antibodies in the CSF and serum can be different in the same patient (e.g., NMDA receptor in CSF and serum) [52]. By other way, serological tests to detect AA have demonstrated the presence of AA in healthy individuals and in known non-EA patients and approximately half of all autoimmune encephalitis series are Ab-negative cases, so AA is a confirmatory diagnostic test, for this reason the diagnostic tests must be combined. Three basic research techniques are used for this purpose must include: tissue-based assay (TBA), cell-based assay (CBA), and immune-precipitation (IP; in-house). In the TBA, rat or mouse brains are stained with CSF or serum of patients with an indirect immunohistochemistry or immunofluorescence technique or the combination of two fluorophores, one that identifies the autoantibody and the other to the antigen and use of confocal microscopy (**Figure 1(C)–(F)**).

In the cell brain adhesion test (CBA), cells (e.g., HEK293 cells) are transfected with the respective neural antigens (receptors, channels, etc.) and incubated with the CSF or serum of patients with an indirect immunofluorescence technique. Autoantibodies to the specifically expressed receptor result in the cell membrane marking cells, similar, primary cultures of hippocampal neurons can be used, with these methods autoantibodies are displayed on the surface of the neuronal membrane [53].

For the detection of classical intracellular and cytoplasmic antibodies, the immunoblot technique is used. Immunoblotting is the method that uses Abs to detect a specific protein from a mixture of several unrelated proteins separated by molecular weight. The diagnosis of antibodies with this technique involves several steps, including protein extraction of mice brain tissue followed by (30–50 μg) spitted proteins through electrophoresis, and transfer of a nitrocellulose membrane and overlapping of the primary antibody (the serum or CSF of the patient) and secondary on the membrane labeled with enzymes (**Figure 1(G)**) or fluorescent antibodies [54]. Recently, we introduced flow cytometry and have confirmed that in those patients with AE, a large presence of activated T and B cells is observed; in some cases, the CD8+ cells are dominated and in negative cases, there is no activation of lymphocytes (unpublished data); the results suggest that this tool could provide additional information on the patient's immune response (**Figure 1(B)**). On the basis of this data, the recommendation is to include both CSF and serum for citometric testing in patients with suspected autoimmune encephalitis.

6. Concluding remarks

Recently, several reports that associate CNS disorders with autoantibodies are directed against cell surface proteins, which are likely to be pathogens. Many of these conditions have seizures as an early and prominent feature, which are commonly refractory to conventional drugs. In contrast, a good response with immunotherapy is often observed. The studies in patients coincide in clinical manifestations, but not in autoantibodies. For this reason, CSF is crucial in the identification of new antigens, including NMDAR, AMPAR, GABABR, GABAARr, mGluR5, DPPX and LGI1, and Caspr2. Serum negativity is more likely with a milder form of the disease, presenting with clinical pictures of psychosis but not requiring intensive care, particularly if the antibodies are generated predominantly in the brain, which makes it necessary to standardize the diagnostic methods in order to be safer and to offer a timely diagnosis. The effects of antibodies on children (the effects of antibodies on hippocampal synapses) are different from that of adults; this may explain some of the differences in clinical pictures between adults and children. For this reason, the selection of patients for the autoimmune evaluation requires a high level of suspicion in the initial consultation. Since there have been currently no universally agreement upon diagnostic criteria for autoimmune epilepsies, the clinical evidence, such as the high frequency of seizures, psychiatric co-morbidity and resistance to AEDs, are important indicators to decide it. More studies are needed to identify early autoantibodies and to perform preventive treatments.

Author details

Sandra Orozco-Suarez[1]*, Angélica Vega-Garcia[1,2], Iris Feria-Romero[1], Lourdes Arriaga-Pizano[3], Emmanuel Rodriguez-Chavez[4] and Israel Grijalva[1]

*Address all correspondence to: sorozco5@hotmail.com

1 Unidad de Investigación Médica en Enfermedades Neurológicas, Hospital de Especialidades "Dr. Bernardo Sepúlveda", Centro Médico Nacional Siglo XXI, Instituto Mexicano del Seguro Social, Mexico City, Mexico

2 Universidad Autónoma Metropolitana (UAM), Mexico City, Mexico

3 Unidad de Investigación Médica en Inmunología, Hospital de Especialidades "Dr. Bernardo Sepúlveda", Centro Médico Nacional Siglo XXI, Instituto Mexicano del Seguro Social, Mexico City, Mexico

4 Servicio de Neurología, Hospital de Especialidades "Dr. Antonio Fraga Mouret", Centro Médico Nacional, La Raza, Instituto Mexicano del Seguro Social, Mexico City, Mexico

References

[1] Fisher RS, Boas WVE, Blume W, Elge C, Genton P, Lee P, Engel J Jr. Epileptic seizures and epilepsy: Definitions proposed by the International League Against Epilepsy (ILAE) and the International Bureau for Epilepsy (IBE). Epilepsia. 2005;**46**:470-472. DOI: 10.1111/j.0013-9580.2005. 66104.x

[2] Rogers SW, Andrews PI, Gahring LC, Whisenand T, Cauley K, Crain B, Hughes TE, Heinemann SF, McNamara JO. Autoantibodies to glutamate receptor GluR3 in Rasmussen's encephalitis. Science. 1994;**265**(5172):648-651

[3] Bien CG, Urbach H, Schramm J, Soeder BM, Becker AJ, Voltz R, Vincent A, Elger CE. Limbic encephalitis as a precipitating event in adult-onset temporal lobe epilepsy. Neurology. 2007;**69**(12):1236-1244. DOI: 10.1212/01.wnl.0000276946.08412.ef

[4] Brenner T, Sills GJ, Hart Y, Howell S, Waters P, Brodie MJ, Vincent A, Lang B. Prevalence of neurologic autoantibodies in cohorts of patients with new and established epilepsy. Epilepsia. 2013;**54**(6):1028-1035. DOI: 10.1111/epi.12127

[5] Adams DD, Knight JG, Ebringer A. Autoimmune diseases: Solution of the environmental, immunological and genetic components with principles for immunotherapy and transplantation. Autoimmunity Reviews. 2010;**9**(8):525-530. DOI: 10.1016/j.autrev.2009.12.012

[6] Ermann J, Fathman CG. Autoimmune diseases: Genes, bugs and failed regulation. Nature Immunology. 2001;**2**(9):759-761. DOI: 10.1038/ni0901-759

[7] Torres Odio S, Martínez Córdova Z. Genetic, immunological and environmental factors associated with autoimmunity. Revista Cubana de Investigaciones Biomedicas. 2011;**30**(4):501-510

[8] Undlien DE, Lie BA, Thorsby E. HLA complex genes in type 1 diabetes and other autoimmune diseases. Which genes are involved?. Trends in Genetics. 2001;**17**(2):93-100. DOI: http://dx.doi.org/10.1016/S0168-9525(00)02180-6

[9] Arnold B. Levels of peripheral T cell tolerance. Transplantation Immunology. 2002; **10**(2-3):109-114. DOI: 10.1001/archneurol.2010.317

[10] Thorsby E, Lie BA. HLA associated genetic predisposition to autoimmune diseases: Genes involved and possible mechanisms. Transplantation Immunology. 2005;**14** (3-4):175-182. DOI: 10.1016/j.trim.2005.03.021

[11] Lie BA, Thorsby E. Several genes in the extended human MHC contribute to predisposition to autoimmune diseases. Current Opinion in Immunology. 2005;**17**(5):526-531. DOI: 10.1016/j.coi.2005.07.001

[12] Cassinotti A, Birindelli S, Clerici M, Trabattoni D, Lazzaroni M, Ardizzone S, Colombo R, Rossi E, Porro GB. HLA and autoimmune digestive disease: A clinically oriented review for gastroenterologists. Am J Gastroenterol. 2009;**104**(1):195-217; quiz 194, 218. DOI: 10.1038/ajg.2008.10.

[13] Shin YW, Lee ST, Shin JW, Moon J, Lim JA, Byun JI. VGKC-complex/LGI1-antibody encephalitis: Clinical manifestations and response to immunotherapy. Journal of Neuroimmunology. 2013;**265**(1-2):75-81. DOI: 10.1016/j.jneuroim.2013.10.005

[14] Caillat-Zucman S. Molecular mechanisms of HLA association with autoimmune diseases. Tissue Antigens. 2008;**73**:1-8. DOI: 10.1111/j.1399-0039.2008. 01167.x

[15] Waldner H. The role of innate immune responses in autoimmune disease development. Autoimmunity Reviews. 2009;**8**:400-404. DOI: 10.1016/j.autrev.2008.12.019

[16] Dandekar S, Wijesuriya H, Geiger T, Hamm D, Mathern GW, Owens GC, Shared HLA, Class I, Alleles II. Clonally restricted public and private brain-infiltrating αβ T cells in a cohort of Rasmussen encephalitis surgery patients. Frontiers in Immunology. 2016;**7**:608. DOI: 10.3389/fimmu.2016.00608. eCollection 2016

[17] Kim TJ, Lee ST, Moon J, Sunwoo JS, Byun JI, Lim JA, Shin YW, Jun JS, Lee HS, Lee WJ, Yang AR, Choi Y, Park KI, Jung KH, Jung KY, Kim M, Lee SK, Chu K. Anti-LGI1 encephalitis is associated with unique HLA subtypes. Annals of Neurology. 2017;**81**(2):183-192. DOI: 10.1002/ana.24860

[18] Doria A, Sarzi-Puttini P, Shoenfeld Y. Infections, rheumatism and autoimmunity: The connecting relationship between humans and their environment. Autoimmunity Reviews. 2008;**8**(1):1-4. DOI: 10.1016/j.autrev.2008.07.014

[19] Ryan KR, Patel SD, Stephens LA, Anderton SM. Death, adaptation and regulation: The three pillars of immune tolerance restrict the risk of autoimmune disease caused by molecular mimicry. Journal of Autoimmunity. 2007;**29**(4):262-271. DOI: 10.1016/j.jaut.2007.07.014

[20] Proal AD, Albert PJ, Marshall T. Autoimmune disease in the era of themetagenome. Autoimmunity Reviews. 2009;**8**(8):677-681. DOI: 10.1016/j.autrev.2009.02.016

[21] Lai M, Huijbers MG, Lancaster E, Graus F, Bataller L, Balice-Gordon R, Cowell JK, Dalmau J. Investigation of LGI1 as the antigen in limbic encephalitis previously attributed to potassium channels: A case series. Lancet Neurology. 2010;**9**(8):776-785

[22] Hansen KB, Ogden KK, Yuan H, Traynelis SF. Distinct functional and pharmacological properties of Triheteromeric GluN1/GluN2A/GluN2B NMDA receptors. Neuron. 2014;**81**(5):1084-1096. DOI: 10.1002/ana.10280

[23] Dingledine R, Borges K, Bowie D, Traynelis SF. The glutamate receptor ion channels. Pharmacological Reviews. 1999;**51**(1):7-61

[24] Cull-Candy SG, Leszkiewicz DN. Role of distinct NMDA receptor subtypes at central synapses. Science's STKE. 2004;**255**:re16. DOI: 10.1126/stke.2552004re16

[25] Karakas E, Simorowski N, Furukawa H. Structure of the zinc-bound amino-terminal domain of the NMDA receptor NR2B subunit. The EMBO Journal. 2009;**28**(24):3910-3920. DOI: 10.1038/emboj.2009.338

[26] Coyle JT. Glutamate and schizophrenia: Beyond the dopamine hypothesis. Cellular and Molecular Neurobiology. 2006;**26**(4-6):365-384. DOI: 10.1007/s10571-006-9062-8

[27] Dalmau J, Gleichman AJ, Hughes EG, Rossi JE, Peng X, Lai M, Dessain SK, Rosenfeld MR, Balice-Gordon R, Lynch DR. Anti-NMDA-receptor encephalitis: Case series and analysis of the effects of antibodies. Lancet Neurology. 2008;**7**(12):1091-1098. DOI: 10.1016/S14744422(08)70224-2

[28] Gleichman E, Spruce L, Dalmau J, Seeholzer S, Lynch D. Anti-NMDA receptor encephalitis antibody binding is dependent on amino acid identity of a small region within the GluN1 amino terminal domain. The Journal of Neuroscience. 2012;**32**(32):11082-11094. DOI: 10.1523/JNEUROSCI.0064-12.2012

[29] Gresa-Arribas NJ, Torrents A, Aguilar E, McCracken L, Leypoldt F, Gleichman AJ, Balice-Gordon R, Rosenfeld MR, Lynch D, Graus F, Dalmau J. Antibody titres at diagnosis and during follow-up of anti-NMDA receptor encephalitis: A retrospective study. Lancet Neurology. 2014;**13**(2):167-177. DOI: 10.1016/S1474-4422(13)70282-5

[30] Moscato EH, Peng X, Jain A, Parsons TD, Dalmau J, Balice-Gordon RJ. Acute mechanisms underlying antibody effects in anti-N-methyl-D-aspartate receptor encephalitis. Annals of Neurology. 2014;**76**(1):108-119. DOI: 10.1002/ana.24195

[31] Mikasova L, De Rossi P, Bouchet D, Georges F, Rogemond V, Didelot A, Meissirel C, Honnorat J, Groc L. Disrupted surface cross-talk between NMDA and Ephrin-B2 receptors in anti-NMDA encephalitis. Brain. 2012;**135**(Pt 5):1606-1621. DOI: 10.1093/brain/aws092

[32] Lancaster E, Lai M, Peng X, Hughes E, Constantinescu R, Raizer J, Friedman D, Skeen MB, Grisold W, Kimura A, Ohta K, Iizuka T, Guzman M, Graus F, Moss SJ, Balice-Gordon R, Dalmau J. Antibodies to the GABA(B) receptor in limbic encephalitis with seizures:

Case series and characterisation of the antigen. Lancet Neurology. 2010;**9**(1):67-76. DOI: 10.1016/S1474-4422(09)70324-2

[33] Reisel D, Bannerman DM, Schmitt WB, Deacon RM, Flint J, Borchardt T, Seeburg PH, Rawlins JN. Spatial memory dissociations in mice lacking GluR1. Nature Neuroscience. 2002;**5**(9):868-873. DOI: 10.1038/nn910

[34] Sanderson DJ, Gray A, Simon A, Taylor AM, Deacon RM, Seeburg PH, Sprengel R, Good MA, Rawlins JN, Bannerman DM. Deletion of glutamate receptor-a (GluR-A) AMPA receptor subunits impairs one-trial spatial memory. Behavioral Neuroscience. 2007;**121**(3):559-569. DOI: 10.1037/0735-7044.121.3.559

[35] Lai M, Hughes EG, Peng X, Zhou L, Gleichman AJ, Shu H, Matà S, Kremens D, Vitaliani R, Geschwind MD, Bataller L, Kalb RG, Davis R, Graus F, Lynch DR, Balice-Gordon R, Dalmau J. AMPA receptor antibodies in limbic encephalitis alter synaptic receptor location. Annals of Neurology. 2009;**65**(4):424-434. DOI: 10.1002/ana.21589

[36] Oguro K, Oguro N, Kojima T, Grooms SY, Calderone A, Zheng X, Bennett MV, Zukin RS. Knockdown of AMPA receptor GluR2 expression causes delayed neurodegeneration and increases damage by sublethal ischemia in hippocampal CA1 and CA3 neurons. The Journal of Neuroscience. 1999;**19**(21):9218-9227

[37] Feldmeyer D, Kask K, Brusa R, Kornau HC, Kolhekar R, Rozov A, Burnashev N, Jensen V, Hvalby O, Sprengel R, Seeburg PH. Neurological dysfunctions in mice expressing different levels of the Q/R site-unedited AMPAR subunit GluR-B. Nature Neuroscience. 1999;**2**(1):57-64

[38] Vitaliani R, Mason W, Ances B, Zwerdling T, Jiang Z, Dalmau J. Paraneoplastic encephalitis, psychiatric symptoms, and hypoventilation in ovarian teratoma. Annals of Neurology. 2005;**58**(4):594-604. DOI: 10.1002/ana.20614

[39] Florance NR, Davis RL, Lam C, Szperka C, Zhou L, Ahmad S, Campen CJ, Moss H, Peter N, Gleichman AJ, Glaser CA, Lynch DR, Rosenfeld MR, Dalmau J. Anti-N-methyl-D-aspartate receptor (NMDAR) encephalitis in children and adolescents. Annals of Neurology. 2009;**66**(1):11-18. DOI: 10.1002/ana.21756

[40] Lizuka T, Sakai F, Ide T, Monzen T, Yoshii S, Iigaya M, Suzuki K, Lynch DR, Suzuki N, Hata T, Dalmau J. Anti-NMDA receptor encephalitis in Japan: Long-term outcome without tumor removal. Neurology. 2008;**70**(7):504-511. DOI: 10.1212/01.wnl.0000278388.90370.c3

[41] Wandinger KP, Saschenbrecker S, Stoecker W, Dalmau J. Anti-NMDAreceptor encephalitis: A severe, multistage, treatable disorder presenting with psychosis. Journal of Neuroimmunology. 2011;**231**(1-2):86-91. DOI: 10.1016/j.jneuroim.2010.09.012

[42] Niehusmann P, Dalmau J, Rudlowski C, Vincent A, Elger CE, Rossi JE, Bien CG. Diagnostic value of N-methyl-D-aspartate receptor antibodies in women with new-onset. Archives of Neurology. 2009;**66**(4):458-464. DOI: 10.1001/archneurol.2009.5

[43] Boronat A, Sabater L, Saiz A, Dalmau J, Graus F. GABA(B) receptor antibodies in limbic encephalitis and anti-GAD-associated neurologic disorders. Neurology. 2011;**76**(9):795-800. DOI: 10.1212/WNL.0b013e31820e7b8d

[44] Bataller L, Galiano R, García-Escrig M, Martínez B, Sevilla T, Blasco R, Vílchez JJ, Dalmau J. Reversible paraneoplastic limbic encephalitis associated with antibodies to the AMPA receptor. Neurology. 2010;**74**(3):265-267. DOI: 10.1146/annurev.immunol.18.1.767

[45] Mitoma H, Adhikari K, Aeschlimann D, Chattopadhyay P, Hadjivassiliou M, Hampe CS, Honnorat J, Joubert B, Kakei S, Lee J, Manto M, Matsunaga A, Mizusawa H, Nanri K, Shanmugarajah P, Yoneda M, Yuki N. Consensus paper: Neuroimmune mechanisms of cerebellar ataxias. Cerebellum. 2016;**15**(2):213-232. https://doi.org/10.1007/s12311-015-0664-x

[46] Stagg CJ, Lang B, Best JG, McKnight K, Cavey A, Johansen-Berg H, Vincent A, Palace J. Autoantibodies to glutamate acid decarboxylase in epilepsy patients are associated with a low cortical GABA levels. Epilepsia. 2010;**51**(9):1898-1901. DOI: 10.1111/j.1528-1167.2010.02644.x

[47] Saiz A, Blanco Y, Sabater L, Gonzalez F, Bataller L, Casamitjana R, Ramió-Torrentà L, Graus F. Spectrum of neurological syndromes associated with glutamic acid decarboxylase antibodies: Diagnostic clues for this association. Brain. 2008;**131**(Pt 10):2553-2563. DOI: 10.1093/brain/awn183

[48] Solimena M, Folli F, Aparisi R, Pozza G, De Camilli P. Autoantibodies to GABA-ergic neurons and pancreatic beta cells in stiff-man syndrome. The New England Journal of Medicine. 1990;**322**(22):1555-1560

[49] Honnorat J, Saiz A, Giometto B, Vincent A, Brieva L, de Andres C, Maestre J, Fabien N, Vighetto A, Casamitjana R, Thivolet C, Tavolato B, Antoine J, Trouillas P, Graus F. Cerebellar ataxia with anti-glutamic acid decarboxylase antibodies: Study of 14 patients. Archives of Neurology 2001;**58**(2):225-230. DOI: 10.1001/archneur.58.2.225

[50] Malter MP, Helmstaedter C, Urbach H, Vincent A, Bien CG. Antibodies to glutamic acid decarboxylase define a form of limbic encephalitis. Annals of Neurology. 2010;**67**(4):470-478. DOI: 10.1002/ana.21917

[51] Bien CG, Vincent A, Barnett MH, Becker AJ, Blümcke I, Graus F, Jellinger KA, Reuss DE, Ribalta T, Schlegel J, Sutton I, Lassmann H, Bauer J. Immunopathology of autoantibody-associated encephalitis : Clues for pathogenesis. Brain. 2012;**135**(Pt 5):1622-1638. DOI: 10.1093/brain/aws082

[52] Andrade DM, Tai P, Dalmau J, Wennberg R. Tonic seizures: A diagnostic clue of anti-LGI1 encephalitis? Neurology. 2011;**76**(15):1355-1357. DOI: 10.1212/WNL.0b013e3182152808

[53] Graus F, Titulaer MJ, Balu R, Benseler S, Bien CG, Cellucci T, Cortese I, Dale RC, Gelfand JM, Geschwind M, Glaser CA, Honnorat J, Höftberger R, Iizuka T, Irani SR, Lancaster E, Leypoldt F, Prüss H, Rae-Grant A, Reindl M, Rosenfeld MR, Rostásy K, Saiz A, Venkatesan A, Vincent A, Wandinger KP, Wate P, Dalmau J. A clinical approach to diagnosis of autoimmune encephalitis. Lancet Neurology. 2016;**15**(4):391-404. DOI: 10.1016/S1474-4422(15)00401-9

[54] Irani SR, Alexander S, Waters P, Kleopa KA, Pettingill P, Zuliani L, Peles E, Buckley C, Lang B, Vincent A. Antibodies to Kv1 potassium channel-complex proteins leucine-rich, glioma inactivated 1 protein and contactin-associated protein-2 in limbic encephalitis,

Morvan's syndrome and acquired neuromyotonia. Brain. 2010;**133**(9):2734-2748. DOI: 10.1093/brain/awq213

[55] Höftberger R, van Sonderen A, Leypoldt F, Houghton D, Geschwind M, Gelfand J. Encephalitis and AMPA receptor antibodies: Novel findings in a case series of 22 patients. Neurology. 2015;**84**(24):2403-2412. DOI: 10.1212/WNL.0000000000001682

[56] Lee SK, Lee ST. The laboratory diagnosis of autoimmune encephalitis. Journal of Epilepsy Research. 2016;**6**(2):45-50. DOI: 10.14581/jer.16010. eCollection 2016

[57] Gu W, Brodtkorb E, Steinlein OK. LGI1 is mutated in familial temporal lobe epilepsy characterized by aphasic seizures. Annals of Neurology. 2002;**52**(3):364-367. DOI: 10. 1002/ana.10280

[58] Kalachikov S, Evgrafov O, Ross B, Winawer M, Barker-Cummings C, Martinelli Boneschi F, Choi C, Morozov P, Das K, Teplitskaya E, Yu A, Cayanis E, Penchaszadeh G, Kottmann AH, Pedley TA, Hauser WA, Ottman R, Gilliam TC. Mutations in LGI1 cause autosomal-dominant partial epilepsy with auditory features. Nature Genetics. 2002;**30**(3):335-341. DOI: 10.1038/ng832

[59] Lim JA, Lee ST, Jung KH, Kim S, Shin JW, Moon J, Byun JI, Kim TJ, Shin YW, Lee KJ, Kim YS, Park KI, Lee SK, Chu K. Anti-N-methyl-D-aspartate receptor encephalitis in Korea: Clinical features, treatment, and outcome. Journal of Clinical Neurology. 2014;**10**(2):157-161. DOI: 10.3988/jcn.10.2.157

[60] Suleiman J, Brenner T, Gill D, Brilot F, Antony J, Vincent A, Lang B, Dale RC. VGKC antibodies in pediatric encephalitis presenting with status epilepticus. 2011;**76**(14):1252-1255. DOI: 10.1212/WNL.0b013e3182143552

[61] Dogan Onugoren M, Deuretzbacher D, Haensch CA, Hagedorn HJ, Halve S, Isenmann S, Kramme C, Lohner H, Melzer N, Monotti R, Presslauer S, Schäbitz WR, Steffanoni S, Stoeck K, Strittmatter M, Stögbauer F, Trinka E, von Oertzen TJ, Wiendl H, Woermann FG, Bien CG. Limbic encephalitis due to GABAB and AMPA receptor antibodies: A case series. Journal of Neurology, Neurosurgery, and Psychiatry. 2015;**86**(9):965-972. DOI: 10.1136/jnnp-2014-308814

[62] Viaccoz A, Desestret V, Ducray F, Picard G, Cavillon G, Rogemond V, Antoine JC, Delattre JY, Honnorat J. Clinical specificities of adult male patients with NMDA receptor antibodies encephalitis. Neurology. 2014;**82**(7):556-563. DOI: 10.1212/ WNL.0000000000000126

[63] Malter MP, Frisch C, Schoene-Bake JC, Helmstaedter C, Wandinger KP, Stoecker W, Urbach H, Surges R, Elger CE, Vincent AV, Bien CG. Outcome of limbic encephalitis with VGKC complex antibodies: Relation to antigenic specificity. Journal of Neurology. 2014;**261**(9):1695-1705. DOI: 10.1007/s00415-014-7408-6

[64] Lilleker JB, Jones MS, Mohanraj R. GKC complex antibodies in epilepsy: Diagnostic yield and therapeutic implications. Seizure. 2013;**22**(9):776-779. DOI: 10.1016/j.seizure. 2013.06.004

[65] Haberlandt E, Bast T, Ebner A, Holthausen H, Kluger G, Kravljanac R, Kröll-Seger J, Kurlemann G, Makowski C, Rostasy K, Tuschen-Hofstätter E, Weber G, Vincent A, Bien CG. Limbic encephalitis in children and adolescents. Archives of Disease in Childhood. 2010;**96**(2):186-191. DOI: 10.1136/adc.2010.183897

[66] Höftberger R, Titulaer MJ, Sabater L, Dome B, Rózsás A, Hegedus B, Hoda MA, Laszlo V, Ankersmit HJ, Harms L, Boyero S, de Felipe A, Saiz A, Dalmau J, Graus F. Encephalitis and GABAB receptor antibodies: Novel findings in a new case series of 20 patients. Neurology. 2013;**81**(17):1500-1506. DOI: 10.1212/WNL.0b013e3182a9585f

[67] Joubert B, Kerschen P, Zekeridou A, Desestret V, Rogemond V, Chaffois MO, Ducray F, Larrue V, Daubail B, Idbaih A, Psimaras D, Antoine JC, Delattre JY, Honnorat J. Clinical spectrum of encephalitis associated with antibodies against the α-amino-3-hidroxy-5-methyl-4-isoxazolepropionic acid receptor: Case series and review of the literature. JAMA Neurology. 2015;**72**(10):1163-1169. DOI: 10.1001/jamaneurol.2015.1715

6

Epilepsy as a Pyridoxine-Dependent Condition: Quantitative Urinary Biomarkers of Epilepsy-Family Disorders of Pyridoxine Metabolism

Svetlana A. Dolina

Abstract

The affected pyridoxine metabolism is discussed as an inborn genetic sign of epilepsy. In children with different forms of epilepsy and matched healthy controls, the urinary parameters of pyridoxal phosphate–dependent tryptophan degradation were measured by high-performance liquid chromatography (HPLC) method with simultaneous ultraviolet and fluorimetric detection. Concentrations of compounds, which are formed in the course of tryptophan degradation, and correlations between them turned out to be quantitative biomarkers useful for evaluation of patient's condition and monitoring individualized antiepileptic treatment. Accumulation of tryptophan, kynurenine, and neurotoxic 3-hydroxykynurenine, along with reduced kynureninase activity, is characteristic of epileptic patients. Growing progressively worse, epilepsy is accompanied by aggravation of pyridoxal phosphate–dependent disturbances of tryptophan metabolism and further inhibition of kynureninase.

In asymptomatic first-degree relatives of epileptic probands, disorders of pyridoxine metabolism are of the same (or even higher) extent as in probands. Long-term pyridoxine treatment (7–10 mg/kg daily) is suggested as safe and effective protective replacement therapy. The protocols of this study have been approved by the ethics committee of Kaplan Hospital (Israel).

Keywords: epilepsy, epileptic families, tryptophan metabolism, vitamin B6 (pyridoxine)-dependent enzymes

1. Quantitative urinary biomarkers for evaluation of patient's state and monitoring antiepileptic treatment

1.1. Introduction

Sixty years ago Hunt et al. [1] described pyridoxine-dependent epilepsy (PDE), which until now is considered as a rare (1:100.000) autosomal recessive genetic disorder, occurring in the uterus, or later in infancy, or early childhood. Most often seizures are observed within the first month of life, even within hours of birth. In atypical (late-onset) PDE seizures start later (up to 2 years). After the first year of life autistic features are often revealed. The resistance to conventional antiepileptic drugs (AEDs) and response to vitamin B6 administration (5–10 mg/kg/day) are accepted as the main characteristic features of PDE [2–5].

Vitamin B6 consists of six different vitamers: pyridoxine (PN), pyridoxal (PL), pyridoxamine (PM), and their phosphate-esterified forms. Pyridoxal phosphate (PLP) is the active B6 vitamer, which is produced from its precursor vitamers (PN, PM, and PL) by phosphorylation and oxidation (PN phosphate, PLP, and PM phosphate) through the actions of pyridoxal kinase and pyridox(am)ine oxidase (PNPO), respectively (**Figure 1**) [6]. Vitamin B6 is broken down to pyridoxic acid (4PA), which is excreted in the urine.

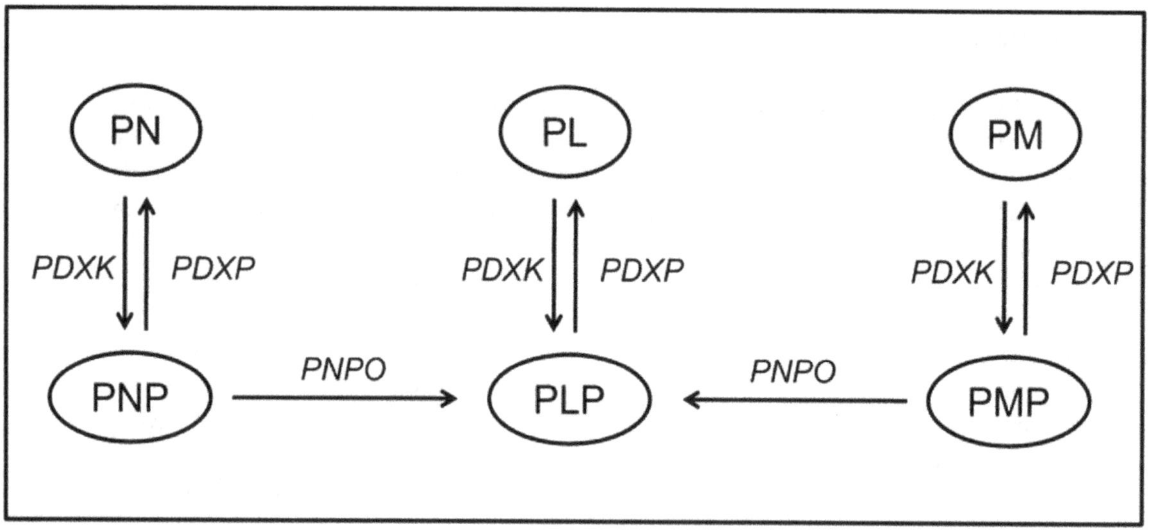

Figure 1. Human vitamin B6 metabolism. PDXK, pyridoxal kinase; PDXR, vitamin B6-specific phosphatase; PNPO, pyridox(am)ine phosphate oxidase.

PLP is a cofactor for numerous enzymatic reactions in the central nervous system (CNS). An inborn abnormality of PLP-dependent GABA synthesis induced by glutamate decarboxylase (GAD) deficiency earlier was postulated as a cause of epilepsy, and lifelong pyridoxine administration was recommended. Later on in the search for the PDE-responsible gene, the primary involvement of the GAD 1 gene on chromosome 2q31 and the GAD 2 on 10p23 was discussed and excluded [7, 8].

At present, PDE is considered as a result of mutations in the ALDH7A1 gene, encoding antiquitin. Antiquitin deficiency in the lysine degradation pathway leads to the accumulation of piperidein-6-carboxylic acid, which inactivates PLP [9, 10]. Recently, several cases of other inborn errors of vitamin B6 metabolism, that is, pyridox(am)ine 5-phospate oxidase deficiency and type 2 hyperprolinemia, have also been described. So, the accumulated data have shown that autosomal recessive pyridoxine-dependent seizures are genetically heterogeneous [11–13].

Nevertheless, neither data accumulation, nor recommendations for pyridoxine administration in early cases of intractable epilepsy [3, 14, 15], or pyridoxine applicability as the first-line drug for infantile spasms [16–19] have changed conventional perception of the strictly limited role of pyridoxine in the pathogenesis of *epilepsy as a whole*.

Meanwhile, disturbances in the metabolism of glutamate, GABA, tryptophan (TRP), serotonin, taurine, dopamine, and norepinephrine, which are synthesized and/or metabolized by PLP-dependent enzymes [20–32], have been repeatedly found in epileptic patients. The increased levels of excitatory amino acids—glutamate, aspartate, and glycine [21–27] along with the reduced levels of inhibitory amino acids and amines—GABA, serotonin, and taurine [28–32] were detected in the plasma, cerebrospinal fluid (CSF), and epileptogenic foci of patients with different forms of epilepsy. Moreover, a moderate increase in the activity of glutamic acid dehydrogenase, the glutamate-synthesizing enzyme, which is specifically inhibited by PLP, has been found in epileptic foci [33].

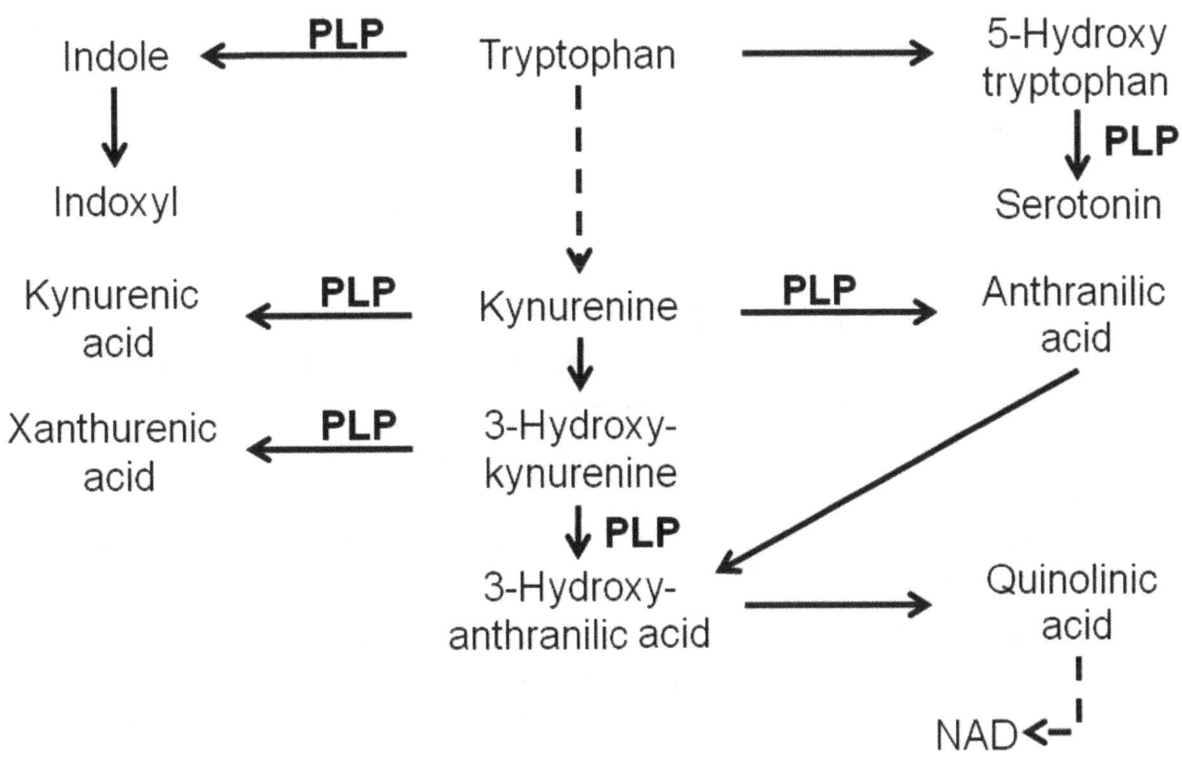

Figure 2. Outline of kynurenic pathway of tryptophan degradation.

These clinical data along with experimental results obtained in genetically epilepsy-prone seizure-naive animals, in comparison with genetically epilepsy resistant [34–37], enable us to hypothesize that an inborn error of pyridoxine metabolism (accentuated by high pyridoxine requirement during early development) is inherent in epilepsy. Being a starting point for neurotransmitter disorders, such an error may be a key determinant of epileptic diathesis. An impairment of GABA (as well as serotonin and taurine)-mediated inhibition along with an enhancement of glutamate (and aspartate)-mediated excitatory transmission evidently facilitates spreading of ictal activity throughout the brain and thereby generation of seizures.

Disturbances of PLP-dependent tryptophan degradation, in particular over-excess of neurotoxic 3-HOKYN, have been repeatedly shown in epileptic patients starting from 50-s [38–41]. Summarizing the data obtained [42–44], we suggested that quantitative correlations between metabolites formed in the course of TRP degradation (**Figure 2**) might be indicative of clinical status in epileptic patients.

Specifically, the ratio of KYN to TRP serves as an index of activity of indoleamine-2, 3-dioxygenase (IDO), the rate-limiting enzyme of TRP degradation, initiating the pathway. (Being heme-containing enzyme, IDO is apparently PLP dependent, inasmuch as heme synthesis is PLP dependent).

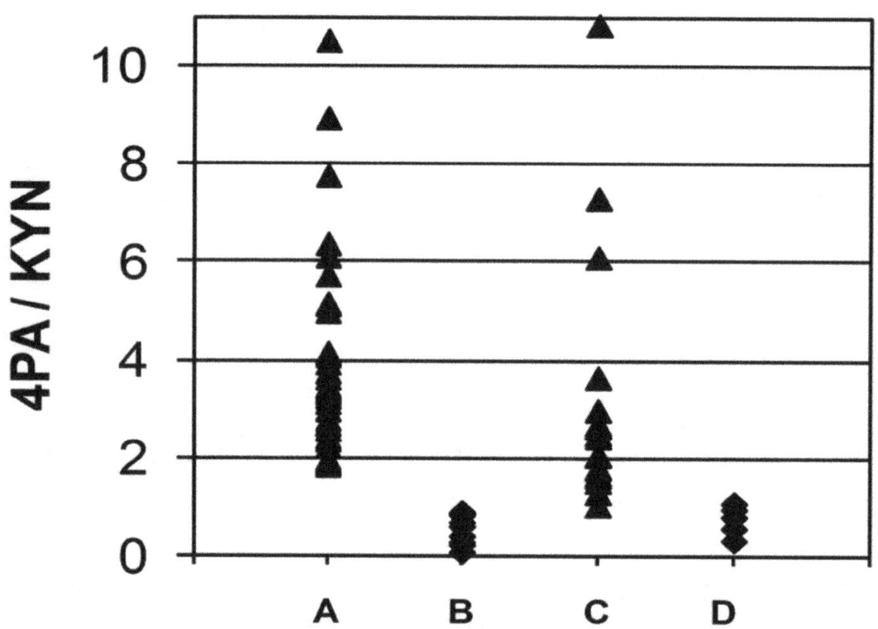

Figure 3. The value of 4PA/KYN ratios in healthy controls (A); patients experienced the first seizure attack (B); AED-treated seizure-free patients (C); partially AED-controlled epileptic patients (D).

The ratio between the levels of 3-HOAA and 3-HOKYN is considered as an index of kynureninase activity, the enzyme of critical sensitivity to PLP supply [45–47]. The ratio between 4-PA and KYN turned out to be an indicator of recently experienced seizure attack (**Figure 3**).

We have used these and other quantitative urinary biomarkers for clarification of patient's state in epilepsy and for tailoring of individual AED treatment.

1.2. Materials and methods

1.2.1. Subjects

Urine samples were analyzed in children of 4–17 years of age with different clinical forms and stages of epilepsy, excluding absence and atonic seizures, healthy in all other respects. Altogether, 109 subjects divided into following groups were comparatively studied:

1. Newly diagnosed epileptic patients, who had experienced their first epileptic attack on the previous day(s) and were never treated with AEDs ($n = 11$);
2. Epileptic patients regardless of the type of epilepsy successfully treated with AED and at present seizure-free for at least 3 months, regardless of the type of epilepsy ($n = 19$);
3. Epileptic patients partially responsive to AED treatment, that is, those having repeated seizure attacks in spite of antiepileptic treatment ($n = 19$);
4. Control group of healthy children matched by sex and age ($n = 37$).

About 270 urine samples were analyzed. Control samples were collected from healthy children in local kindergartens and elementary schools.

1.2.2. Determination of tryptophan and its metabolites in urine by high-performance liquid chromatography with simultaneous ultraviolet and fluorimetric detection

Urinary TRP and its metabolites were determined by high-performance liquid chromatography (HPLC) modified in our laboratory by Rabinkov, Pressman, and Malitsky. In addition to KYN, 3-HOKYN and 3-HOAA detected by Herve et al. [48]; some other TRP metabolites, that is, anthranilic acid (AA), kynurenic acid (KA), indoxyl sulfate (IND), and 4-PA, were also measured [36, 49].

All standards were purchased from Sigma. All solvents were of HPLC grade. The same method of TRP metabolite detection has been used by our collaborators in patients with attention deficit hyperactivity disorder (ADHD), the disease mutually interconnected with epilepsy [50].

1.2.2.1. Sample preparation

Mixed standard solutions (1 mM of each compound) were stored at −80°C for up to 3 months. Urine samples were collected into 20-mL glass scintillation vials and stored in aliquots at −80°C. Samples were acidified by the addition of 100 μL of 2.4 M perchloric acid to 900 μL of urine. After centrifugation (5000 g, 15 min, 4°C), supernatants were filtered (0.22-μL Millipore filter) into HPLC vials and analyzed the same day.

1.2.2.2. Chromatography

Reverse phase HPLC analysis was performed with an Inertsil (C-18, 5 μm) column (250 × 4.6 mm) and Merck Hitachi system equipped with a Quaternary Pump L-7100 and interface D-7000.

Peaks detection and quantification were carried out using a scanning fluorescence detector L-7485 connected to the programmable photodiode array detector L-7450A. Samples were analyzed using the following gradient: 28-min isocratic elution of 100% solvent A, 6-min linear gradient from 100 to 75% of solvent A, 61-min isocratic elution of 75% of solvent A, 2-min linear gradient from 75 to 100% of solvent A, and 8-min isocratic elution of 100% solvent A. Solvent A was 1 M ammonium acetate buffer, pH 5.2. Solvent B was 6% acetonitrile in 1 M ammonium acetate buffer, pH 5.2. The mobile phase was prepared on the day of analysis. Acquisition and processing of chromatograms were performed using HSM software (Merck-Hitachi). Standard compounds showed linearity range from 0.03 to 10 μM. Concentrations were calculated on the basis of peak areas of external standards. TRP, its metabolites, and 4-PA were determined with UV and fluorescence detection at two different excitation and emission wavelengths: 3-HOKYN and KYN were detected by UV absorption at 365 nm and eluted at 14.3, 41.4, and 87.0 min, respectively, while 3-HOAA, 4-PA, AA, TRP, IND, and KA were detected by fluorescence and eluted at 31.6, 58.9, 72.4, 84.5, 92.8, and 99.9 min, respectively.

For 3-HOAA and 4-PA, fluorescence excitation and emission wavelengths were set up as 320/420 nm during the first 60 min of elution; for AA, TRP, IND, and KA the wavelengths were 254/404 nm during the following 45 min of elution.

1.2.3. Statistical analysis

The data were expressed as mean ± SEM. Paired Student's *t*-test was used to assess the difference between groups; $p < 0.05$ was considered as statistically significant difference between values of parameters.

1.3. Urinary biomarkers for detection of the endured first seizure attack

In patients who endured seizures for the first time before admission to the ward, the mean level of TRP, and especially of KYN were sharply increased in comparison with healthy control group, thus providing the elevated mean value of KYN/TRP ratio and decreased value of 3-HOKYN/KYN ratio. The level of KA was twofold elevated, while the IND level was almost twice reduced.

Taken together, these changes in "first seizure attack" children formed a pattern strongly distinguishable from that of healthy controls (**Table 1**). The level of urinary 4-PA was statistically indistinguishable from healthy controls (though in four out of 11 patients it was reduced to 1μM or even lower). The mean value of 4-PA/KYN ratio in children of this group turned out to be almost sevenfold less than in healthy controls (**Table 1** and **Figure 3**) and appeared to be the marker of seizure attack occurred (regardless of its type).

The alterations in the urinary levels of TRP and KYN lead to a rightward shift in the histogram of distribution of the KYN/TRP ratio and a strong leftward shift in the histogram of distribution of the ratio 3-HOKYN/KYN (**Figures 4** and **5**).

Parameters	Epileptic patients								P values between compared groups $^{*}p < 0.1$; $^{**}P \le 0.05$; $^{***}P \le 0.01$				
			Non treated		AED treated								
	Group 1: healthy controls (*n* = 37)		Group 2: after first seizure attack (*n* = 11)		Group 3: seizure-free (*n* = 19)		Group 4: partially controlled (*n* = 19)						
	Mean	SEM	Mean	SEM	Mean	SEM	Mean	SEM	1–2	1–3	2–3	2–4	3–4
TRP, (μM)	23	2	57	20	36	7	58	15	***	**			
KYN, (μM)	1.7	0.2	5.7	1.4	2.4	0.2	3.3	0.3	***	**	***		**
3-HOKYN, (μM)	1.1	0.1	1.8	0.5	1.1	0.2	4.6	0.8	*			**	****
3-OHAA, (μM)	4.5	0.7	3.5	0.6	4.4	1.0	2.4	0.5					*
AA, (μM)	0.20	0.02	0.26	0.09	0.20	0.06	0.30	0.11					
KA, (μM)	3.3	0.4	6.3	1.1	5.3	1.3	8.4	1.3	***	**			*
4PA, (μM)	6.0	0.9	5.0	1.3	6.8	1.2	5.5	1.0					
IND, (μM)	576	53	294	70	289	50	460	77	**	***			*
4PA/KYN	4.1	0.5	0.6	0.1	3.1	0.6	2.5	0.7	***		***	**	
4PA/3HOKYN	8.42	1.45	3.85	0.94	8.6	1.26	4.12	1.53	*		***		**
4PA/(KYN + 3HOKYN)	2,5	0.35	0.76	0.24	1.94	0.28	1.3	0.35	***		***		
KYN/TRP	0.08	0.005	0.226	0.086	0.116	0.029	0.116	0.034	***	*			
3HOKYN/KYN	0.72	0.08	0.35	0.09	0.56	0.12	1.57	0.29	**			***	***
3HOAA/ 3HOKYN	6.0	1.1	4.4	1.3	5.9	1.5	0.9	0.2				***	***
KA/3HOAA	2.2	0.6	2.9	0.8	1.8	0.3	4.9	1.2					**
KYN/ (3HOAA/ 3HOKYN)	1.06	0.27	4.16	1.74	0.91	0.19	9.73	2.65	***		**	***	****
KA/(3HOAA/ 3HOKYN)	2.0	0.5	5.3	2.3	1.5	0.3	20.4	4.8	**		*	**	***
TRP/(3HOAA/ 3HOKYN)	14	3	38	15	13	3	155	53	**		***	**	****
IND/TRP	29.4	2.8	6.7	1.4	13.1	2.3	14.1	5.4	****	***	**		
IND/KYN	433	50	78	23	164	26	210	42	***	***	**	**	

Table 1. Urinary metabolites of tryptophan and correlations between them in epileptic patients in comparison with healthy controls.

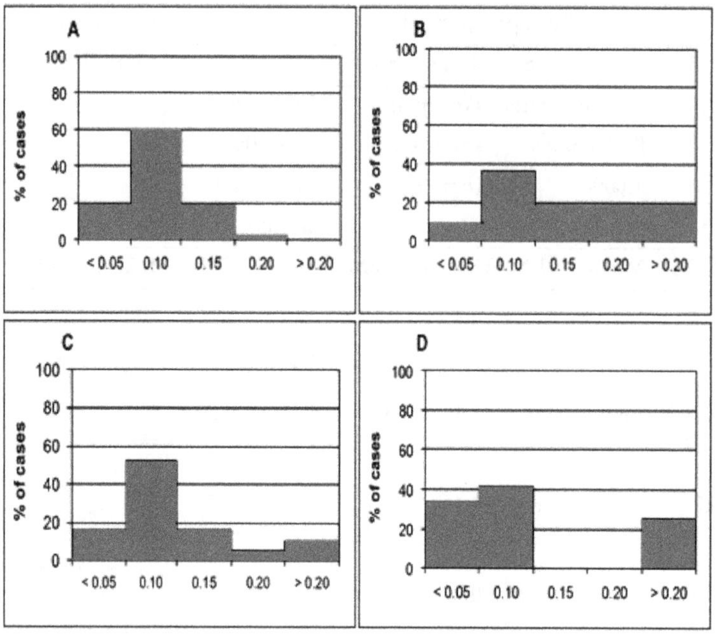

Figure 4. Distribution of KYN/TRP values in epileptic patients, in comparison with healthy controls. Designations: healthy controls (A); patients experienced the first seizure attack (B); AED-treated seizure-free patients (C); partially AED-controlled patients (D).

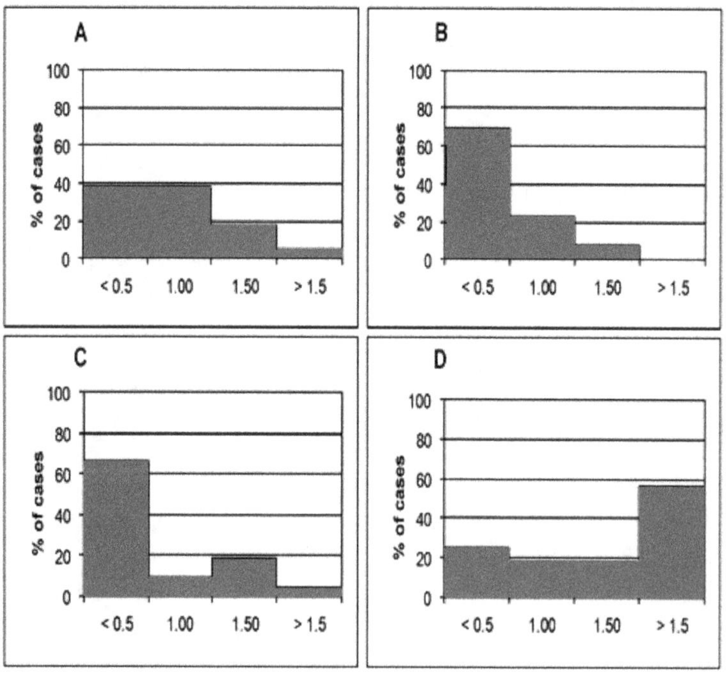

Figure 5. Distribution of 3HOKYN/KYN values in epileptic patients, in comparison with healthy controls. Designations: healthy controls (A); patients experienced the first seizure attack (B); AED-treated seizure-free patients (C); partially AED-controlled patients (D).

At the same time, the histogram of distribution of the 3-HOAA/3-HOKYN ratio tends distinctly to the left (**Figure 6**), reflecting some reduction in kynureninase activity, though the mean value of this ratio is decreased insignificantly (**Table 1**). The correlations between concentrations of TRP (as well as KYN) and the ratio indicative of kynureninase activity, that is, TRP: (3-HOAA/ 3-HOKYN) and KYN: (3-HOAA/3-HOKYN), are strongly higher in "first-attack" children than in the control group.

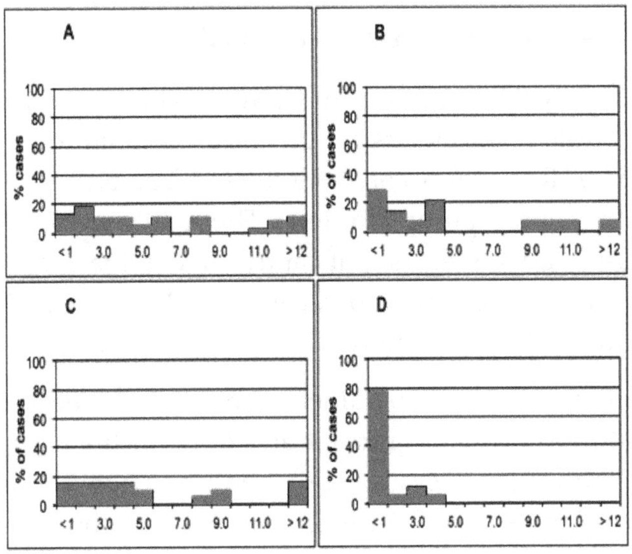

Figure 6. Distribution of 3HOKYN/3HOAA values in epileptic patients, in comparison with healthy controls. Designations: healthy controls (A); patients experienced the first seizure attack (B); AED-treated seizure-free patients (C); partially AED-controlled patients (D).

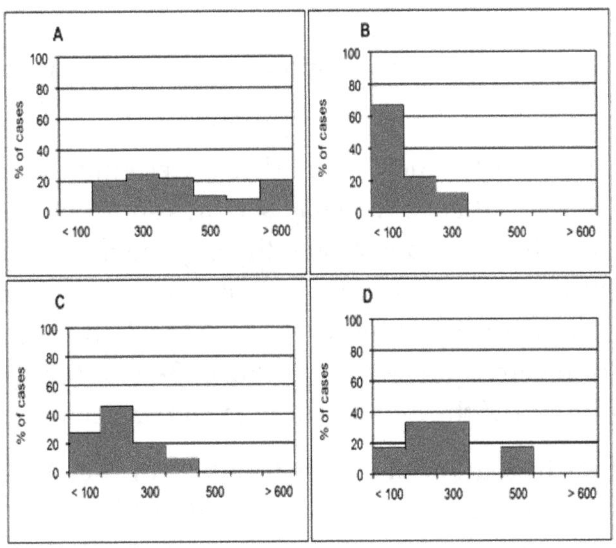

Figure 7. Distribution of IND/KYN values in epileptic patients, in comparison with healthy controls. Designations: healthy controls (A); patients experienced the first seizure attack (B); AED-treated seizure-free patients (C); partially AED-controlled patients (D).

The low value of IND/TRP and especially IND/KYN are also the markers, distinguishing first-attack children from healthy controls. The combination of increased concentrations of TRP and

KYN with decreased concentrations of IND provides drastic diminution in both IND/TRP and IND/KYN ratios in patients who endured the first attack. In approximately 70% of these patients, the IND/KYN ratio is lower than 100, while in healthy children these ratios are always higher than 100; in 60% of the healthy group, these ratios are even higher than 300 (**Table 1** and **Figure 7**).

1.4. Urinary markers in AEDs treated seizure-free patients

In patients well controlled by AEDs (in our study, those who has been seizure-free for at least 3 months) most of the studied parameters are practically similar to those in healthy controls. The mean values of KYN/TRP, 4-PA/KYN, 3- HOKYN/KYN, and 3-HOAA/3-HOKYN ratios coincide with those in the control group (**Table 1**). Though the urinary concentrations of TRP and KYN in seizure-free patients are significantly higher than in the healthy group, the correlations TRP: (3HOAA/3-HOKYN) and KYN: (3HOAA/3-HOKYN) practically coincide with corresponding values in healthy controls.

Histograms of distribution of studied parameters in AED-treated seizure-free children are similar to those in healthy controls (**Figures 4** and **6**), with the exception of histograms of distribution of 3-HOKYN/KYN ratios (**Figure 5**). Similarity between the histogram of distribution of these ratios in seizure-free AED-treated children and the group experienced the first attack signifies that kynureninase activity is not yet restored in AED-treated patients.

The mean concentration of IND in these patients remains as low as in "first-attack" group, but values of IND/TRP and IND/KYN ratios—due to reduction of TRP and KYN levels—are higher than in first-attack group, but far lower than in healthy group. The histogram of the distribution of IND/KYN ratios remains still shifted to the left (**Figure 7**).

1.5. Urinary markers in patients partially responsive to AED treatment

Repeated convulsive attacks, which occur in epileptic patients in spite of AED treatment, result in decreased values of 4-PA/KYN ratio, the marker of recently experienced seizure attacks (**Figure 3**). In three out of five patients, who had seizures shortly before the admission to the hospital, this ratio was less than one, decreasing thereby the mean value of the group (**Table 1**). The fourfold elevated concentration of toxic 3-HOKYN, the twofold elevated ratio of 3-HOKYN/KYN, and the dramatically reduced value of the 3-HOAA/3-HOKYN ratio are the most remarkable signs of the group. The mean value of 3-HOAA/3-HOKYN ratio is reduced to 0.9 and represents only 15% of the corresponding value in seizure-free patients (**Table 1**).

The strongly right-shifted histogram of the distribution of 3-HOKYN/KYN ratios and the strongly left-shifted histogram of the distribution of 3-HOAA/3-HOKYN ratios are apparently the signs of severe disturbances of kynureninase activity in partially AED-controlled patients (**Figures 5** and **6**).

Reduction in the kynureninase activity results also in the accumulation of TRP, KYN, and KA. Accordingly, the correlation of each of these compounds to the 3-HOAA/3-HOKYN ratio, that is, KYN: (3-HOAA/3-HOKYN), KA: (3-HOAA/3-HOKYN), and TRP: (3-HOAA/3-HOKYN), reaches extremely high values in patients partly responsive to AEDs (**Table 1**).

The intensive inpatient AED treatment distinctly changes the examined parameters. First of all, the value of 4-PA/KYN ratio is increased. The value of 3-HOAA/3-HOKYN ratio is also increased, reflecting an increase in kynureninase activity. Accordingly, values of KYN: (3-HOAA/3-HOKYN), KA: (3-HOAA/3-HOKYN), and TRP: (3-HOAA/3-HOKYN) are significantly diminished. In successful cases, favorable changes, once attained, remain stable (**Figure 8**; patients E and K). In unsuccessful cases, the initial increase in the 3-HOAA/3-HOKYN ratio suddenly reverts back, and the related parameters are accordingly changed (**Figure 8**, patient D).

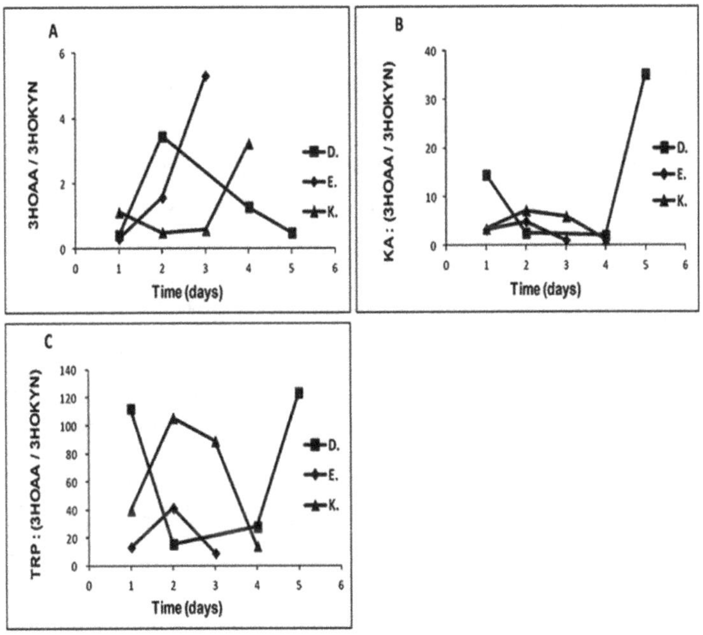

Figure 8. Dynamics of correlations between TRP metabolites under intensive AED treatment in partially AED-controlled patients. Note the difference between successfully (E and K) and unsuccessfully (case D) treated patients.

1.6. Discussion

Disturbances of PLP-dependent TRP degradation revealed in children with different forms of epilepsy confirm the suggestion that **epilepsy as a whole is PLP-dependent disorder**. The data obtained testify that concentrations of compounds formed or metabolized in the course of PLP-dependent TRP degradation, as well as correlations between them, are quantitative urinary biomarkers for the determination of clinical status—from the first seizure attack up to progressively worsening condition. These biomarkers are also indicative for the evaluation of AED treatment effectiveness and its individual monitoring. The parameters reflecting kynureninase activity turned out to be the most sensitive link of this chain.

Once the initial seizure attack has occurred, the drastically increased levels of TRP, KYN, and toxic 3HOKYN, and the drastically reduced level of IND pointed to the disordered PLP-dependent TRP degradation. Low values of IND/TRP and IND/KYN, as well as 4-PA/KYN and 4PA/3-HOKYN ratios, completely change the pattern of TRP metabolites (**Table 1**).

Specifically, the low value of 4-PA/KYN ratio (**Figure 3**) distinguishes an epileptic episode from paroxysmal loss of consciousness of nonepileptic origin. It is important to trace how long this index remains at such a low level after a single seizure episode.

The effective AED treatment normalizes most of the discussed parameters (**Table 1**). The ratio 4-PA/KYN is increased almost up to its control value. We believe that maintaining this ratio within the range between two and four (**Figure 3**) would help to provide adequate seizure control and reduce a risk of pharmacological overtreatment [45, 46]. However, increased levels of TRP, KA, and KYN, reduced concentrations of IND, and diminished IND/TRP and IND/KYN ratios (**Table 1** and **Figure 8**) still clearly distinguish AED-treated seizure-free patients from healthy controls.

The values of IND/KYN and IND/TRP ratios require an additional consideration. Intestinal PLP-dependent tryptophanase of bacterial origin is the key enzyme of alternative IND pathway of TRP degradation, which is inhibited by KYN [20]. A drastic drop in the levels of IND along with increased concentrations of KYN results in diminished IND/KYN and IND/TRP ratios in the studied groups.

Parameters reflecting the activity of kynureninase at the different stages of disease indicate that aggravation of epilepsy is accompanied by expanding inhibition of the enzyme activity [51–53]. The accumulation of toxic 3-HOKYN, along with twofold increase in the 3HOKYN/KYN ratio and sixfold decrease in the 3-HOAA/3-HOKYN ratio, appear to be the most characteristic signs of sharply reduced kynureninase activity in patients partially controlled AEDs (**Table 1**). The decrease in the value of 3HOAA/3HOKYN ratio leads to the accumulation of TRP, KYN, and KA (**Table 1**). The similar pattern is reproduced by kynureninase inhibitors, once even considered as possible anticonvulsants [54].

The intensive inpatient AED treatment of partially controlled patients decreases the 3-HOKYN/KYN ratio and increases the ratio 3-HOAA/3-HOKYN. Stability of attained parameters signifies successful treatment (**Figure 8**). The data obtained indicate that indices of kynureninase activity are the reliable markers for evaluation of clinical status and effectiveness of individual AED therapy.

The effective AED treatment increases alkaline phosphatase (ALP) activity [55–58], the enzyme which dephosphorylates PLP, and thus provides pyridoxal transport through membranes. Intensification of pyridoxine transport normalizes PLP-dependent systems (more details in part 2).

In summary, the suggested quantifiable urinary biomarkers, based on dynamic alterations of TRP metabolites in the course of the disease and antiepileptic treatment, are potentially helpful for

1. Identifying the patients who recently experienced seizure episode regardless of seizure type;
2. Detecting minimal effective doses of AED and gradual improvement of clinical status in the course of AED treatment;

3. Evaluating seizure-free status with greater precision;
4. Identification of inadequate seizure control, and rapid evaluation of the effectiveness of the novel treatment regimen;
5. Tracing the stability of results attained in the course of individualized AED treatment.

Taking into account the overall misdiagnosis rate of epilepsy (26%) and the rate of seizure recurrence after discontinuation of AED treatment ranging from 12 to 66% [59, 60], the use of suggested biomarkers seems to be expedient.

2. Family disorders of pyridoxine metabolism: Urinary TRP metabolites in asymptomatic first-degree relatives of epileptic probands

2.1. Introduction

The results obtained gave us an opportunity to discuss the nature of pyridoxine metabolism derangements in epilepsy. Are they a part of etiology of the disease [61], or consequences of seizures? Namely, are they an inborn error of metabolism, or epiphenomena of seizures, or possibly epiphenomena of seizures superimposed on inherently dysfunctional system of pyridoxine metabolism?

To understand whether dysfunctional vitamin B6 metabolism is an inborn error of metabolism inherent in epileptic families, and thereby a part of etiology of the disease, urinary parameters of vitamin B6–dependent TRP metabolism were HPLC detected in epileptic probands and their first-degree asymptomatic relatives in comparison with healthy controls.

Two non-sanguineous families were studied. Samples of each person were repeatedly analyzed over several (2–8) consecutive days. The mean value of each parameter is presented in **Table 2**.

Family one consisted of AED-treated proband D, an 8-year-old boy with a 3-s/spike-wave epilepsy (the only patient with absence epilepsy included into our study), his asymptomatic 13-year-old sibling brother, their mother affected with bronchial asthma [62], and the healthy stepfather of both children.

Grossly abnormal TRP metabolism in all three closely interconnected relatives, that is, the proband, his sibling (note especially his data), and their mother, clearly distinguished them from healthy controls and their healthy stepfather. Severe hypertryptophanuria and strongly reduced ratio KYN/TRP reflected the low activity of PLP-dependent IDO in all these three relatives. The values of 3-HOAA/3-HOKYN ratios in the proband, his mother, and especially in his asymptomatic sibling brother were 10–25% of the corresponding mean value in healthy controls, coinciding with the mean value of this parameter in epileptic patients ineffectively treated with AED *(see part 1)*. Extremely low values of 3HOAA/3HOKYN ratios along with increased levels of toxic 3-HOKYN testified kynureninase inhibition in all these three interconnected relatives. High levels of urinary 4-PA in siblings apparently meant the elevated PLP plasma level [63]. The combination of hypertryptophanuria (and increased KA levels) with extremely low values of 3-HOAA/3-HOKYN ratios provides drastically increased correlations between these indices. In each of the relatives from this family ratios TRP: (3-HOAA/3-HOKYN) and KA: (3-HOAA/3-HOKYN) were much higher than in control patients. Low concentrations of IND and low values of IND/TRP ratios in all three interconnected relatives (**Table 2**) attest to familial disruption of alternative pathway of TRP degradation as well.

Family two included AED-resistant proband (Sh-T), a 10-year-old boy with frontal lobe epilepsy and secondary generalized convulsions unsuccessfully treated with carbamazepine, phenytoin, and valproic acid, and his asymptomatic sibling brother of 7 years. Diversity of proband's data made us repeat his analyses every 5 consecutive days and to demonstrate the ranges of them.

Parameters		Family 1			Family 2	
	Healthy controls (n = 37)	Proband D. (n = 8)	Proband's mother M. (n = 8)	Proband's sibling Y. (n = 2)	Proband Sh.-T (n = 5)	Proband's sibling (n = 1)
	Average ± SE	Average ± SE	Average ± SE	Average	Range	
TRP (μM)	23 ± 2	**135** ± 27	**166** ± 17	**180**	23.6–61.8	25
KYN (μM)	1.7 ± 0.2	1.5 ± 0.23	1.8 ± 0.30	2.8	1.2–2.0	1.7
3HOKYN (μM)	1.1 ± 0.1	1.7 ± 0.41	1.5 ± 0.37	3.6	1.2–2.8	0.80
3HOAA (μM)	4.5 ± 0.7	5.0 ± 2.1	**2.4** ± 0.67	**2.3**	1.3–30.0	1.8
KA (μM)	3.3 ± 0.4	4.3 ± 1.2	5.0 ± 0.95	7.1	2.3–4.6	3.6
4PA (μM)	6.0 ± 0.9	**11.1** ± 2.1	5.3 ± 0.49	**14.3**	**0.6–3.5**	**2.1**
IND (μM)	576 ± 53	**182** ± 38	**365** ± 33	660	446–767	74
4PA/TRP	0.29 ± 0.03	**0.136** ± 0.05	**0.04** ± 0.005	**0.087**	**0.02–0.06**	**0.08**
4PA/KYN	4.1 ± 0.5	**8.3** ± 2.1	3.4 ± 0.46	**8.2**	**0.03–2.69**	**1.3**
4PA/3HOKYN	8.42 ± 1.45	9.4 ± 3.4	**4.5** ± 0.81	**4.2**	**0.3–2.3**	**2.6**
4PA/(KYN + 3HOKYN)	2.5 ± 0.35	4.0 ± 0.96	1.7 ± 0.21	2.7	**0.16–0.85**	**0.86**
KYN/TRP	0.08 ± 0.005	**0.016** ± 0.005	**0.01** ± 0.003	**0.014**	**0.02–0.06**	**0.06**
3HOKYN/KYN	0.72 ± 0.08	**1.14** ± 0.21	0.72 ± 0.14	**1.80**	1.0–2.12	0.48
3HOAA/3HOKYN	6.0 ± 1.1	**2.6** ± 0.87	**1.2** ± 0.21	**0.7**	**0.58–2.7**	**2.3**
KA/KYN	2.5 ± 0.4	2.8 ± 0.64	2.9 ± 0.39	2.8	1.5–3.54	2.2
KA/3HOAA	2.2 ± 0.6	1.9 ± 0.63	3.5 ± 1.1	3.0	0.7–2.6	2.0
KYN/(3HOAA/3HOKYN)	1.06 ± 0.27	1.16 ± 0.48	1.48 ± 0.52	5.03	0.46–3.5	0.73
KA/(3HOAA/3HOKYN)	2.0 ± 0.5	**3.8** ± 1.5	**3.9** ± 1.2	**12.4**	0.9–6.5	1.6
TRP/(3HOAA/3HOKYN)	14 ± 3	**65** ± 17	**106** ± 29	**305**	9.1–57.9	11
IND/TRP	29.4 ± 2.8	**1.8** ± 0.60	**2.3** ± 0.29	**3.4**	**7.9–23.2**	**2.9**
IND/KYN	433 ± 50	**128** ± 21	**225** ± 25	**272**	372–432.8	**45**

Parameters similarly altered in family members are shown in bold.

Table 2. Urinary tryptophan metabolites and correlations between them in epileptic families compared to healthy controls.

In both brothers, the values of 3HOAA/3HOKYN ratios were low, reflecting the low kynureninase activity; the value of this ratio in the asymptomatic brother did not exceed one-third of that in healthy controls (**Table 2**). The IND levels, as well as IND/TRP ratios, were also strongly diminished in both siblings, indicating severe disruption of the alternative route of TRP metabolism.

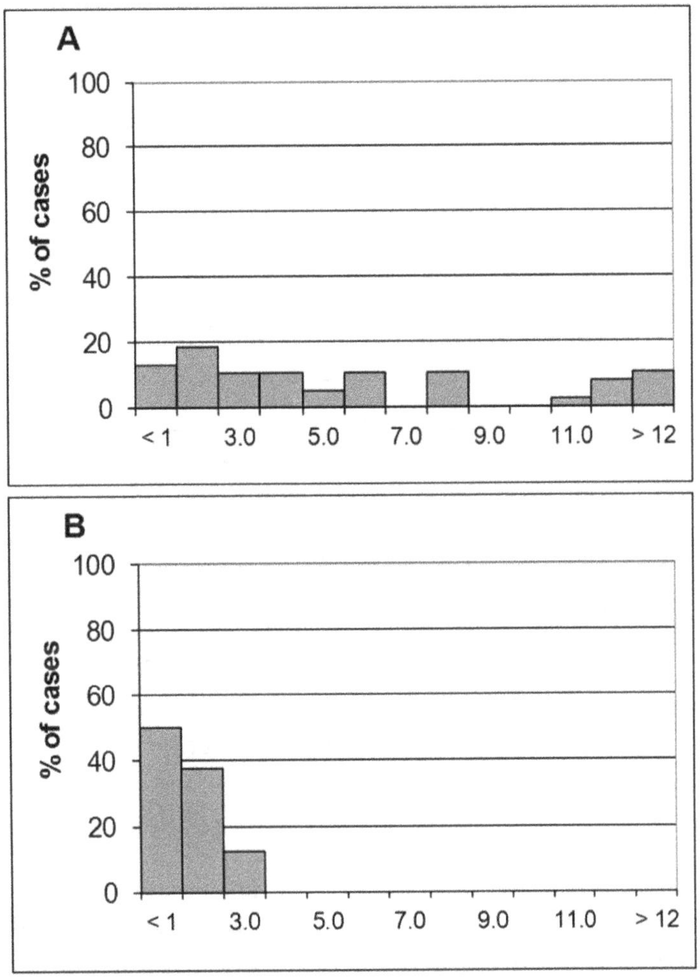

Figure 9. Distribution of 3HOAA/3HOKYN ratios in healthy controls (A) in comparison with epileptic families (B).

2.2. Discussion

Thus, the low activity of kynureninase (mirrored by 3-HOAA/3-HOKYN ratios) and disordered alternative route of TRP metabolism turned out to be the common hidden signs of asymptomatic relatives in both epileptic families, whereas hypertryptophanuria and the elevated level of 4-PA (signifying the increased plasma PLP level) [63] were inherent only in members of the first family (**Table 2**).

Histograms of the distribution of KYN/TRP and 3HOAA/3HOKYN ratios summarized in both families (**Figures 9** and **10**) reveal the reduced activity of both IDO and kynureninase in epileptic families, in comparison with healthy controls.

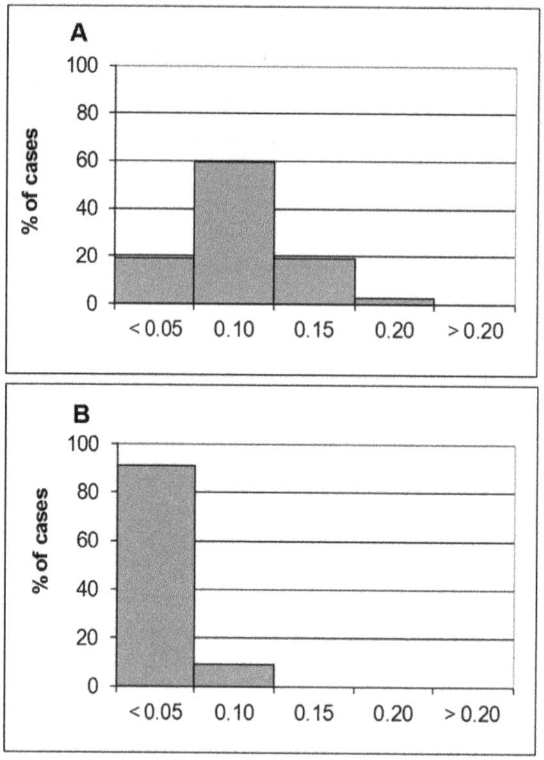

Figure 10. Distribution of the KYN/TRP ratios in healthy controls (A) in comparison with epileptic families (B).

This similarity of studied PLP-dependent disorders in epileptic probands and their asymptomatic first-degree relatives allows considering these disorders as inherent hidden traits of such families. Moreover, in clinically unaffected relatives these disorders are sometimes even more severe than in probands themselves (**Table 2**). The term "endophenotype" [64], as a heritable biochemical sign, which manifests in an individual whether or not illness is active and "co-segregated" with illness within the family, seems the most adequate definition of the state.

Judging by data obtained, *The inherent derangement of pyridoxine metabolism is a part of epilepsy etiology*. Repeated seizure attacks, superimposed on an inherently dysfunctional system of pyridoxine metabolism, may apparently provide extreme diversity of repeated results.

Van Gelder et al. [21–23, 65] were the first to find increased plasma levels of glutamate in first-degree relatives of epileptic patients just as in the patients themselves. The authors, however, considered their finding as a single symptom, rather than the manifestation of pyridoxine metabolism disorders. Later, these results were repeated, and plasma excess of aspartate and glycine along with the reduced level of urinary taurine was found in asymptomatic first-degree relatives of epileptic patients [66, 67], as well as in probands themselves. And again, the combination of biochemical alterations common to epileptic families was not explained, though PLP-dependent metabolism of amino acids pointed to the etiology of these familiar disorders.

We believe that reduced activity of alkaline phosphatase, the enzyme which dephosphorylates PLP and thus provides pyridoxal transport through membranes, may be the main factor of pyridoxine disorders in epileptic patients and their first-degree relatives.

In our experiments carried out in genetically epilepsy-prone and control epilepsy-resistant BALB/c mice (selectively bred from BALB/c strain for susceptibility or resistance to audiogenic seizures) [35, 36, 49], ALP activity in the cortex and hippocampus of seizure-naïve epilepsy-prone mice amounted to only 77.2 ± 6.7 and 74.1± 6.1% of activity inherent in epilepsy-resistant controls (Bresler a. Dolina, unpublished). In agreement with these data, the elevated PLP level was found in the brain of epilepsy-prone DBA/2 mice, in comparison with control epilepsy-resistant animals of the same strain [68].

Recently, it was shown that mice with a splice site mutation in the Akp2 gene for tissue nonspecific isoenzyme of ALP (TNSALP) have approximately 50% of normal plasma ALP activity and possess the elevated PLP plasma level, but do not manifest spontaneous seizures [69]. Unlike them, TNSALP knockout mice have 20-fold elevation of serum PLP level, large reduction in the intracellular brain PLP and lethal convulsions relieved by pyridoxal administration [70, 71].

We believe that disorders of pyridoxine metabolism in epileptic families are the consequences of inborn hypophosphatasia caused by a low activity of TNSALP. Mutations in *ALPL* gene, which encodes TNSALP, are responsible for the reduction of enzymatic activity [71–73]. The clinical spectrum of congenital hypophosphatasia presents a wide variety of phenotypes—from newborn, or infant convulsions controlled by pyridoxine [74–79] to their asymptomatic parents [80–84], whose ALP deficiency may be manifested, for example, by osteoarthropathy and/or odontohypophosphatasia. Diversity of these manifestations may depend on the extent of ALP activity reduction which, in its turn, depends on the variability of mutations in "candidate" ALP genes. Mutations in candidate genes may become the determining factor of pyridoxine metabolism disorders in epileptic families.

In their turn, disruptions of pyridoxine metabolism affect the production of PLP-dependent neurotransmitters. The imbalance of excitatory and inhibitory neurotransmitters becomes the neurochemical background of enhanced familial seizure predisposition.

We believe that *long-term* pyridoxine treatment started at early development (7–10 mg/kg daily) is safe and effective protective replacement therapy for a child born in epileptic families.

3. Conclusion

The pilot clinical trial carried out in children with different forms of epilepsy has confirmed our previous assumption of affected pyridoxine metabolism as an inborn genetic sign in epilepsy [35, 61]. We believe that clinical manifestations of inborn errors of pyridoxine metabolism are a kind of clinical continuum, ranging from severe convulsions resistant to AEDs to more common AEDs correctable forms of epilepsy, and up to remote symptoms in asymptomatic relatives of epileptic probands. This clinical continuum is open to *long-term high dose pyridoxine replacement therapy*. According to our experience, prolonged (over the years) pyridoxine treatment in pharmacological doses (10 mg/kg not exceeding 200 mg/daily) is valuable for different types of epilepsy (excluding—at least at present—absence and atonic forms). Being started at early stages of the disease and targeted at the stable correction of PLP-dependent metabolic disturbances, such a treatment will be effective by itself, and also as a background for AED management. It seems reasonable to suggest the same **long-term** pyridoxine treatment as a safe and effective protective replacement therapy for a child born in epileptic families.

Acknowledgements

The author is indebted to Dr. J. Levin for invaluable editorial corrections and wishes to acknowledge Mr. P. Danichev's excellent technical assistance and graphic presentation. The study was funded by Advance Neuroprotective System (ANS) sources.

Abbreviations

PDE	pyridoxine-dependent epilepsy
PLP	pyridoxal-5-phosphate
AED	antiepileptic drug(s)
GAD	glutamic acid decarboxylase
TRP	tryptophan
KYN	kynurenine
IDO	indoleamine 2, 3-dioxygenase (IDO)
3-HOKYN	3-hydroxykynurenine
3-HOAA	3-hydroxyanthranilic acid
KA	kynurenic acid
IND	indoxyl sulfate
4-PA	4-pyridoxic acid
ALP	alkaline phosphatase
TNSALP	tissue nonspecific isoenzyme of ALP

Author details

Svetlana A. Dolina

Address all correspondence to: dolina.svetlana@gmail.com

Advanced Neuroprotective Systems LTD., Ness-Ziona, Israel

References

[1] Hunt AD, Stokes JM, Crory Jr W, Stroud HH. Pyridoxine-dependency: report of a case of intractable convulsions in an infant controlled by pyridoxine. Paediatrics 1954;13:140–5. DOI:10.1177/088307389200700104.

[2] Surtees RA, Mills PB, Clayton P. Inborn errors affecting vitamin B6 metabolism. Future Neurol 2006;1(5):61520. DOI:10.2217/14796708.1.5.615.

[3] Mills PB, Footitt EJ, Mills KA, et al. Genotypic and phenotypic spectrum of pyridoxine-dependent epilepsy (ALDH7A1 deficiency). Brain 2010;133(7):2148–59. DOI:10.1093/brain/awq143 2148-2159.

[4] Bankier A, Turner M, Hopkins JJ. Pyridoxine-dependent seizures-a wider clinical spectrum. Arch Dis Child 1983;58:415–8. DOI:10.1016/S1570-9639(03)00045-1.

[5] Baxter P. Pyridoxine-dependent seizures: a clinical and biochemical conundrum. Biochim Biophys Acta 2003;1647(1–2):36–41. DOI:10.1016/S1570-9639(03)00045-1.

[6] Albersen M, Bosma M, Jans J, et al. Vitamin B6 in plasma and cerebrospinal fluid of children. PLoS One 2015;10(3):e0120972. DOI:10.1371/journal.pone.0120972.

[7] Gospe Jr SM, Olin KL, Keen CL. Reduced GABA synthesis in pyridoxine-dependent seizures. Lancet 1994;343(8906):7910233. DOI:10.1016/S0140-6736(94)90236-4.

[8] Cormier-Daire V, Dagoneau N, Nabbout R, et al. A gene for pyridoxine-dependent epilepsy maps to chromosome 5q31. Am J Hum Genet 2000;67:991–3. DOI: 10.1086/303087.

[9] Plecko B, Hikel C, Korenke GC, et al. Pipecolic acid as a diagnostic marker of pyridoxine-dependent epilepsy. Neuropediatrics 2005;36(3):200–5. DOI:10.1055/s-2005-865727.

[10] Plecko B, Paul K, Paschke E, et al. Biochemical and molecular characterization of 18 patients with pyridoxine-dependent epilepsy and mutation of the antiquitin (ALDH7A1) gene. Hum Mutat 2007;28(1):19–26. DOI:10.1002/humu.20433.

[11] Bennett CL, Huynh HM, Chance PF. Genetic heterogeneity for autosomal recessive pyridoxine-dependent seizures. Neurogenetics 2005;6:143–9. DOI:10.1007/s10048-005-0221-8.

[12] Walker V, Mills GA, Peters SA, Merton WL. Fits, pyridoxine and hyperprolinemia type two. Arch Dis Child 2000;82(3):236–7.

[13] Scriver CR, Beaudet AL, Sly WS, Valle D, editors. The metabolic and molecular bases of inherited disease. 8th ed. New York, NY: McGraw-Hill; 2001. p. 2863–913.

[14] Clayton PT. B6-responsive disorders: a model of vitamin dependency. J Inherent Metab Dis 2006;29(2–3):317–26. DOI:10.1007/s10545-005-0243-2.

[15] Goutieres F, Aicardi J. Atypical presentations of pyridoxine-dependent seizures: a treatable cause of intractable epilepsy in infants. Ann Neurol 1985;17(2):117–20.

[16] Yamamoto H, Murakami H, Horiguchi K, et al. Studies on the cerebrospinal fluid kynurenic acid concentration in epileptic children. Brain Dev 1995;17(5):327–9. DOI: 10.1016/j.visres.2003.11.003.

[17] Langlais PJ, Wardlow ML, Yamamoto H. Changes in CSF neurotransmitters in infantile spasms. Pediatr Neurol 1991;7(6):440–5.

[18] Yamamoto H, Shindo I, Egawa B, et al. Kynurenic acid is decreased in cerebrospinal fluid of patients with infantile spasms. Pediatr Neurol 1994;10(1):9–12.

[19] Appleton RE. Infantile spasms. Arch Dis Child 1993;69(5):614–8.

[20] Metzler DE. Biochemistry. The chemical reactions of living cells. New York, San Francisco, London: Academic Press; 2003.

[21] Van Gelder NM. Epilepsy and glutamic acid. Union Med Can 1980;109(7):996–1003.

[22] Van Gelder NM, Janjua NA, Metrakos K, et al. Plasma amino acids in 3/sec spike-wave epilepsy. Neurochem Res 1980;5(6):659–71.

[23] Perry TL, Hansen S. Amino acid abnormalities in epileptogenic foci. Neurology 1981;31(7):872–6.

[24] Sherwin AL, Van Gelder NM. Amino acid and catecholamine markers of metabolic abnormalities in human focal epilepsy. Adv Neurol 1986;44:1011–32.

[25] Sherwin A, Robitaille Y, Quesney F, et al. Excitatory amino acids are elevated in human epileptic cerebral cortex. Neurology 1988;38(6):920–3.

[26] Labiner DM, Yan CC, Weinand ME, et al. Disturbances of amino acids from the temporal lobe synaptosomes in human complex partial epilepsy. Neurochem Res 1999;24(11):1379–83.

[27] Ito M. Neurochemical approach to epilepsy. No To Hattatsu 1994;26(2):101–10.

[28] Bonhaus DW, Laird H, Mimaki T, Jamamura HI, Huxtable R. Possible bases for the anticonvulsant action of taurine. Prog Clin Biol Res 1983;125:195–209.

[29] Van Gelder NM. Pathologies of the CNS and associated taurine changes. Adv Exp Med Biol 1992;315:253–61.

[30] Yamamoto M, Takahashi S, Otsuki S, et al. GABA levels in cerebrospinal fluid of patients with epilepsy. Folia Psychiatr Neurol Jpn 1985;39(4):515–9.

[31] Pearl PL, Gibson KM. Clinical aspects of the disorders of GABA metabolism in children. Curr Opin Neurol 2004;17(2):107–113.

[32] Crawford PM, Chadwick DW. GABA and amino acid concentrations in lumbar CSF in patients with treated and untreated epilepsy. Epilepsy Res 1987;1(6):328–38.

[33] Spector R, Johanson CE. Vitamin transport and homeostasis in mammalian brain: focus on vitamins B and E. J Neurochem 2007;103:425–38.

[34] Dolina S. Is pyridoxine dependency an inborn error of metabolism triggering enhanced convulsibility in different animal models of genetic epilepsy? A commentary. Neurosciences 1992;18(Suppl. 2):153–62.

[35] Dolina S, Peeling J, Sutherland G, Pillay N, Greenberg A. Effect of sustained pyridoxine treatment on seizure susceptibility and regional brain amino acid levels in genetically epilepsy-prone BALB/c mice. Epilepsia 1993;34:33–42.

[36] Dolina S, Rabinkov A, Pressman E. Pyridoxal-5-phospate dependent kynurenine pathway in genetic epilepsy. Effect of persistent high dose pyridoxine treatment. In: 10th International Symposium on Vitamin B6 and Carbonyl Catalysis, Santa Fe, New Mexico, USA; 1999. p. 32.

[37] Dailey JW, Mishra PK, Ko KH, Penny JE, Jobe PC. Serotonergic abnormalities in the central nervous system of seizure-naive genetically epilepsy-prone rats. Life Sci 1992;50(4):319–26.

[38] Dalgliesh CE, Tekman S. The excretion of kynurenine and 3-hydroxykynurenine by man. Biochem J 1954;56:458–63.

[39] Hughes PAM, Bower BD, Raine DN, Syed N. Metabolism of tryptophan in childhood epilepsy. Arch Dis Child 1966;4:1642–51.

[40] Hughes PAM, Bower BD, Raine DN, Syed N. Effect of treatment on the metabolism of tryptophan in childhood epilepsy. Arch Dis Child 1967;42:281–8.

[41] Hansson O. Tryptophan loading and pyridoxine treatment in children with epilepsy. Ann NY Acad Sci 1969;166:306–9.

[42] Bender DA. The kynurenine pathway of tryptophan metabolism. In: Stone TW, editor. Quinolinic acid and the kynurenines. Boca Raton, FL: CRC Press, Inc.; 1989. p. 3–39.

[43] Stone TW. Endogenous neurotoxins from tryptophan. Toxicon 2001;39(1):61–73.

[44] Allegri G, Costa C, Baccichetti F, Biasiolo M. Effects of two different loading doses of L-tryptophan on the urinary excretion of tryptophan metabolites in rats, mice and guinea pigs. Correlation with the enzyme activities. Ital J Biochem 1987;36(3):194–203.

[45] Holmes GL. How to evaluate the patient after a first seizure. Postgrad Med 1988;83(2): 199–209.

[46] Holmes GL. Overtreatment in children with epilepsy. Epilepsy Res 2002;52(1):35–42.

[47] Connick JH, Heywood GC, Sills GJ, et al. Nicotinylalanine increases cerebral kynurenic acid content and has anticonvulsant activity. Gen Pharmacol 1992;239(2):235–9.

[48] Herve C, Beyne P, Jamault H, Delacoux E. Determination of tryptophan and its kynurenine pathway metabolites in human serum by high-performance liquid

chromatography with simultaneous ultraviolet and fluorimetric detection. J Chromatogr 1996;675:157–61.

[49] Dolina S, Margalit D, Malitsky S, Pressman E, Rabinkov A. Epilepsy as pyridoxine-dependent condition: Quantified urinary biomarkers for status evaluation and monitoring antiepileptic treatment. Med Hypothes 2012;79:157–64.

[50] Dolina S, Margalit D, Malitsky S, Rabinkov A. Attention-deficit hyperactivity disorder (ADHD) as a pyridoxine-dependent condition: Urinary diagnostic biomarkers. Med Hypothes 2014;82:111–16.

[51] Braunstein AE, Goryachenkova EV, Paskina TS. Enzymatic formation of alanine from l-kynurenine and l-tryptophan, and role of vitamin B6 in this process. Biokhimya (Russ) 1949;14:163–71.

[52] Soda K, Tanazawa K. Kynureninases: enzymological properties and regulation mechanism. Adv Enzymol 1979;49:1–40.

[53] Walsh HA, Bottling NP. Purification and biochemical characterization of some of the properties of recombinant human kynureninase. Eur J Biochem 2002;269:2069–74.

[54] Carpendo R, Chiardi A, Russi P, et al. Inhibitors of kynurenine hydroxylase and kynureninase increase cerebral formation of kynureninate and have sedative and anticonvulsant activities. Neuroscience 1994;61(920):237–43.

[55] Kazamatsuri H. Elevated serum alkaline phosphatase levels in epilepsy during diphenylhydantoin therapy. N Engl J Med 1970;283(25):1411–2.

[56] Kruse K, Bartels H, Gunter H. Serum alkaline phosphatase isoenzymes in epileptic children receiving anticonvulsant drugs. Eur J Pediatr 1977;126(4):237–42.

[57] Vouldris K, Moustaki M, Zies PM, et al. Alkaline phosphatase and its isoenzyme activity for the evaluation of bone metabolism in children receiving anticonvulsant monotherapy. Seizure 2002;11(6):377–80.

[58] Smith D, Defalla BA, Chadwick DW. The misdiagnosis of epilepsy and the management of refractory epilepsy in a specialist clinic. QJM 1999;92(1):15–23.

[59] Schmidt D, Löscher W. Uncontrolled epilepsy following discontinuation of antiepileptic drugs in seizure-free patients: a review of current clinical experience. Acta Neurol Scand 2005;111(5):291–300.

[60] Schmidt D, Schachter SC, editors. Epilepsy problem solving in clinical practice. Martin Dunitz; 2000.

[61] Dolina S. Is pyridoxine dependency an inborn metabolism error in genetic epilepsy? Pediatric epileptology. Cleveland, OH: Book of Abstracts; 1988. p. 35.

[62] Ubbink JB, Vermaak WJ, Delport R, et al. The relationship between vitamin B6 metabolism, asthma, and theophyllin therapy. Ann N Y Acad Sci 1990;585:285–94.

[63] Lumeng L, Aronoff GR, et al. Relationship between body store of vitamin B6 and plasma pyridoxal-P clearance: metabolic balance studies in humans. J Lab Clin Med 1985;106(5):491–7.

[64] Gottesman I, Gould TD. The endophenotype concept in psychiatry: etymology and strategic intentions. Am J Psych 2003;160:636–45.

[65] Janjua NA, Itano T, Kugoh T, et al. Familial increase in plasma glutamic acid in epilepsy. Epilepsy Res 1992;11(1):37–44.

[66] Haines JL, Panter SS, Rich SS, Eaton JW, Tsai MY, Anderson E, Opitz JM. Reduced plasma haptoglobin and urinary taurine in familial seizures identified through the multisib strategy. Am J Med Genet 1986;24(4):723–34.

[67] Monako F, Gianelli M, Scviavell MP, et al. Plasma amino acid alterations in idiopathic generalized epilepsy: an investigation in probands and their first degree relatives. Ital J Neurol Sci 1994;15(3):137–44.

[68] Chung SH, Cox RA. Determination of pyridoxal phosphate levels in the brain of audiogenic and normal mice. Neurochem Res 1983;8(10):1245–59.

[69] Polewski M, Johnson K, et al. Novel mouse model of autonomic semidominant adult hypophosphatasia has a splice site mutation in the tissue nonspecific alkaline phosphatase gene Akp2. J Bone Miner Res 2007;22(9):1397–407.

[70] Waymire KG, Mahuren JD, Jaje JM, et al. Mice lacking tissue non-specific alkaline phosphatase die from seizures due to defective metabolism of vitamin B-6. Nat Genet 1995;11:45–51.

[71] Narisawa S, Wennberg C, Millan JL. Abnormal vitamin B6 metabolism in alkaline phosphatase knock-out mice causes multiple abnormalities, but not the impaired bone mineralization. Pathology. 2001;193(1):125–33.

[72] Bloch-Zupan A. Hypophosphatasia: diagnosis and clinical signs-adental surgeon perspective. Int J Pediatr Dentistry 2016;83(3), 346–8. DOI: 10.1016.

[73] Henthorn PS, Whyte MP. Missense mutations of the tissue-nonspecific alkaline phosphatase gene in hypophosphatasia. Clin Chem 1992;38(12):2501–5.

[74] Baumgartner-Sigl S, Haberlandt E, Mumm S, et al. Pyridoxine-responsible seizures as the first symptom of infantile hypophosphatasia caused by two novel missense mutations (c.677T>C, p.M226T; c.1112C>T, p.T731I) of the tissue-nonspecific alkaline phosphatase gene. Bone 2007;40(6):1655–61.

[75] Nunes ML, Mugnol F, Bica I, et al. Pyridoxine-dependent seizures associated with hypophosphatasia in a newborn. J Child Neurol 2002;17(3):222–4.

[76] Yamamoto H, Sasamoto Y, Miyamoto Y, et al. A successful treatment with pyridoxal phosphate for west syndrome in hypophosphatasia. Pediatr Neurol 2004;30(3):216–8.

[77] Litmanovitz I, Reish O, Dolfin T, et al. Glu274Lys/Gly309Arg mutation of the tissue-nonspecific alkaline phosphatase gene in neonatal hypophosphatasia associated with convulsions. J Inherit Metab Dis 2002;25(1):35–40.

[78] Ozono K, Yamagata M, Michigami T, et al. Identification of novel missense mutations (Phe310Leu and Gly439Arg) in a neonatal case of hypophosphatasia. J Clin Endocrinol Metab 1996;81(12):4458–61.

[79] Smilari P, Romeo DM, Palazzo P, et al. Neonatal hypophosphatasia and seizures. A case report. Minerva Pediatr 2005;57(5):319–23.

[80] Stoll C, Fishbach M, Terzic J, et al. Severe hypophosphatasia due to mutations in the tissue-nonspecific alkaline phosphatase (TNSALP) gene. Genet Couns 2002;13(3):289–95.

[81] Sugimoto N, Iwamoto S, Hoshino Y, et al. A novel missense mutation of the tissue-nonspecific alkaline phosphatase gene detected in a patient with hypophosphatasia. Hum Genet 1998;43(3):160–4.

[82] Taillandier A, Cozien E, Muller F, et al. Fifteen new mutations (-195C>T, L-12X, 298-2A>G, T117N, A159T, R229S, 997+2T>A, E274X, A331T, H364R, D389G, 1256delC, R433H, N461I, C472S) in the tissue-nonspecific alkaline phosphatase (TNSALP) gene in patients with hypophosphatasia. Hum Mutat 2000;15(3):293.

[83] Watanabe H, Takinami H, Goseki-Sone M, et al. Characterization of the mutant (A115V) tissue-nonspecific alkaline phosphatase gene from adult-type hypophosphatasia. Biochem Biophys Res Commun 2005;327(1):124–9.

[84] Khandwala HM, Mumms S, Whyte MP. Low serum alkaline phosphatase activity and pathologic fracture: case report and brief review of hypophosphatasia diagnosed in adulthood. Endocr Pract 2006;12(6):676–81.

7

Self-Reporting Technologies for Supporting Epilepsy Treatment

Jonathan Bidwell, Eliana Kovich, Cam Escoffery,
Cherise Frazier and Elizabeth D. Mynatt

Abstract

Epilepsy diagnosis and treatment relies heavily on patient self-reporting for informing clinical decision-making. These self-reports are traditionally collected from handwritten patient journals and tend to be either incomplete or inaccurate. Recent mobile and wearable health tracking developments stand to dramatically impact clinical practice through supporting patient and caregiver data collection activities. However, the specific types and characteristics of the data that clinicians need for patient care are not well known. In this study, we conducted interviews, a literature review, an expert panel, and online surveys to assess the availability and quality of patient-reported data that is useful but reported as being unavailable, difficult for patients to collect, or unreliable during epilepsy diagnosis and treatment, respectively. The results highlight important yet underexplored data collection and design opportunities for supporting the diagnosis, treatment, and self-management of epilepsy and expose notable gaps between clinical data needs and current patient practices.

Keywords: health tracking, patient self-reporting, clinical data indicators, neurocognitive, neurophysiological, implications for design

1. Introduction

Health tracking technologies such as wrist-worn seizure detection devices stand to play an increasingly important role in epilepsy diagnosis and treatment as tools that can assist patients with reporting physical [1] and psychiatric symptoms [2]. Neurologists rely on patient self-reporting to document a wide range of symptoms and triggers [3, 4] such as medication intake, sleep, exercise, missed meals and stress levels. In practice, most patients struggle with reporting these types of information [5], and these reports are known to be highly inaccurate [6–10].

These shortcomings present two sets of challenges for technology developers and healthcare providers alike. First, the type, priority, and characteristics of clinically relevant patient data are not well documented. This presents problems for technology developers, who must understand these needs for establishing appropriate technology design requirements. Second, the performance of health tracking devices is not well explored with respect to clinical seizure reporting needs. This presents problems for healthcare providers, who require an understanding of current reporting capabilities for recommending appropriate patient self-reporting tools.

In this chapter, we present our research with clinicians to first establish clinical patient self-reporting needs with respect to clinical decision-making during epilepsy diagnosis and treatment, and second to investigate the extent that the performance of current seizure detection and classification devices may be suitable for addressing these needs.

Our study included a literature review and interviews with clinicians to identify relevant epilepsy-related symptoms and triggers; a card sorting session to prioritize these symptoms and triggers; a technology review of seizure detection devices; and finally, a pair of online surveys was administered for establishing further characteristics of clinical patient self-reporting needs during epilepsy diagnosis and treatment, respectively.

Our results include a consensus on the types, priorities, and characteristics of clinical patient self-reporting needs during anti-epileptic drug (AED) selection and treatment along with a comparison of seizure detection devices and patient self-reporting performance. These findings are intended to provide a useful reference for both developing future patient self-reporting tools and to highlight the extent that current technologies may be suitable for addressing the clinical needs that we identified within the practice. Finally, we conclude with a discussion of technology recommendations that could stand to benefit mainstream epilepsy treatment.

The main contribution of this work is a "roadmap" for developing technologies that support epilepsy treatment. The results include:

1. Identification of the **type, priority,** and **characteristics** of self-reported data that clinicians need from patients as a reference for technology developers.
2. Evaluation of current device and patient seizure reporting performance as a reference for providers.
3. Identification of **self-reporting challenges** associated with current reporting as a starting point for developing future patient self-reporting and data collection tools.

Moreover, our study demonstrated the importance of stakeholder engagement. The role of clinical patient self-reporting is important yet often undocumented in literature. In our findings, we help to address this gap by presenting specific data collection strategies to help providers to collect high priority patient self-reports that are not well supported by current health reporting mechanisms and technologies. This research is unique in that we investigate both the information needs of neurologists during clinical treatment and the performance statistics that technologists need for guiding development efforts.

2. Related work

2.1. Patient self-reporting challenges

Health information can also be challenging for patients to collect and therefore be unreliable even when available, or it may not be collected frequently enough to be informative [9, 11]. Handwritten and electronic patient "seizure diaries" tends to be either incomplete or inaccurate [5, 12]. In practice, many patients (30–50%) fail to report seizures during the day [6–9] while most patients fail to report seizures at night (85.8%) [9]. Eyewitness accounts often disagree on important details of how a seizure presents [9, 13], and observation is often difficult at night [5, 14]. Reminding patients to fill in reports may be ineffective as consciousness can be impaired both during and following a seizure [9]. These collective challenges present problems for clinicians as important patient information is often unavailable, unreliable, or not collected frequently enough to be informative during diagnosis and treatment [9, 11].

The **types** and **priorities** of patient self-reporting information are therefore important to understand for informing care along with the following self-reporting **characteristics**:

1. **Reporting availability:** Self-reports may not be available due to patient non-compliance, inability to document or observe the requested data [9], or limited awareness regarding the types of information that would be most relevant to collect in preparation for appointments.
2. **Reporting usefulness:** Self-reports may not be useful for clinical management. For example, patients may be unsure of what data to collect and fail to report important indicators [15] while devices may report data in a manner that requires considerable interpretation for answering clinical questions.
3. **Reporting reliability:** Self-reports may not be reliable due to issues such as recall bias [16]. Moreover, self-reporting performance can be difficult to assess given the absence of readily quantified measurements or validated study designs [5].
4. **Reporting difficulty:** Self-reporting may be too difficult or burdensome for patients to collect between appointments [17]. Neurologists often ask patients to document and report data such as the time, date, and a description of symptoms before, during, and after clinical presentations of symptoms [5, 18–20].
5. **Reporting frequency:** Finally, patient health data must be sampled or collected at an appropriate frequency for clinical interpretation. For example, clinicians require frequent and detailed seizure and developmental reports when treating patients with infantile spasms [24].

2.2. Health tracking design challenges

Health tracking technologies could help answer these questions but many practical challenges remain [17]. Health tracking priorities among clinicians and the patient's role in self-reporting are each often under-specified in the literature. There is considerable interest in behavioral surveillance [21] as input for both assessing chronic conditions and evaluating self-management during treatment [22].

These advancements stand to greatly inform traditional diagnosis and treatment, but current health tracking measurements only touch on a small subset of health indicators that are relevant for patient care. The Chronic Care Model [23] is helpful in describing the role of clinical systems, healthcare communications, and self-management in patient care, but it is not instructive in terms of describing what clinical, self-management, and electronic health record (EHR) information is most important to keep track of for achieving positive long-term outcomes.

Current developments can be leveraged for greatly enhancing the capabilities of the existing systems. For example, inertial-based seizure detection wristbands are increasingly capable of detecting convulsive seizures [24]. Most patients have access to smartphones with increasingly powerful sensing capabilities [9, 10]. Well-designed health tracking [25] and health reporting tools [26] have the potential to greatly reduce the burden placed on patients to collect clinically significant health information [27]. It is, therefore, important for researchers to establish an understanding of clinical information needs and health tracking performance for developing appropriate and effective health tracking tools.

3. Methods

In this section, we present a multiphase, sequential mixed method study design. The study included a total of 16 clinicians who specialized in pediatric and adult epilepsies.

Our study included two main parts: The first part of the study investigated the **types, priorities,** and **characteristics** of useful clinical indicators during epilepsy diagnosis and treatment, respectively; while the second part investigated the **performance of current seizure detection technologies** as compared with current patient self-reporting.

3.1. Part 1: establishing self-reporting types, priorities, and characteristics

The first step was establishing the **types, priorities,** and **characteristics** of useful patient indicators that clinicians need during diagnosis and treatment. This included

- Interviews and a literature review to identify symptoms and triggers.
- Interviews with subject matter experts to identify five **characteristics of** self-reporting challenges.

The complete list of symptoms and triggers is available upon request. The resulting findings are intended to provide technology developers with insights for anticipating clinical patient self-reporting needs.

3.1.1. *Investigating self-reporting needs*

We conduct interviews over a 2-month period. The interviews included one-on-one meetings with one nurse practitioner specializing in pediatric epilepsy at the Children's Healthcare of Atlanta (CHOA), Georgia and two attending specializing in adult epilepsy at Emory University Hospital, Georgia. These meetings highlighted important patient self-reporting characteristics that we would later include in our online survey.

Next, we conducted a literature review to generate a list of patient symptoms and triggers that clinicians might find as useful feedback during diagnosis and treatment. Inclusion criteria for the symptoms included any health indicators that described a specific aspect of the condition such as duration and quality; while triggers included any factors that were known to impact the likelihood of symptoms such as physical activity, sleep quality [28], and self-management behaviors [29, 30]. The literature review resulted in a list of 48 symptoms and 11 triggers that may be of interest during either diagnosis or treatment.

3.1.2. *Investigating self-reporting priorities*

The next step was to establish the clinical priority of these symptoms and triggers during diagnosis and treatment. A one-hour card sorting session was conducted with six pediatric epilepsy care specialists at CHOA. Informed consent was obtained from all participants. The participants included four nurse practitioners and two epileptology attendings.

The card sorting was conducted as follows. First, we printed the list of symptoms and triggers from the literature review on two separate stacks of notecards. The same card sorting exercise was conducted twice, with one stack of cards being sorted in terms of usefulness to prioritize data needs during diagnosis, and the second stack of cards being sorted to prioritize the same data during treatment. Each card contained a single symptom or trigger, and each set of notecards was shuffled beforehand.

The clinicians were asked to order the notecards in terms of "most-to-least" useful patient-reported symptoms and triggers during diagnosis and treatment, respectively. Notecards of equal importance were stacked on top of one another. New note cards were added to both piles if the clinicians believed we had overlooked any important symptoms and triggers from our literature review. Likewise, irrelevant or difficult to understand notecards were discarded from both piles, as shown in **Figure 1**.

The priority ranking for each card was then computed transcribing the notecards into a three-columned Excel spreadsheet that contained: (1) symptom/triggers names, (2) notecard positions during diagnosis, and (3) notecard positions during treatment, respectively and then summing the two sorted card indices for diagnosis and treatment as shown in Eq. (1).

$$\text{Priority ranking} = \text{diagnosis card index} + \text{treatment card index} \tag{1}$$

The spreadsheet was then sorted by our resulting priority ranking column from least to greatest for establishing a list of clinical data indicators that were considered important during both diagnosis and treatment. It should be noted that the exercise could have been accomplished

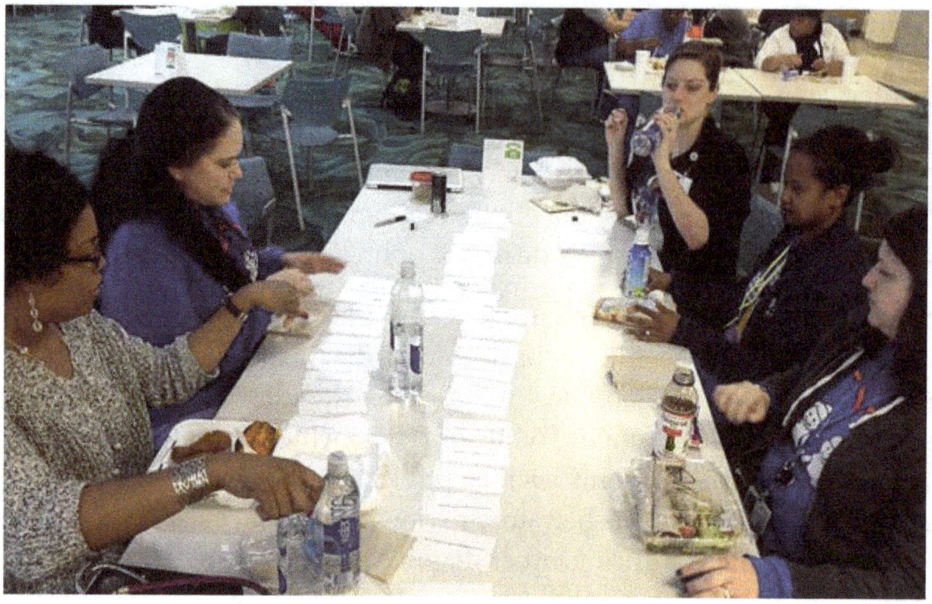

Figure 1. Expert panel card sorting exercise with four nurse practitioners and two epileptology attendings who specialized in diagnosing and treating pediatric epilepsy.

by using a single set of notecards, however, we opted to use two sets of cards to avoid having to document the cards before moving onto the second sorting session.

3.1.3. *Establishing self-reporting consensus*

Next, we conducted an online survey with the aim of further understanding several practical characteristics of these clinical data collection needs. The survey was administered to 6 clinicians over a 5-week period and included the following 5 questions for each of the "top 20" highest ranked symptoms and triggers:

1. Availability	Is this information available?
2. Reliability	Is this information useful?
3. Usefulness	Is this information reliable in your opinion?
4. Difficulty	Is it easy or hard for patients to report?
5. Frequency	How frequently would you ideally like this information to be collected?

The survey had two pages and was designed to take less than 15 min. The first page included demographics questions. The second page contained a 20 row by 5 column table of multiple-choice questions with symptoms and triggers as rows and questions as columns.

3.2. Part 2: investigating seizure reporting performance and capabilities

The second part of our study specifically investigated clinical patient self-reporting needs surrounding patient seizure reporting. This included:

- Interviews and a literature review to identify aspects of seizure reporting.
- Technology review and a meta-analysis to present common performance statistics.

Moreover, we discussed our findings with clinicians. This feedback highlighted several important yet underexplored data collection opportunities for supporting diagnosis, treatment, and self-management.

The findings are intended to help providers to assess the extent that current seizure detection devices may be suitable for complementing patient self-reporting capabilities.

3.2.1. *Investigating seizure reporting needs*

Interviews, a literature review, and an online survey were conducted as background for establishing clinical seizure reporting needs during diagnosis and treatment.

The interviews included two fellows and one attending at the Emory School of Medicine and provided us with an opportunity to discuss seizure reporting practices among current patients and caregivers. The literature review included 27 papers and focused on identifying seizure reporting needs for informing clinical decision-making. The most common clinical information needs were seizure frequency, duration, type, and ability to observe seizure progression over time.

Next, we administered an online survey among an additional group of clinicians to further assess the perceived importance and accuracy of these seizure reporting measures. The survey was administered to 10 epileptologists at Emory (5 residents, 1 fellow, and 4 attendings) and included 23 Likert scale ratings. The Likert ratings were presented on a scale from 1 to 5 with 1 being "not important" and 5 being "most important" while ratings of self-reporting accuracy ranged between <20 and >80% with 5 even intervals. The respondents were also asked which type of patient reporting error would be the most detrimental during treatment and then given three choices: (a) patient over reporting, (b) patient underreporting, or (c) both errors are equally detrimental.

The online survey results highlighted the need for a follow-on technology review. Most notably, while survey respondents indicated a strong need for more accurate patient and caregiver seizure movements and seizure counts, limited research was available regarding the applicability of current technologies for addressing these needs. In addition, the literature did not specifically compare patient self-reporting to system performance [37].

3.2.2. *Evaluating seizure reporting technologies*

The technology review addressed these shortcomings by evaluating the performance of current systems for detecting and counting seizures, characterizing patient seizure motion, and comparing performance against that of current patient self-reporting capabilities.

Inclusion criteria included all systems that had been evaluated within a home or clinical setting. Exclusion criteria included vagus nerve [31] and brain stimulation [32] systems that required permanent surgeries and electroencephalogram (EEG) systems that can be burdensome for patients during long-term use [33, 34].

The first step was to choose performance measures that would address two sets of findings from our earlier research. First, our survey respondents showed no consensus regarding the relative impact of over or under reporting seizures. Second, our interviews with clinicians indicated that most patients and caregivers report seizures themselves without the help of seizure detection devices [3, 5]. It was, therefore, important for us to choose performance metrics that would both quantify over and under reporting as well as support comparison between seizure reporting systems and patient self-reporting rates from the literature [9].

To address these requirements, we evaluated each system in terms of three statistics: precision, recall, and F-score. Recall or sensitivity is the fraction of all seizures that were detected. High recall values reflect a low chance of under reporting or missing a seizure. Missed seizure events are problematic as untreated seizures can have serious long-term health consequences.

$$\text{Recall} = \frac{\text{true positives}}{\text{true positives} + \text{false negatives}} \tag{2}$$

Precision is the fraction of all relevant seizures that are detected. High precision values reflect a low chance of over reporting seizures or triggering false alarms. Low false alarm rates are important to avoid changing already effective medication.

$$\text{Precision} = \frac{\text{true positives}}{\text{true positives} + \text{false positives}} \tag{3}$$

The F-score balances over and under reporting and is expressed as:

$$F = \frac{2 * \text{precision} * \text{recall}}{\text{precision} + \text{recall}} \tag{4}$$

In practice, notable inconsistencies between studies required making several assumptions. Many systems did not report precision and recall directly. In some cases, these rates had to be calculated based on information in the papers. Next, several studies presented statistics in terms of only those patients with seizures (PWS) [38–40] while other studies reported statistics for all patients in a study [41–43]. Including all patients meant that some patients without seizures might also contribute false positives. To address this discrepancy, we recomputed precision to include only those false positives from patients with seizures. For example, Poh et al. [41] reported performance for all patient and precision subsequently increased 24.54% when calculated among only those patients with seizures.

Next, we calculated patient self-reporting performance based on previous studies [18]. In this case, we assumed perfect self-reporting precision. Blum et al. [7, 9] evaluated seizure awareness among 31 patients with partial and generalized type epilepsies and observed that patients never falsely reported seizures. Next, we calculated based on observations from a similar study from Hoppe et al. [9] in which 91 patients with focal type epilepsies failed to report 32.0% of seizures during the day and 85.8% of seizures while asleep at night. This resulted in a precision of 100% for both day and night time reporting, recall values of 68.0 and 14.5% and F-scores of 0.25 and 0.81 for day and night time reporting, respectively.

4. Results

4.1. Part 1: self-reporting types, priorities, and characteristics

This section summarizes our key research findings. **Figure 2** presents the type, priority, and characteristics of important information that clinicians need patients to report along with notable perceived patient self-reporting challenges and agreement between participants.

4.1.1. *Self-reporting types*

The first step for our analysis was establishing the types of patient self-reported data that clinicians need from patients. The bottom row of **Figure 2** shows a sorted list with highest to lowest priority clinical information needs.

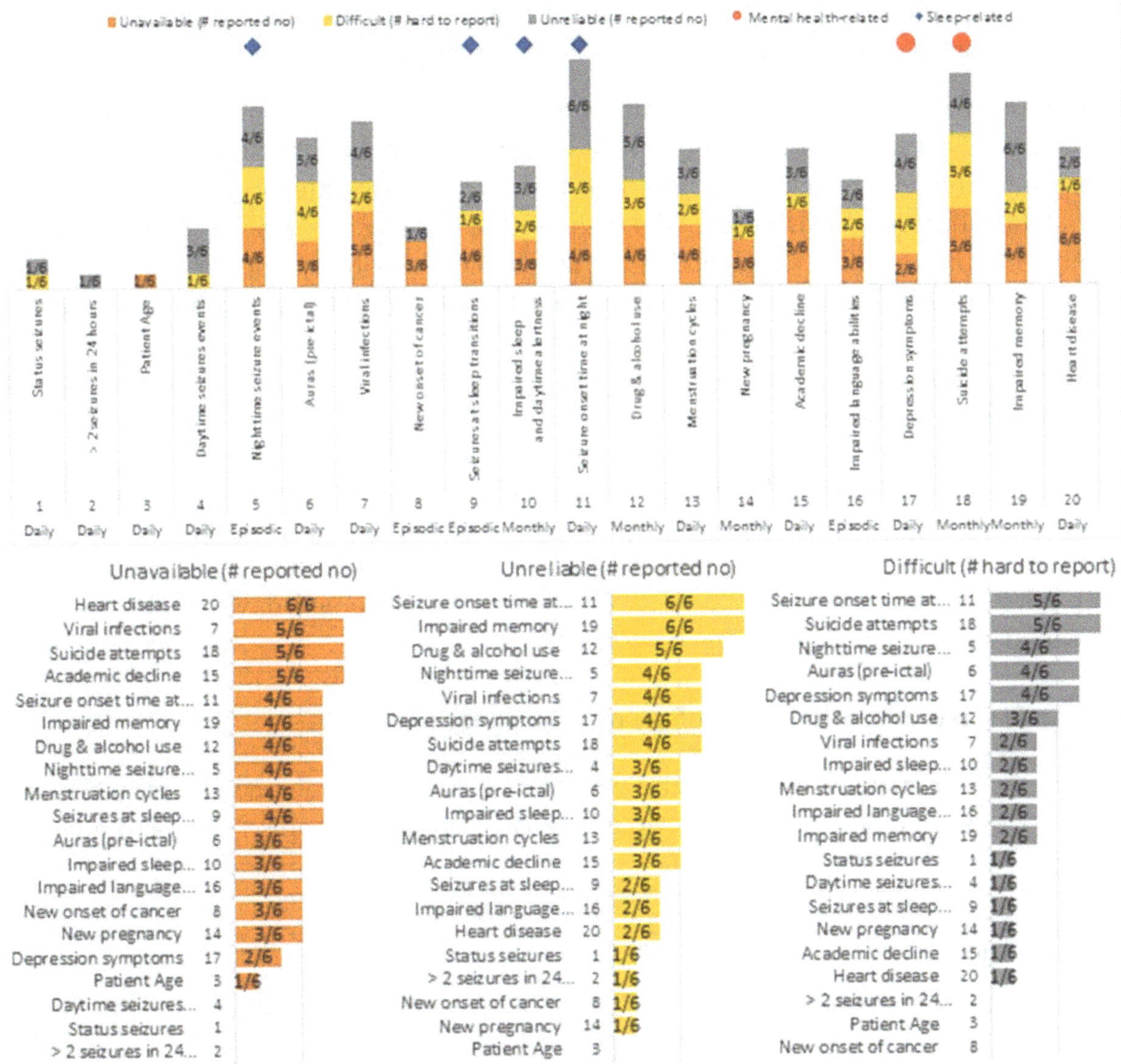

Figure 2. "Top 20" types, priorities, and characteristics of neurocognitive self-reporting needs (top row) and specific self-reporting challenges (sorted from greatest to least importance) (bottom row).

4.1.2. Self-reporting priorities

Next, we investigated the priority of the patient self-reported data that clinicians need from patients. The "top 20" highest priority symptoms and triggers are shown in **Figure 2**.

4.1.3. Self-reporting characteristics

The online survey established a consensus regarding several important self-reporting characteristics. The top row of **Figure 2** shows clinician perceptions regarding the "top 20" highest ranked symptoms and triggers in terms of availability, reliability, difficulty and desired frequency; while the bottom row shows the same characteristics but categorized in terms of "unavailable", "difficult" for patients to collect" or "unreliable", respectively.

4.1.4. Self-reporting challenges

Next, we identified the pair of symptoms and triggers with the highest number of critical clinical responses. The most frequent clinician survey responses are shown in **Table 1**.

The first row in **Table 1** highlights patient reporting challenges associated with information access. This includes the symptom or trigger with the greatest number of "unavailable" and "difficult" responses. The second row, further accounts for problems associated with data collection performance. This includes the symptom or trigger with the greatest number of "unavailable", "difficult", and "unreliable" responses, respectively. The results highlight "suicide attempts" and "seizure onset time at night" as two important unmet clinical needs.

4.1.5. Self-reporting themes

Mental health and sleep-related symptoms and triggers each appeared among the "top 20" highest ranked symptoms and triggers. Icons above the bar graphs in **Figure 2** denote mental health-related symptoms and triggers such as "depression symptoms" with red circles and sleep-related symptoms and triggers such as "impaired sleep and daytime alertness" and "impaired sleep quality" with blue diamonds.

4.2. Part 2: seizure reporting technology review capabilities

This section summarizes our research findings and highlights how inaccurate patient and caregiver seizure reporting impacts clinical decision-making for prescribing and adjusting

	Epilepsy
Unavailable + dfficult	Suicide attempts
Unavailable + difficult + unreliable	Seizure onset time at night

Table 1. Most frequent clinician reported survey responses.

AEDs. Here our key findings were that limited technologies exist for supporting the process of characterizing patient seizure type, and while most seizure detection devices are more accurate than patients for nighttime reporting, these devices must be made more accurate to be beneficial for daytime use.

The results in **Figure 3** provide a comparison of seizure detection device and patient self-reporting capabilities on an F-score axis between 0 and 1. The results also account discrepancies in study population size by computing performance for only those patients with seizures (PWS) as opposed to all patients that participated in each study. The following subsections describe inertial systems, video systems, and multimodal systems.

4.2.1. *Inertial systems*

Inertial systems utilize one or more wrist and/or chest-worn motion sensor [36, 44] and detect seizure-like convulsions as intense, repetitive limb, and torso movements with F-scores ranging from 0.133 to 0.990. These systems offer the benefit of being able to measure motion under blankets for nighttime use [36] and typically measure limb motion using an accelerometer [42], and/or gyroscope [45]. The two highest performing research systems in our review were from Schulc et al. [45] and Dalton et al. [46]. Schulc et al. [45] instrumented patients with a

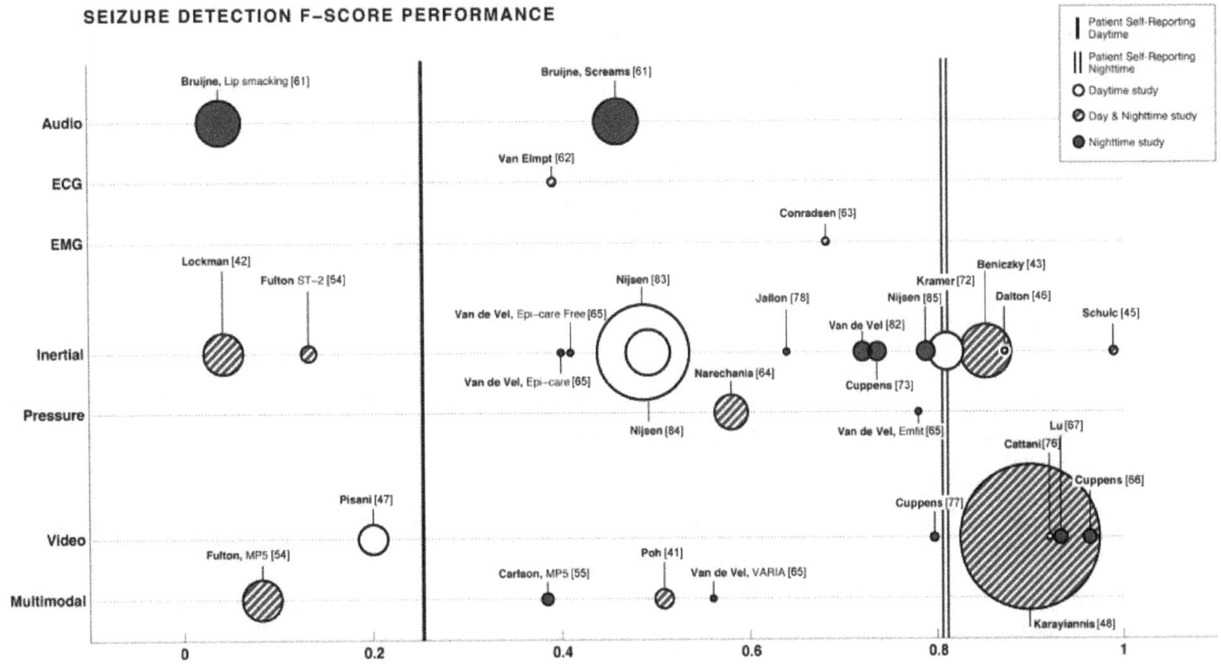

Figure 3. Seizure reporting performance comparison: multiple types of non-EEG seizure detection systems are compared against patient self-reporting on a continuous F-score scale from 0.0 to 1.0, read left to right, where 0.0 is worst and 1.0 is shows the best performance. Each seizure detection system is represented as a circle for given class technology. The circle texture indicates the time of day that the system was evaluated and diameter reflects the relative number of patients that had at least one seizure during each study. Self-reporting performance is shown using vertical lines. Daytime performance is shown as a vertical white line with a black border while nighttime performance is shown as a solid black line, respectively.

single sensor on the forearm (98.00% precision, 100.00% recall) while Dalton et al. [46] instrumented patients with a pair of wrist-worn sensors (84.0% precision, 91% recall). The highest performing commercial product is Epi-care Free. Epi-care Free is a single wrist sensor with similar performance (81.95% precision, 89.74% recall) [43]. High false positive rates remain a challenge as rhythmic activities such as brushing teeth [42, 43] and exercise [41] are often responsible for triggering false alarms.

4.2.2. *Video systems*

Marker and markerless video systems been developed for detecting and classifying a range of seizure types [39] with F-scores between 0.201 and 0.964. These systems had lower overall performance than other alternatives such as inertial systems, but modern computer vision techniques are making these systems increasingly flexible and attractive for long-term use.

Markerless video systems can be trained to reliably detect patient seizure movement without the need to wear sensors on the body. For example, while prior systems were restricted to specific settings such as specific Neonatal Intensive Care Units [47, 48], more recent systems such as the one from Cuppens et al. [77] use image features that are more robust to lighting and viewpoint changes and thus applicable to different bedrooms.

Marker-based video systems, by contrast, require patients to wear active or passive markers for measuring patient motion but provide among the few examples of systems that also classify types of detected seizures [35, 38, 51]. Rémi et al. [35] used an infrared camera and retroreflective markers to track and classify different types of patient limb movements during seizures. The video recordings were analyzed to track the position of each marker over time. The relative movement of these markers between video frames was then used to discriminate between motor characteristics during different types of convulsive seizures.

4.2.3. *Multimodal systems*

Multimodal systems utilize inputs from multiple types of sensors thereby improving seizure detection performance with F-scores ranging from 0.083 to 0.560. Poh et al. [41] showed that electrodermal activity (EDA), in conjunction with an accelerometer, could detect seizures better than using accelerometry alone [41]. EDA measures autonomic arousal and could play a role in detecting seizures with subtle motor movement. In addition, future research may highlight differences between EDA responses on both wrists and legs for differentiating generalized and partial seizures, and for characterizing seizure laterality [52].

The MP5 system [54, 55] consisted of an under mattress microphone and accelerometer according to Ref. [56], although performance was comparatively poor (average F-score = 0.234). More recently, Pavlova et al. showed that respiration can complement video EEG during seizure diagnosis [57]. Heart rate variability [58], EDA, and respiration may enable systems to recognize life-threatening postictal depression following seizures [59, 60].

4.2.4. Audio, ECG, EMG, pressure systems

van Elmpt et al. [62] used ECG measurements for detecting the onset of heart rate changes associated with seizures and achieved competitive performance with inertial sensors (F-score = 0.391). Heart rate was observed to increase (tachycardia) at the onset of seizures and decrease following seizures (postictal bradycardia). Muscle activated sensors have been used to detect seizures [63], however, no further efforts have been made, perhaps due to adhesive EMG sensors being cumbersome to wear for long periods of time.

Mattress pressure pads have achieved mid-level performance for generalized tonic clonic (GTC) seizures [64, 65] with F-scores ranging from 0.580 to 0.78. These sensors present the added benefit of not requiring patients to wear sensors and increased privacy over having a camera installed in bedrooms. Most mattress systems, however, report false positive rates that are notably higher than inertial and video-based systems [66], due to pillows dampening pressure readings or the patient sitting up in bed [64].

4.2.5. Seizure reporting comparison between devices and patient self-report

Table 2 presents a set of statistics for comparing each system to patient [9] seizure reporting performance. Each row contains an F-score along with precision, recall, and number of patients with seizures and modality or type of system and is sorted by descending F-score for reference. Next, **Table 3** presents statistics for comparing performance between each type of system. Each row includes the mean, standard deviation, minimum and maximum values together with two sets of p-values from a one-sided t-test. The p-values report the likelihood that each type of system would achieve a higher average F-score performance than that of patient self-reporting [9]. It should be noted that the t-test could not be computed for EMG and ECG as we only evaluated a single system from each of these categories.

Systems	F-score	Precision	Recall	PWS	Modality
Schulc [45]	0.990	0.980	1.000	3	Inertial
Cuppens [66]	0.964	0.931	1.000	5	Video
Lu [67]	0.933	0.933	0.933	5	Video
Cattani [76]	0.921	0.932	0.910	1	Video
Karayiannis [48]	0.900	0.900	0.900	54	Video
Dalton [46]	0.874	0.840	0.910	5	Inertial
Beniczky [43]	0.854	0.814	0.897	20	Inertial
Kramer [72]	0.811	0.714	0.938	15	Inertial
Cuppens [77]	0.797	0.850	0.750	3	Video
Nijsen [85]	0.788	0.650	1.000	7	Inertial
Van de Vel, Emfit [65]	0.780	0.780	0.780	1	Pressure
Cuppens [73]	0.737	0.600	0.952	7	Inertial

Systems	F-score	Precision	Recall	PWS	Modality
Van de Vel [82]	0.721	0.578	0.957	7	Inertial
Conradsen [63]	0.682	0.750	0.625	2	EMG
Jallon [78]	0.639	0.717	0.577	2	Inertial
Narechania [64]	0.580	0.430	0.890	13	Pressure
Van de Vel, VARIA [65]	0.560	0.560	0.560	1	Multimodal
Poh [41]	0.508	0.349	0.938	7	Multimodal
Nijsen [84]	0.492	0.350	0.830	18	Inertial
Nijsen [83]	0.487	0.350	0.800	36	Inertial
Bruijne Screams [61]	0.459	0.300	0.980	17	Audio
Van de Vel, Epi-care Free [65]	0.410	0.410	0.410	1	Inertial
Van de Vel, Epi-care [65]	0.400	0.400	0.400	1	Inertial
van Elmpt [62]	0.391	0.900	0.250	3	ECG
Carlson MP5 [55]	0.385	0.278	0.625	4	Multimodal
Pisani [47]	0.201	0.117	0.714	12	Video
Lockman [42]	0.133	0.072	0.875	6	Inertial
Fulton MP5 [54]	0.083	1.000	0.043	15	Multimodal
Fulton ST-2 [54]	0.043	1.000	0.022	15	Inertial
Bruijne Lip smacking [61]	0.039	0.020	0.980	17	Audio
Self-reporting					
Daytime reporting [9]	0.810	100.00	68.00	91	Patient
Nighttime reporting [9]	0.253	100.00	14.50	91	Patient

Table 2. System and patient self-reporting performance comparison.

Modality	Mean	SD	Min	Max	Right-tail hypothesis test	
					p-Value day	p-Value night
Inertial	0.598	0.282	0.043	0.99	0.008	1
Video	0.786	0.292	0.201	0.964	0.426	0.997
Pressure	0.68	0.142	0.58	0.78	0.209	0.927
EMG	0.682	0	0.682	0.682	–	–
Multimodal	0.384	0.214	0.083	0.56	0.014	0.846
Audio	0.249	0.297	0.039	0.459	0.114	0.494
ECG	0.391	0	0.391	0.391	–	–
All systems	0.585	0.288	0.039	0.99	0	1

Table 3. System F-score and p-value statistics by modality.

The resulting tables can then be used for more closely examining system performance with respect to under and over reporting. High recall systems with low precision [41, 61] seldom miss seizures for addressing the concern of underreporting yet tend to overcompensate and over report seizures due to false alarms. High-precision systems with low recall [54, 62] have the opposite problem and address the concern of over reporting seizures at the risk of missing seizures. High F-score systems [45, 66, 67] have high-precision and recall values and therefore perform well without over or under reporting.

5. Discussion

5.1. Part 1: self-reporting types, priorities, and characteristics

The multiphase structure of our study was instrumental in translating our interviews, literature review, and expert panel findings into effective online survey questions. The key findings included the types, priorities, and characteristics of self-reported data that clinicians need from patients as shown in **Figure 2**.

The remainder of this section highlights notable patient self-reporting challenges as well as subsequent feedback after sharing these findings with clinicians.

5.1.1. Self-reporting availability

Many symptoms and triggers were reported as "useful" but "unavailable" as shown in orange in **Figure 2**. "Academic decline" was said to be unavailable (five out of six respondents). These findings highlight the need for patient data that may already be collected but unavailable to clinicians. Improved interoperability between electronic health records (EHRs) and electronic grading systems could alert clinicians to changes in patient grades during appointments.

5.1.2. Self-reporting difficulty

There were several symptoms and triggers that were reported as "difficult" for patients to report as shown in yellow in **Figure 2**. Notably, "Seizure onset at night" and "excessive sleep movements" were said to be "difficult" to report among most epilepsy specialists (five out of six respondents). These findings highlight the inherent difficulty of patient data collection while sleeping or unconscious. Introducing automated wrist-worn devices such as the Empatica E4 [68] and ActiGraph Link [69] could stand to increase patient self-reporting performance by detecting events such as seizure and unusual sleep movements, while also reducing patient and caregiver data collection burden.

5.1.3. Self-reporting reliability

Next, many symptoms and triggers were reported as being useful but unreliable when self-reported as shown in gray in **Figure 2**. All epilepsy specialists (six out of six respondents) agreed that patient and caregiver reports of patient "memory impairment" were "unreliable".

These findings suggest a need for more reliable and simple patient data collection tools. For example, introducing automated data collection tools could help to increase reliability for clinicians by making data collection more accurate and consistent. The forward auditory Digit Span task, WISC-R subtest [70] could be administered as a smartphone unlock screen for periodically assessing short-term memory.

5.1.4. *Self-reporting desired frequency*

Finally, the majority response for desired patient self-reporting frequency is shown in each column of **Figure 2**. Epilepsy clinicians desired daily reports for over half of all "top 20" indicators (11 out of 20 items). New onset "viral infections" and "status seizures" require immediate medical attention for managing seizure control medications.

Finally, "episodic" patient self-reporting was most frequently desired by psychologists. Many patient behavior changes are highly context driven such as "loss of interest in activities". These findings have implications for displaying patient health dashboards for clinicians within these respective specialties as episodic changes may be more difficult to anticipate than daily, weekly, and monthly data collection on a pre-defined schedule.

5.1.5. *Self-reporting challenges*

Mental health indicators and patient seizure reports may not always be available to clinicians during pediatric epilepsy treatment.

Most notably, suicide attempts were reported as useful, unavailable, and difficult for patients to collect at monthly intervals by all but one clinician. Medication side effects can often trigger depression and there is a high prevalence of depression among patients with epilepsy. If symptoms are known, then clinicians can consider prescribing a seizure control medication that may be less effective but help to stabilize mood. The main challenge for clinicians is that this type of data is often not available or difficult to collect depending on the patient's age and caregiver situation. For example, a primary caregiver may be knowledgeable of the patient's mental health but a patient may be accompanied by an uninformed family member.

The onset of nighttime seizure reports was also reported as useful, unavailable, and difficult for patients to collect at daily intervals by most clinicians. All respondents indicated that patient reports were unreliable due to age and cognition. This reliability is important for treating and thereby helping to reduce the risk of a condition called sudden unexpected death in epilepsy (SUDEP).

These results suggest the need for more reliable and easy to use mental health and seizure reporting tools. For example, automated weekly or monthly validated mental health surveys such as the Personal Health Questionnaire PHQ-9 [71] could be emailed or assessed in clinic on a tablet to increase reliability when it comes to screening for suicide attempts and depression. Finally, clinicians could suggest that patients wear seizure detection wristbands at night for detecting and reporting convulsive type seizures [41].

5.2. Part 2: seizure reporting performance and capabilities

Interviews and our literature review and card sorting exercise with clinicians helped us characterize the types of information that neurologists deem to be the most important during typical stages of epilepsy treatment, how likely they are to have access to this information, and the perceived accuracy of patient reports.

Most neurologists reported having access to EEG reports and verbal descriptions of seizures during treatment. However despite this information, neurologist also expressed a need for more and more detailed characterization of patient movement during seizures and more accurate seizure counts over time.

These needs were then further reflected in our literature review as we explored current methods for characterizing motion during seizures and compared existing patient seizure counting performance to current seizure detection systems. Moreover, our online survey results highlighted two important self-reporting challenges. First, there are limited recording and annotation tools available for characterizing patient motion during seizures. Second, seizure detection systems tend to have false positives and therefore over report seizures. Introducing video capture systems that are triggered by wearable seizure detection sensors may prove beneficial in both cases. More accurate seizure data could, therefore, present new opportunities for informing clinical decisions.

5.2.1. Self-reporting needs

Neurologists reported mixed reliance on patient and caregiver reports when making decisions during treatment. In our questionnaire, 70% of neurologists rated patient and caregiver self-reporting as playing a significant role when determining the best course of AED treatment (4 or greater on a scale of 5), however there was considerable in terms of how frequently these initial self-reports included patient movement characteristics during seizures (SD = 1.10) and/or described the evolution of the seizure over time (SD = 0.78). This finding suggests that, while neurologists perceive self-reporting as important, they also emphasize the need for evaluating the validity of patient reports.

5.2.1.1. Informing initial AED selection

Neurologists from our survey indicated that support for characterizing patient seizure type could be beneficial for selecting the most suitable initial AED based on the patient's seizure symptoms. The survey respondents ranked seizure type and movement characterization as the most important information during the initial diagnosis and AED selection phase. Most respondents had access to EEG reports (7/10) and MRI reports (5/10) and verbal accounts of seizures (80%). Less than one-third of neurologists had access to hospital records, imaging records, blood work, seizure diaries, and video of patient seizure events. Most notably, while all neurologists (10/10) expressed a desire for supplemental video only 3/10 respondents had regular access to such video for informing diagnosis and treatment.

These findings stress a need for capturing additional patient information prior to diagnosis and have implications for patient and caregiver data collection efforts. MRI and EEG may not be available for first-time general practitioner referrals. Initial outpatient EEG sessions tend to be short, ~20 min. Moreover, even with routine activation procedures such as patient hyperventilation, photic stimulation, and sleep withdrawal, many patients may not show symptoms during a single visit and require further observation. It may, therefore, be helpful for patients to collect additional seizure observations such as video recordings prior to initial appointments.

5.2.1.2. Informing AED adjustment

Neurologists ranked seizure frequency as the most important patient self-reported information available to them (100% rated 5 out of a scale of 5) for making AED adjustments. Most neurologists (8/10) estimated that patients failed to report between 40 and 60% of seizures overall (given 5 uniform ranges between 0 and 100%). This estimate agreed with Hoppe et al.'s findings that 55% of patients failed to document 55% of seizures overall [9]. Most neurologists also agreed that an ictal description of a seizure is the most difficult for a patient to report, and 66% of the surveyed neurologists said that patients or caregivers report less than 60% of their seizures. It may, therefore, be helpful to introduce seizure detection devices that address specific patient challenges such as nighttime reporting.

5.2.2. Seizure reporting shortcomings

Major shortcomings of current seizure classification and detection technologies include (1) limited capture and playback solutions for characterizing seizure type and (2) inaccurate seizure detection for counting seizures and limited support for identifying seizure types that do not exhibit limb movement.

5.2.2.1. Limited tools for AED selection

The prospect of developing motion characterization tools for informing initial AED selection remains largely unexplored. Efforts have been limited to active and passive motion tracking as additional feedback for EEG technicians [38, 51]. To date, existing research and commercial systems have not focused on the problem of motor characterization for initial partial versus generalized seizure characterization. There is, therefore, a need to utilize additional video and motion tracking technologies for informing AED selection.

5.2.2.2. Inaccurate seizure counts for AED adjustment

Neurologists from our survey agreed that accurate seizure counts are the most important feedback. In our review, inertial seizure detection systems [43, 45, 46, 72] achieved higher performance than embedded mattress devices [55, 65] and multimodal devices [41]. Inertial devices also tend to support daytime use, while mattress and video systems are often limited nighttime use within bedrooms [47, 65].

High false positive rates remain a problem. More accurate seizure counts could better inform AED treatment. We contend that false positives remain a problem despite studies with higher precision, but fewer numbers of patients [45, 46, 73]. In turn, more work is needed for reducing false positives among all classes that we surveyed. **Table 3** shows that many of the best performing systems utilize video with an average F-score of 0.79 (SD = 0.29) while audio-based systems performed the worse with an average F-score performance of 0.25 (SD = 0.30) with precision as low as 2% for detecting audible lip smacking [61]. High p-values above 0.05 in **Table 3** suggest that mean F-scores for each type of system share a greater than chance probability of performing better than self-reporting at night while low p-values suggest that systems will perform worse than patients during the day on average.

Most systems performed better than patient reporting during the night but notably worse than patients during the day. In our review, all but two systems achieved higher F-score performance at night while only four inertial systems performed better during the day. The average F-score for all systems was 0.59 (SD = 0.29); this reflects a notable improvement over patient self-reporting at night (F-score 0.25) yet remains significantly worse than self-reporting during the day (F-score 0.81). Inertial systems are shown to perform well across both day and nighttime studies [41, 43], however, as noted more work must be done for reducing false alarms during daily activities [40].

High-performance variability was observed between the same types of systems. These discrepancies can largely be explained by the following four contributing factors:

1. **Day versus night:** Many systems were only evaluated at night [55, 65, 73], or strictly during the day, [36] while others were evaluated during the night and day [41–43]. Nighttime studies tended to perform better than daytime studies with an average F-score of 0.62 as compared to 0.56 during studies that included daytime monitoring. This makes direct comparison difficult because daytime seizure detectors must also distinguish non-seizure events such as exercise and teeth brushing which were less prevalent at night. For example, Van De Vel et al.'s [65] evaluation of the Emfit pressure mat highlighted false positives when sitting up in bed, Pisani et al. [47]'s video analysis confused random infant movements, Lockman et al.'s inertial wristband [42] reported false positives during rhythmic activities such as brushing teeth and pen tapping while Poh et al. [41] reported similar false positives during dice rolling and video game activities.

2. **Alerting versus reporting:** Many systems are primarily designed for alerting caregivers rather than accurately reporting seizure counts. Existing commercial systems are designed for alerting caregivers to ongoing seizures [43, 53, 67]. The caregiver is often burdened with adjusting system-specific threshold settings for minimizing false positives [51, 74–75]. This, in turn, may result in missing facial tics and other less apparent symptoms.

3. **Patient age:** We observed considerable variation between the age and number of patients enrolled in studies. For example, Cuppens et al. [73] and Lockman et al. [42] each developed similar inertial-based systems, however, Cuppens et al. [73] studied patients aged 5–16 while Lockman et al. [35] studied ages 3–85. It may be reasonable to expect that differences in muscle development and limb length between these age groups could have resulted in slightly different movement characteristics during seizures.

4. **Patient count:** The number of patients with seizures also varied between studies with a single patient having seizures at night. For example, seven studies had less than four

participants [45, 62, 63, 65, 76–78]. Van De Vel et al. [65] and Narechanie et al. [64] each evaluated pressure sensing mattress inserts, however, Van De Vel et al. [65] included only 1 patient with an F-score of 0.78 while Narechanie et al. [64] included 51 patients with a perfect F-score of 1.0 for reporting seizure counts at night.

5.2.2.3. Limited diversity of seizure types

Most patients have focal types seizures (70%>50%) [80, 81]; however, only some but not all focal seizures involve limb movement. This presents a challenge as most systems to date are limited to measuring seizures based on limb movements. More reliable metrics or a combination of metrics should be studied for capturing non-motor seizure symptoms.

To date, there has been limited work on detecting seizures using non-inertial and video sensors. Bruijne et al. analyzed [61] audio for detecting "lip smacking" and "screams" however; the performance was among the poorest of all the systems that we evaluated (F-score = 0.04). To the best of our knowledge, there are no non-EEG devices for detecting symptoms (e.g. subtle face or hand movement during partial seizures or behavioral arrest).

Inertial seizure detection wristbands [43] and nighttime video recording could provide a promising short-term solution for increasing the accuracy of patient reporting. Most patients are seen by a general practitioner and are later referred to see a neurologist [79]. This gap presents an opportunity to equip patients with data collection systems for detecting and recording patient seizures in the home prior to an initial neurology visit. For example, the open source OpenSeizureDetector [52] inertial wristband could be used in conjunction with an already available and bedroom instrumented camera such as the SAMi [49] or OpenSeizureDetector [50] detect seizures and trigger video recording. In turn, neurologists could review video for characterizing the seizure prior to treatment. Movements during seizures could be captured and reviewed.

Finally, seizure reporting video annotation tools could enable patients, caregivers, and neurologists to label the start and stop of seizure events could improve seizure detection performance over time and address the problem of having to manually adjust thresholds as in commercial products [42, 43] as the system will be trained for a particular individual.

6. Conclusions

The role of clinical patient self-reporting is important yet often undocumented in literature. Health tracking technologies such as wrist-worn seizure detection devices stand to play an increasingly important role in epilepsy treatment and diagnosis as data collection tools that can help patients and caregivers to collect self-report seizure counts and other high priority health indicators for informing clinical decision-making.

In this paper, we conducted a multiphase study that included interviews with clinicians, two literature reviews, a card sorting exercise and online surveys for investigating clinical patient self-reporting needs within the context of epilepsy diagnosis and treatment. In our work with clinicians, we identified a need for more reliable mental health reporting and sleep indicators during epilepsy treatment. In our technology review, we surveyed seven types of seizure detection sensing modalities and identified a strong need for more accurate and reliable seizure reporting and motion characterization during diagnosis and treatment.

The key challenges faced by technology developers and providers are:

1. Identifying the specific types, priorities, and characteristics of data that clinicians need from patients.
2. Establishing the extent that current health tracking devices are suitable for addressing these needs is similarly unknown.

The findings from our research highlighted important patient self-reporting needs among a diverse set of clinicians for epilepsy diagnosis and treatment and in turn, may provide clinicians and technology developers with a useful reference for aligning development efforts with clinical information needs within epilepsy treatment. High false positives remain a problem for seizure detection devices; however low-cost hardware may be able to mitigate these issues. For example, inertial sensors [42] and the bedroom instrumented camera [49] could be sent home with patients prior to treatment; such a combination of tools could be vital information aiding neurologist in how best to treat the patient.

Acknowledgements

This chapter is taken in part from our paper on, "Seizure reporting technologies for epilepsy treatment: A review of clinical information needs and supporting technologies" [24].

Author details

Jonathan Bidwell[1]*, Eliana Kovich[2], Cam Escoffery[3], Cherise Frazier[2] and Elizabeth D. Mynatt[1]

*Address all correspondence to: bidwej@gatech.edu

1 Georgia Institute of Technology, School of Interactive Computing, Atlanta, GA, USA

2 Children's Healthcare of Atlanta, GA, USA

3 Emory University, Rollins School of Public Health, Atlanta, GA, USA

References

[1] Kooiman TJM, Dontje ML, Sprenger SR, Krijnen WP, van der Schans CP, de Groot M. Reliability and validity of ten consumer activity trackers. BMC Sports Science, Medicine and Rehabilitation Oct 2015;7:24

[2] Sayar GH, Tarhan N. Future of psychiatry: Mobile health and social sensing. Journal of Neurobehavioral Sciences. 2016;**3**(2):76-80

[3] Fisher RS. Tracking epilepsy with an electronic diary. Acta Paediatrica. Apr 2010;**99**(4): 516-518

[4] Riviello JJ Jr. Classification of seizures and epilepsy. Current Neurology and Neuroscience Reports. Jul 2003;**3**(4):325-331

[5] Fisher RS, et al. Seizure diaries for clinical research and practice: Limitations and future prospects. Epilepsy and Behavior. Jul 2012;**24**(3):304-310

[6] Blumenfeld H. Impaired consciousness in epilepsy. Lancet Neurology. Sept 2012;**11**(9): 814-826

[7] Blum DE, Eskola J, Bortz JJ, Fisher RS. Patient awareness of seizures. Neurology. Jul 1996;**47**(1):260-264

[8] Kerling F, Mueller S, Pauli E, Stefan H. When do patients forget their seizures? An electroclinical study. Epilepsy and Behavior. Sept 2006;**9**(2):281-285

[9] Hoppe C, Poepel A, Elger CE. Epilepsy: Accuracy of patient seizure counts. Archives of Neurology. Nov 2007;**64**(11):1595-1599

[10] Tatum WO 4th, et al. Outpatient seizure identification: Results of 502 patients using computer-assisted ambulatory EEG. Journal of Clinical Neurophysiology. Jan 2001;**18**(1): 14-19

[11] Shiffman S, Stone AA, Hufford MR. Ecological momentary assessment. Annual Review of Clinical Psychology. 2008;**4**:1-32

[12] Sabaz M, Cairns DR, Lawson JA, Nheu N, Bleasel AF, Bye AM. Validation of a new quality of life measure for children with epilepsy. Epilepsia. Jun 2000;**41**(6):765-774

[13] Rugg-Gunn FJ, Harrison NA, Duncan JS. Evaluation of the accuracy of seizure descriptions by the relatives of patients with epilepsy. Epilepsy Research. Mar 2001;**43**(3):193-199

[14] Detyniecki K, Blumenfeld H. Consciousness of seizures and consciousness during seizures: Are they related?. Epilepsy Behaviour. Jan 2014;**30**:6-9

[15] Fiore-Gartland B, Neff G. Communication, mediation, and the expectations of data: Data valences across health and wellness communities. International Journal of Communication Systems. May 2015;**9**:19

[16] Gorin AA, Stone AA. Recall biases and cognitive errors in retrospective self-reports: A call for momentary assessments. Handbook of Health Psychology. 2001;**23**:405-413

[17] Berenson RA, Horvath J. Confronting the barriers to chronic care management in Medicare. Health Aff. Jan 2003;Suppl Web Exclusives:W3-37-53

[18] Thiele C, Laireiter A-R, Baumann U. Diaries in clinical psychology and psychotherapy: A selective review. Clinical Psychology & Psychotherapy. Jan 2002;**9**(1):1-37

[19] Rogers AE, Caruso CC, Aldrich MS. Reliability of sleep diaries for assessment of sleep/wake patterns. Nursing Research. Nov 1993;**42**(6):368-372

[20] Park SY, Chen Y. Individual and social recognition: Challenges and opportunities in migraine management. In: Proceedings of the 18th ACM Conference on Computer Supported Cooperative Work & Social Computing; Vancouver, BC, Canada; 2015. pp. 1540-1551

[21] Appelboom G, et al. The promise of wearable activity sensors to define patient recovery. Journal of Clinical Neuroscience. Jul 2014;**21**(7):1089-1093

[22] Loring DW, et al. Common data elements in epilepsy research: Development and implementation of the NINDS epilepsy CDE project. Epilepsia Jun 2011;**52**:1186-1191

[23] Coleman K, Austin BT, Brach C, Wagner EH. Evidence on the chronic care model in the new millennium. Health Affairs. Jan 2009;**28**(1):75-85

[24] Bidwell J, Khuwatsamrit T, Askew B, Ehrenberg JA, Helmers S. Seizure reporting technologies for epilepsy treatment: A review of clinical information needs and supporting technologies. Seizure Nov 2015;**32**:109-117

[25] Le S, Shafer PO, Bartfeld E, Fisher RS. An online diary for tracking epilepsy. Epilepsy and Behavior. Dec 2011;**22**(4):705-709

[26] DiIorio C, et al. Evaluation of WebEase: An epilepsy self-management web site. Health Education Research. Apr 2009;**24**(2):185-197

[27] Almalki M, Gray K, Sanchez FM. The use of self-quantification systems for personal health information: Big data management activities and prospects. Health Information Science and Systems. Feb 2015;3(Suppl 1) HISA Big Data in Biomedicine and Healthcare 2013 Conference:S1

[28] Strine TW, Chapman DP. Associations of frequent sleep insufficiency with health-related quality of life and health behaviors. Sleep Medicine. Jan 2005;**6**(1):23-27

[29] Cutting S, Lauchheimer A, Barr W, Devinsky O. Adult-onset idiopathic generalized epilepsy: Clinical and behavioral features. Epilepsia. Nov 2001;**42**(11):1395-1398

[30] Strine TW, Kobau R, Chapman DP, Thurman DJ, Price P, Balluz LS. Psychological distress, comorbidities, and health behaviors among U.S. adults with seizures: Results from the 2002 National Health Interview Survey. Epilepsia. Jul 2005;**46**(7):1133-1139

[31] DeGiorgio CM, et al. Prospective long-term study of vagus nerve stimulation for the treatment of refractory seizures. Epilepsia. Sept 2000;**41**(9):1195-1200

[32] Theodore WH, Fisher RS. Brain stimulation for epilepsy. Lancet Neurology. Feb 2004;**3**(2):111-118

[33] Cunha JPS, Vollmar C, Li Z, Fernandes J, Feddersen B, Noachtar S. Movement quantification during epileptic seizures: A new technical contribution to the evaluation of seizure semiology. Proceedings of the 25th Annual International Conference of the IEEE Engineering in Medicine and Biology Society. 2003;**1**:671-673

[34] Dash D, Hernandez-Ronquillo L, Moien-Afshari F, Tellez-Zenteno JF. Ambulatory EEG: A cost-effective alternative to inpatient video-EEG in adult patients. Epileptic Disorders. Sept 2012;**14**(3):290-297

[35] Rémi J, et al. Quantitative movement analysis differentiates focal seizures characterized by automatisms. Epilepsy and Behavior. Apr 2011;**20**(4):642-647

[36] Nijsen TME, Arends JBAM, Griep PAM, Cluitmans PJM. The potential value of three-dimensional accelerometry for detection of motor seizures in severe epilepsy. Epilepsy and Behavior. Aug 2005;**7**(1):74-84

[37] Panayiotopoulos CP. A Clinical Guide to Epileptic Syndromes and their Treatment. London: Springer; 2010

[38] Li Z, da Silva AM, Cunha JPS. Movement quantification in epileptic seizures: A new approach to video-EEG analysis. IEEE Transactions on Biomedical Engineering. Jun 2002;**49**(6):565-573

[39] Pediaditis M, Tsiknakis M, Leitgeb N. Vision-based motion detection, analysis and recognition of epileptic seizures: A systematic review. Computer Methods and Programs in Biomedicine. Dec 2012;**108**(3):1133-1148

[40] Van de Vel A, et al. Non-EEG seizure-detection systems and potential SUDEP prevention: State of the art. Seizure. Jun 2013;**22**(5):345-355

[41] Poh M-Z, et al. Convulsive seizure detection using a wrist-worn electrodermal activity and accelerometry biosensor. Epilepsia. May 2012;**53**(5):e93-e97

[42] Lockman J, Fisher RS, Olson DM. Detection of seizure-like movements using a wrist accelerometer. Epilepsy and Behavior. Apr 2011;**20**(4):638-641

[43] Beniczky S, Polster T, Kjaer TW, Hjalgrim H. Detection of generalized tonic-clonic seizures by a wireless wrist accelerometer: A prospective, multicenter study. Epilepsia. Apr 2013;**54**(4):e58-e61

[44] Poh M-Z. Continuous Assessment of Epileptic Seizures with Wrist-Worn Biosensors. Massachusetts Institute of Technology; 2011

[45] Schulc E, et al. Measurement and quantification of generalized tonic-clonic seizures in epilepsy patients by means of accelerometry: An explorative study. Epilepsy Research. Jun 2011;**95**(1-2):173-183

[46] Dalton A, et al. Development of a body sensor network to detect motor patterns of epileptic seizures. IEEE Transactions on Biomedical Engineering. Nov 2012;**59**(11):3204-3211

[47] Pisani F, et al. Real-time automated detection of clonic seizures in newborns. Clinical Neurophysiology: Official Journal of the International Federation of Clinical Neurophysiology. 2014;**125**(8):1533-1540

[48] Karayiannis NB, Tao G, Frost JD Jr, Wise MS, Hrachovy RA, Mizrahi EM. Automated detection of videotaped neonatal seizures based on motion segmentation methods.

Clinical Neurophysiology: Official Journal of the International Federation of Clinical Neurophysiology. Jul 2006;**117**(7):1585-1594

[49] SAMi: The Sleep Activity Monitor. July 2014. Available from: https://www.samialert.com/ [Accessed: August: 7, 2017]

[50] Jones G. "OpenSeizureDetector – Free, Open Source Tools to Alert Carers If Someone Suffers an Epileptic Seizure." 2017. Accessed August 7. http://www.openseizuredetector.org.uk/. Jun 2014

[51] Yang X, et al. Motor trajectories in automatisms and their quantitative analysis. Epilepsy Research. Feb 2009;**83**(2-3):97-102

[52] Mangina CA, Beuzeron-Mangina JH. Direct electrical stimulation of specific human brain structures and bilateral electrodermal activity. International Journal of Psychophysiology. Apr 1996;**22**(1-2):1-8

[53] Monitor Stress, Seizures, Activity, Sleep. 2017. Empatica. Accessed August 7. https://www.empatica.com/product-embrace.

[54] Fulton S, Poppel KV, McGregor A, Ellis M, Patters A, Wheless J. Prospective study of 2 bed alarms for detection of nocturnal seizures. Journal of Child Neurology. Nov 2013;**28**(11):1430-1433

[55] Carlson C, Arnedo V, Cahill M, Devinsky O. Detecting nocturnal convulsions: Efficacy of the MP5 monitor. Seizure. Apr 2009;**18**(3):225-227

[56] Ramgopal S, et al. Seizure detection, seizure prediction, and closed-loop warning systems in epilepsy. Epilepsy and Behavior. Aug 2014;**37**:291-307

[57] Pavlova M. et al. Advantages of respiratory monitoring during video-EEG evaluation to differentiate epileptic seizures from other events. Epilepsy and Behavior. Mar 2014;32142-32144

[58] Jeppesen J, et al. Heart rate variability analysis indicates preictal parasympathetic overdrive preceding seizure-induced cardiac dysrhythmias leading to sudden unexpected death in a patient with epilepsy. Epilepsia. Jul 2014;**55**(7):e67-e71

[59] Lamberts RJ, Thijs RD, Laffan A, Langan Y, Sander JW. Sudden unexpected death in epilepsy: People with nocturnal seizures may be at highest risk. Epilepsia. Feb 2012;**53**(2):253-257

[60] Poh M-Z, et al. Autonomic changes with seizures correlate with postictal EEG suppression. Neurology. Jun 2012;**78**(23):1868-1876

[61] de Bruijne GR, Sommen PCW, Aarts RM. Detection of epileptic seizures through audio classification. In 4th European Conference of the International Federation for Medical and Biological Engineering, Springer Berlin Heidelberg; 2009. pp. 1450-1454

[62] van Elmpt WJC, Nijsen TME, Griep PAM, Arends JAM. A model of heart rate changes to detect seizures in severe epilepsy. Seizure. Sept 2006;**15**(6):366-375

[63] Conradsen I, Beniczky S, Wolf P, Jennum P, Sorensen HBD. Evaluation of novel algorithm embedded in a wearable sEMG device for seizure detection. Conference Proceedings: Annual International Conference of the IEEE Engineering in Medicine and Biology Society. 2012;**2012**:2048-2051

[64] Narechania AP, Garić II, Sen-Gupta I, Macken MP, Gerard EE, Schuele SU. Assessment of a quasi-piezoelectric mattress monitor as a detection system for generalized convulsions. Epilepsy and Behavior. Aug 2013;**28**(2):172-176

[65] Van de Vel A, Verhaert K, Ceulemans B. Critical evaluation of four different seizure detection systems tested on one patient with focal and generalized tonic and clonic seizures. Epilepsy and Behavior. Aug 2014;**37**:91-94

[66] Cuppens K, Lagae L, Ceulemans B, Van Huffel S, Vanrumste B. Automatic video detection of body movement during sleep based on optical flow in pediatric patients with epilepsy. Medical and Biological Engineering and Computing. Sept 2010;**48**(9):923-931

[67] Lu H, Pan Y, Mandal B, Eng H-L, Guan C, Chan DWS. Quantifying limb movements in epileptic seizures through color-based video analysis. IEEE Transactions on Biomedical Engineering. Feb 2013;**60**(2):461-469

[68] Real-time physiological signals—E4 EDA/GSR sensor. Empatica [Online]. Available from: https://www.empatica.com/e4-wristband [Accessed: February 02, 2017]

[69] Enzo RTS, Culiolo A. ActiGraph Link|ActiGraph [Online]. Available from: http://actigraphcorp.com/products-showcase/activity-monitors/actigraph-link/ [Accessed: February 02, 2017]

[70] Wechsler D. Manual for the Wechsler Intelligence Scale for Children, Revised. New York: Psychological Corporation; 1974

[71] Kroenke K, Spitzer RL. The PHQ-9: A new depression diagnostic and severity measure. Psychiatric Annals. 2002;**32**(9):509-515

[72] Kramer U, Kipervasser S, Shlitner A, Kuzniecky R. A novel portable seizure detection alarm system: Preliminary results. Journal of Clinical Neurophysiology. Feb 2011;**28**(1):36-38

[73] Cuppens K, et al.Accelerometry-based home monitoring for detection of nocturnal hypermotor seizures based on novelty detection. IEEE Journal of Biomedical and Health Informatics. May 2014;**18**(3):1026-1033

[74] AREMCO. Disability World. November 2014. Available from: http://www.disability-world.com/co/company.php?ID=3460 [Accessed: August 07, 2017]

[75] Movement Monitor. EMFIT Corporation. July 2014. Available from: http://emfitcorp.com/shop_usa/fin/movement_monitor-p-1-0/ [Accessed: August 07, 2017]

[76] Cattani L, Ntonfo GMK, Lofino F, Ferrari G, Raheli R, Pisani F. Maximum-likelihood detection of neonatal clonic seizures by video image processing. In 2014 8th International Symposium on Medical Information and Communication Technology (ISMICT); 2014. pp. 1-5

[77] Cuppens K, et al. Using spatio-temporal interest points (STIP) for myoclonic jerk detection in nocturnal video. Conference Proceedings: Annual International Conference of the IEEE Engineering in Medicine and Biology Society. 2012;**2012**:4454-4457

[78] Jallon P. A Bayesian approach for epileptic seizures detection with 3D accelerometers sensors. Conference Proceedings: Annual International Conference of the IEEE Engineering in Medicine and Biology Society. 2010;**2010**:6325-6328

[79] McKee PJ, Wilson EA, Dawson JA, Larkin JG, Brodie MJ. Managing seizures in the casualty department. BMJ. Apr 1990;**300**(6730):978-979

[80] Rao, Vikram R, Hixson JD. Acknowledgements. 2017. Focal Seizures. http://bestpractice.bmj.com/best-practice/monograph/544/basics/epidemiology.html [Accessed August 7]

[81] Epilepsy by the Numbers: Facts, Statistics, and You. Healthline. October 20.2014. http://www.healthline.com/health/epilepsy/facts-statistics-infographic

[82] Van de Vel A et al. Long-term home monitoring of hypermotor seizures by patient-worn accelerometers. Epilepsy & Behavior. 2013;**26**(1):118-125

[83] Nijsen TME, Aarts RM, Cluitmans PJM, Griep PAM. Time-frequency analysis of accelerometry data for detection of myoclonic seizures. IEEE Transactions on Information Technology in Biomedicine

[84] Nijsen TME, Aarts RM, Johan BA, Cluitmans PJM. Automated detection of tonic seizures using 3-D accelerometry. In: 4th European Conference of the International Federation for Medical and Biological Engineering; 2009. pp. 188-191

[85] Nijsen TME, Cluitmans PJM, Arends JBAM, Griep PAM. Detection of subtle nocturnal motor activity from 3-D accelerometry recordings in epilepsy patients. IEEE Transactions on Biomedical Engineering. 2007;**54**(11):2073-2081

8

Subarachnoid Cysticercosis and Ischaemic Stroke in Epileptic Patients

Humberto Foyaca-Sibat and
Lourdes de Fátima Ibañez-Valdés

Abstract

Whether subarachnoid neurocysticercosis (SNCC) induces ischaemic stroke (IS) in epileptic patients is not yet confirmed because only short-case series and anecdotal case reports have been published, and no observational studies exist in the literature to date. Our main goals are: to estimate the prevalence of ischaemic stroke in epileptic patients presenting with SNCC and stroke frequency among HIV-positive patients in three subgroups; to determine if the odds of ischaemic stroke are elevated in SNCC-epileptic patients compared to epileptic patients with intraparenchymal NCC (INCC); to determine whether the risk for stroke is elevated in HIV-seropositive patients presenting with SNCC or INCC and epilepsy; and to evaluate if and when the potential interaction varies by location of NCC in the brain (intraparenchymal or subarachnoid). Eligible epileptic patients' seropositive status was recorded, and cross-associations for the independent variables (NCC status and HIV status) and outcome variables (ischaemic stroke event) were performed. Compared to the reference group, the odds of IS in PLWNCC were 2.0 and 2.6 times greater in patients with SNCC and INCC, respectively. The frequency of IS was greater in HIV-positive patients in all three groups, but the risk was especially pronounced when seropositive epileptic patients were both NCC groups when compared with the reference group. Subarachnoid NCC increased the risk of IS three time more.

Keywords: neurocysticercosis, stroke, epilepsy, cross-sectional study, subarachnoid neurocysticercosis, HIV, imagenology

1. Introduction

1.1. Background

Neurocysticercosis (NCC) is a preventable and potentially eradicable neurological disease caused by the larva form of tapeworm *Taenia solium* which primarily affects people living in the developing world. Seizures are widely reported to be the most common symptom, occurring in 70–90% of patients [1]. Most patients respond to praziquantel, if cystic lesions are located in the parenchymal tissue, and albendazole when parasites are located in the ventricular system and subarachnoid space, including patients with an associated HIV infection [2]. A well-designed clinical trial about treatment response in subarachnoid neurocysticercosis (SNCC) has not been published; however, some authors have reported the effectiveness of these drugs in SNCC [3–5], while others have found that parasites remain alive at the subarachnoid space even after high dose of albendazole/praziquantel/prednisone was administered [6–10].

In 1977, Gubbay and Matz [11] reported two cases presenting with intracranial hypertension (ICH) and hydrocephalus in association with chronic meningitis; the authors confirmed that repeated CSF analysis may result in diagnostic confirmation of SNCC causing ICH with hemiparesis, partial seizures, and other neurological signs. Currently, it is well known that SNCC in the basal cisterns may cause inflammatory reaction; the leptomeninges become fibrotic at the base of the brain.

According to Takayanagui and Odashima [12], in approximately 60% of the cases, there is an obstruction of the CSF circulation, resulting in hydrocephalus and raised intracranial pressure. When hydrocephalus secondary to cysticercoid meningitis is present, the mortality rate is high (50%) and most patients die within 2 years after CSF shunting; therefore, ventricular and basal cisternal locations are considered to be malignant forms of NCC. In 2001, Bannur and Rajshekhar [13] reported a case as an example of difficulty in confirming diagnosis: this patient had a hypodense non-enhancing mass on CT scan in the regions of quadrigeminal cistern causing obstructive hydrocephalus. He was initially diagnosed with an epidermoid mass but subsequent MRI evaluation and surgery resulted in the diagnosis of a racemose cysticercus cyst. Authors concluded that clinical features of NCC largely depend on the number, type, size, localisation and stage of development of cysticerci, as well as on the host immune response against the parasite [13].

Typical of South Africa, high incidence and prevalence of NCC is found at the former Transkei, currently region C and D of Eastern Cape Province, which is the most disadvantaged region countrywide [14–18].

Many people in the world who suffer a fatal stroke live in developing countries where NCC is endemic. However, prevalence of several tropical diseases, including NCC, is likely to increase in Western, industrialised nations as a result of demographic changes due to migratory flows. It is very well known that stroke is the third most cause of death and the principal cause of adult disability worldwide. Cerebrovascular complications of NCC include transient ischaemic attacks, ischaemic strokes due to infective vasculitis and intraparenchymal haemorrhage [19, 20].

Several case reports about cerebral infarction related to cysticercosis have been published, including angiographic abnormalities [21–27].

In our region, there are other infectious diseases causing infective vasculitis leading to ischaemic stroke such as HIV/AIDS, tuberculosis, INCC and neurosyphilis, but Chagas disease, malaria, haemorrhagic fever, infective endocarditis and mucormycosis are also reported in the medical literature [28, 29].

In 2001, Rocha et al. [30] reported three cases of stroke secondary to NCC. The first one was a 36-year-old man with bilateral middle cerebral artery occlusions presenting an acute right hemiparesis and expressive aphasia. MRI demonstrated several enhancing subarachnoid cysts surrounding the occluded vessels, a right parietal racemose cyst and a left temporal large infarction area. Angiographic study showed total occlusion of left middle cerebral artery and a subtotal occlusion of right middle cerebral artery. The second one was a 42-year-old man with vasculitis of small cortical vessels presenting headache, seizures and focal neurological deficit. CT scan demonstrated several calcifications and a left temporal infarct. Cerebral angiographic study was normal. The third case was a woman, 53 years old, with a past history of six stroke events, behaviour disturbance and seizures. MRI scan demonstrated several cortical and sub-cortical infarcts and cisternal cystic lesions, and angiographic study showed diffuse arteritis of basilar and carotid arterial system. In all three cases, CSF study showed linfomonocitic pleocytosis and positive ELISA for cysticercosis.

Aditya et al. [31] in 2004 reported two autopsied cases of chronic cysticercal basal arachnoiditis causing large arterial territory infarcts and, in the second case, a hypothalamic mass. Both patients were diagnosed and managed, clinically and by neuroimaging, as stroke and neurotuberculosis, respectively. The diagnosis was established only at autopsy, which revealed NCC causing basal arachnoiditis, major vessel vasculitis and infarcts. Histologically, one case showed degenerating racemose cysticercal cyst within the thick basal exudates. In the second case, remnants of the degenerated cysticercal cyst in the form of hooklets and calcareous corpuscles were identified within the giant cell inciting a granulomatous response to form a hypothalamic mass lesion mimicking tuberculoma. They highlighted the importance of considering the non-tuberculous aetiology of chronic basal arachnoiditis like SNCC before initiating therapy, especially in countries where both NCC and tuberculosis are endemic.

Conspicuously absent in the case reports available in the current medical literature are the following research questions: What is the prevalence of SNCC in patients living with neurocysticercosis (PLWNCC)? Is SNCC a risk factor for ischaemic stroke? Does HIV comorbidity increases the stroke frequency in epileptic patients infected with NCC? The main aim of this study is to explore these inquiries and propose new hypotheses for future study.

1.2. Our study

We performed a non-published cross-sectional study of epileptic patients diagnosed with NCC from January 1999 to December 2003 at Umtata General Hospital and from January 2004 to January 2010 at Nelson Mandela Academic Hospital from the rural areas of Mthatha, South Africa. Selected patients for a case–control study under the project: 'Neurocysticercosis' were taken for this research.

All patients were classified into one of the three respective sample groups according to presence and type of NCC or not, collected in groups A, B and C. All patients from Group A met the following selection criteria (inclusion criteria): a positive serology ELISA test for cysticercosis, CT scan of the brain with intravenous contrast enhancement consistent with definitive evidence of cystic lesion (isolate or racemose) in the subarachnoid space without hydrocephalus and suitable to evaluate: (1) focal arachnoiditis when there was contrast enhancement in only one cerebral basal cistern; (2) bilateral cystic lesions with diffuse arachnoiditis, in which contrast enhancement involved several basal cisterns; and (3) ischaemic infarction, in which the number and location of cerebral lesions were analysed and classified as superficial, deep no lacunar (>16 mm), and deep lacunar (<15 mm) at the basal ganglia, without an associated cardiac disease. Demographic and associated stroke were analysed in accordance with the presence of SNCC, and ELISA test for HIV when it was done.

From the large number of epileptic patients with NCC-HIV co-infection in our database, we selected only a few number of epileptic cases for Group B similar to Group A, regarding age and gender to assure a better statistical analysis and under an absolute diagnosis of intraparenchymal NCC (both active and calcified at the same time) with or without ischaemic stroke. The ELISA test for NCC and HIV were both positive. Patients in Group C had no NCC in any presentation and, ELISA test for NCC was negative and HIV test was positive.

Exclusion criteria: All patients with gross modifiable risk factors for stroke such as uncontrolled hypertension and diabetes mellitus, heavy drinkers or smokers, familial hyperlipidaemia, thrombophilia, bleeding disorders and other haematological disorders were excluded. We also excluded patients with heart problems, diagnosis of infective vasculitis apart from those associated with NCC/HIV, suspicion of primary or secondary arterial disease, cognitive or sensory deterioration, patients who have not had check-ups for their NCC/SNCC and stroke for more than 11 months, patients with intraventricular NCC and/or associated hydrocephalus; patients with terminal illnesses, serious psychological illnesses, active addictions to psychoactive substances; patients younger than 13 years old; pregnant patients; patients living with HIV/AIDS in stage IV, patients who have lived more than 6 months outside of our region, the 'first or worst' headache, headaches with increasing frequency or severity, progressive headache, chronic daily headache, headaches always on the same side, headache not responding to treatment, new-onset headaches in patients who have cancer or who were tested positive for HIV infection and new-onset headaches after age 45.

All statistical analyses were conducted using Statistical Package for the Social Sciences (SPSS) version 16.0 for Windows (SPSS Inc., Chicago, Ill). Analyses were performed using an intention to treat bias. A descriptive analysis and an analysis of baseline comparability between the study groups were performed for all study variables. The main variables are INCC, SNCC, IS and headache. All patients were epileptic and HIV reactive. To investigate the potential associations between ischaemic stroke outcomes and the variables of NCC group type and HIV status, prevalence odds ratio and 95% confidence intervals were calculated.

Written consent forms were administered in the first contact with the eligible patients following verbal agreement for participation. For all patients, information on the study's purpose and procedures was provided in addition to ethical considerations, including the participant's right to intimacy, anonymity, confidentiality, withdrawal and information. Due to the large proportion of low literacy among the patient population, oral consent was observed and confirmed by an impartial witness in many cases where necessary. For patients selected between 1999 and 2002 only oral consent was taken.

All investigators completed CITI training course on the protection of human research. All are sworn to the Hippocratic Oath and committed to respecting the norms of good clinical practice, as well as the requirements of the Helsinki Declaration.

Methods for patient selection and information processing were approved by clinical governance at Umtata General Hospital, and the research protocol was evaluated and approved by Mthatha Umtata General Hospital, University of Transkei and Walter Sisulu University IRB and the respective Ethical Committees (UGH:0001/99, UNITRA:0018/05 and WSU:0068/009).

Out of 459 eligible epileptic patients asked to participate, five initially refused to participate for the baseline evaluation. Four out of the five patients agreed to participate during their follow-up appointment and their data are included here.

The proportion of SNCC without hydrocephalus in PLWNCC (Groups A and B) was 4.77%.

Group A (n = 144) and B (n = 153) showed no remarkable differences between age, gender and HIV status. The control group C (n = 161) consisted of 35.1-year-old-mean age (SD 15.4), 43.5% were males (n = 70) and 56.5% were female (n = 91) and the frequency of HIV positive (stage I–II, 11.2%) almost similar to Groups A and B (**Table 1**).

In total, 243 serial CT scans with at least one scan (range = 1–2) per subject were available in Group A, 201 CT scans in Group B and 162 CT scans in Group C, over the 10-year study period.

Table 2 shows the frequencies of ischaemic stroke events in SNCC and INCC (Groups A and B) and the reference sample (Group C) without considering HIV status.

Table 2 shows the frequency and odds ratio of IS events in each NCC group (as previously discussed) now stratified by HIV seropositive status. HIV-positive patients in Groups A and B had greater odds of IS compared to the HIV-positive patients without NCC co-infection as expected. However, the increased odds were more pronounced in those HIV patients with SNCC (OR: 2.66, 95% CI). The risk of IS in HIV-negative patients followed similar trend with the greatest odds occurring in SNCC group patients comparatively. The risk of developing stroke was 2.82 times more probable in Group A compared with Group B. (**Table 2** and **Figure 1**). This suggests that although co-infection with HIV increases risk of IS, the location of NCC in the brain is a

Groups	Age	Gender (%)		HIV (%)		
	Mean (SD)	Male	Female	+	–	Unknown
A (144)	38.2 (16.9)	52.1	47.9	13.9	31.2	54.9
B (153)	36.9 (15.3)	47.7	52.3	15.7	28.8	55.6
C (161)	35.1 (15.4)	43.5	56.5	11.2	28.0	60.9

Table 1. Patient characteristics by sample group.

Groups	Stroke		Total
	Yes	No	
A	23(15.97%)	121(84.02%)	144
B	14(9.15%)	139(90.84%)	153
C	4(2.48%)	157(97.51%)	161

Table 2. Frequency of stroke by groups.

better predictor of IS risk than comorbidity status. This is also evident in a similar difference in odds ratio for HIV- compared HIV+ were exhibited in Groups A and B. These results also suggest that the interactive effect of co-infection is generalised and do not vary significantly for one type of NCC.

Taking into consideration the HIV status of patients by groups, we found that 40% of patients presented ischaemic stroke (Group A) and the risk to develop an IS among Groups A and B is almost three times more.

After comparing all three groups with similar age, gender and HIV-positive status, the risk of developing an IS increases to more than seven times in patients presenting SNCC over the control group and almost four times in patients presenting intraparenchymal NCC, as shown in **Table 4**.

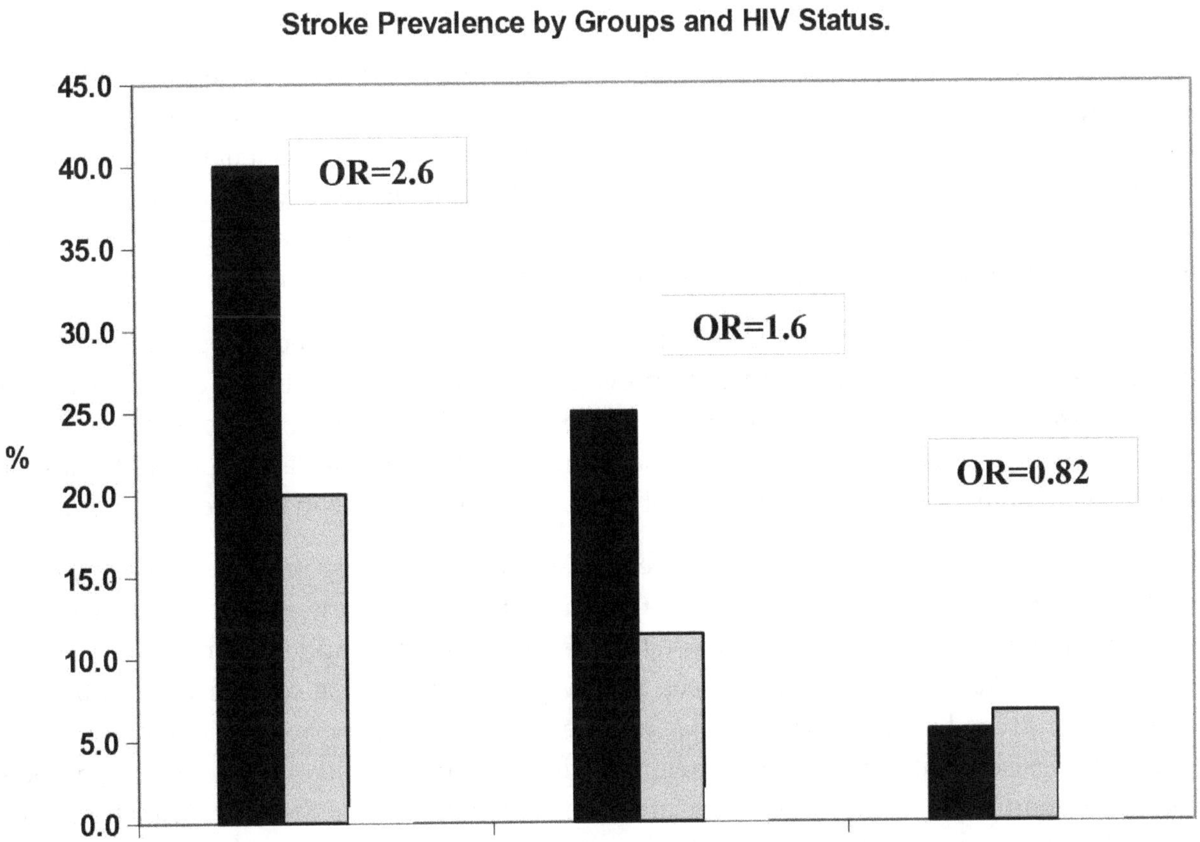

Figure 1. Shows prevalence of stroke by groups and HIV status. *Source*: **Table 3**.

HIV status	Groups	Stroke (%)	OR	
			(95% CI)	
				A vs. B
+	A	40.0 (n = 20)	2.66 (n = 23)	2.82
	B	25.0 (n = 24)	2.60 (n = 14)	
	C	5.6 (n = 18)	0.82 (n = 4)	
–	A	20.0 (n = 121)		
	B	11.4 (n = 139)		
	C	6.7 (n = 157)		

Table 3. Proportion of patients with IS events by groups and HIV status.

Groups	OR	IC 95%	
A vs. C	7.46	2.51	22.1
A vs. B	1.88	1.33	3.82
B vs. C	3.95	1.27	12.2

Table 4. Odds ratio after comparing different groups.

Concurrent infection with *T. solium* and HIV was expected to occur more frequently because of the increasing frequency of HIV infection in endemic areas of cysticercosis like our region. However, little is known about the influence of HIV infection on the frequency and the clinical course of cysticercosis. Delobel et al. [32] established that giant cysts and racemose forms of neurocysticercosis seem to be more frequent in HIV-infected patients and may be secondary to an uncontrolled parasitic growth because of an impaired cell-mediated immune response.

Prevalence on SNCC in patients LWNCC is not as higher as we expected but can represent the frequency of this problem, while the prevalence of HIV is increasing in countries where NCC is also endemic. Therefore, sooner or later SNCC will be highest, if adequate measures are not taken to eradicate NCC at due time. Other co-infection rates are expected to raise it but unfortunately no systematic reviews of the subject are available in the medical literature.

In spite of the variety of ways used by the parasite to modify host immune response, their mechanism of excretory/secretory product fail and its anti-immune properties are weaker, paradoxically these pathologic changes on the parasite membrane and the surrounding tissue (without remarkable oedema) can be seen in HIV patients with CD4 count around 350 cells/mm^3 and viral load around 55,000 copies/ml or even in window period. Therefore, we have had hypothesised that at the colloid stage, there is an increased microglial activation, associated oligodendrocyte, astroglial changes and subsequent damage of the axonal functions and blood–brain barrier, which can explain the well-known mechanism of *pathological concentration of macrophage histocompatibility complex, interleukin-1 and -6 and tumour necrosis factor-alpha among other neurotoxins causing neurovascular lesions, accompanied by increased concentration of pro-inflammatory molecules from meningeal macrophages, choroids plexus macrophages, perivascular macrophages, multinucleated giant cells, according to the number and location of the cysticercus as previously described* [33]. *At the present moment, we believe that toxins released by the T. solium cysticercus cause inflammatory changes on the perforating arteries (toxic vasculitis?) at the subarachnoid space rather than a direct effect on the cluster of parasites (mechanical compression). However, the differential of infective vasculitis should be preserved because pathological source is the presence of intracranial cysticercosis.*

In our series, we did not identify any case presenting immune reconstitution inflammatory syndrome, probably because we selected patients from stage I to III of AIDS not on HAART. It is interesting to know that in the brain of patients with ischaemic stroke-associated deaths, there are abundant CD3+, CD8+ and CD68+ cells in the postmortem autopsy [34]. In our study, only one patient died from Group A. We believe that low mortality rate may be related to the exclusion of patients with subarachnoid cysticercosis growing to giant size causing mass effect and obstructive hydrocephalus with mechanical compression, as already discussed [33]. The disease course in SNCC is often long in duration and cysticerci continue to grow and proliferate through tissue. This increase in volume and mechanical resistance from the brain parenchymal may cause osmotic exchange with the CSF and this one factor that may lead to a poor prognosis [35]. Obviously, selecting patients before this stage can help to investigate the effect of the SNCC on the blood vessels without an effect of associated mechanical compression.

Evidence of carotid occlusion in cysticercosis [23, 36, 37], transient ischaemic attack of the vertebrobasilar territory [38] even in children [39] has been reported as anecdotic cases.

The most common affected vascular territory in our series was middle cerebral artery followed by posterior cerebral artery. We did not confirm any patients with SNCC and ischaemic infarct on the anterior cerebral artery territory and only one case has been reported in the medical literature [40].

Haemorrhagic stroke (intracerebral or subarachnoid) associated with NCC and HIV was not selected in our series and some cases reported in the medical literature are not certain [41, 42]. We will investigate the association of haemorrhagic stroke and SNCC in a forthcoming research. Strengths of our study include the large sample size, geographically distinct locations of the participating clinics from the former Transkei in rural South Africa, and potential feasibility of its replication in similar regions worldwide.

Weaknesses of this study include the exclusion of a number of variables that may have contributed to the analysis, such as patient's response to anti-parasitic treatment and the degree of immune compromise. Better reporting of HIV status is also necessary, as over half of the patients selected were HIV-status unknown. In our study, the prevalence of SNCC without hydrocephalus in patients living with NCC is 4.77%.

Risk for ischaemic stroke in patients with subarachnoid NCC is almost three times more for patients with intraparenchymal NCC. Comorbidity of subarachnoid NCC in HIV-positive patients increases up to 7.6-fold.

2. Racemose neurocysticercosis

Racemose neurocysticercosis (RC) also known as SNCC refers to a very uncommon form of NCC, with the cyst localised mainly in the subarachnoid space and basal cisterns. Usually, the scolex is absent and multiple complex small cysts may form (cluster of grapes), filling the basal cisterns, determining mass effect and distortion of adjacent structures, namely sulci, brainstem and cranial nerves [43–45], these authors consider that in racemose NCC, there is a presence of abnormally large growths of many cystic membranes without a scolex, normally without enhancement, in subarachnoid space and basal cisterns and they found on imagenology that the cysts have a thin wall without a scolex; their signal is isointense or slightly different from CSF, hypointense on T1-weighted images (T1-WIs) and fluid-attenuated inversion recovery (FLAIR), hyperintense on T2-WI, without diffusion restriction, and after contrast there is no wall enhancement. A three-dimensional balanced steady-state free precession sequence (constructive interference in steady state (CISS)), driven equilibrium (DRIVE) or contrast-enhanced MR cisternography helps to detect the underlying cysts [46]. Pamplona et al. [46] reported a case of a *43-year-old woman from Cabo Verde, with an eight-month history of right frontotemporal headaches (without releasing or aggravating factors), ataxia and loss of vision, without significant past medical history of note and no history of head trauma. Home hospital computed tomography (CT) disclosed a large intraventricular cyst, without enhancement after ionic contrast administration, distorting lateral and third ventricles, with obliterations of Monro foramina, determining non-communicating hydrocephalus, with enlargement of occipital and temporal horns of lateral ventricles and ependimary transudation.* They established that *racemose neurocysticercosis (INCC) refers to cysts in the subarachnoid space and is characterised by proliferative lobulated cysts without a scolex.* We also agree with such definition if the presence of scolex is not excluded from the definition, as discussed later. These cysts may vary in size, from 2 to 3 mm in subarachnoid space and basal cisterns, to a few centimetres when intraventricular. Intracranial hypertension and hydrocephalus are two complications that happen when there is a flow obstruction due to intraventricular cysts, arachnoiditis, ependymitis secondary to inflammatory response or mass effect in cases of very large cysts [44, 45].

It is known that in the next several months to years, there is degeneration of the cyst, with associated inflammatory response and peripheral oedema, leading to clinical symptoms and manifestations that may vary according to localisation and mass effect [43–45]. The final stage (calcified) with or without associated oedema is seen in the intraparenchymal presentation and is the main cause of epilepsy in this series; obviously, associated oedema never happens at the subarachnoid space.

The differential diagnosis depends on where the cysts are localised; if in the subarachnoid space and basal cysterns, the differential diagnoses are arachnoid cysts, neuroglial cysts, gliomas, cavernous malformations and echinococcal cysts.

Detection of cysticercal antigens by monoclonal antibody-based enzyme-linked immunosorbent assay (ELISA) in the CSF of clinically suspected patients supports the diagnosis of active SNCC.

3. Stroke

Almost all clinical presentations of stroke can be seen in epileptic patients having SNCC [27, 41, 46–65]. Despite the increasing number of reports on haemorrhagic stroke to the medical literature [19, 20, 23, 24, 26, 27, 29–31, 37–41, 47–62], the prevalence of stroke secondary to NCC remains higher in IS secondary to infectious vasculitis. The most common clinical manifestations of NCC are seizure and headaches. In addition, cysticerci may cause mass effect, obstructive hydrocephalus, intracranial hypertension, cerebral infarction, vasculitis and meningitis [66, 67]. Seizures are more common in intraparenchymal NCC, resulting from cystic perilesional inflammation, new infarcts and vasculitis. Acute encephalitis-like presentation is rare, but can be the first symptom in the paediatric population [66]. Cerebrovascular complications of NCC include lacunar infarction, large-vessel disease, transient ischaemic attacks, progressive midbrain syndrome and brain haemorrhage, resulting from a multiplicity of mechanisms, including luminal narrowing due to sub-intimal cushions, vasospasm due to arteritis in midsized and small perforating vessels of the brain, and fresh thrombi [44, 45].

In our region, the incidence and prevalence of ischaemic stroke due to infectious vasculitis is higher in HIV patients compared with other causes of infectious vasculitis because HIV/AIDS is more common than other mentioned infectious diseases, at the present moment. Tuberculosis (TB) of the CNS and neurosyphilis are not uncommon problems. Unfortunately, the worse prognosis is reserved for HIV/AIDS followed by TB, neurosyphilis and others.

Stroke as a complication of NCC occurs in a very small percentage of cases, mostly involving small perforating vessels while major intracranial vessel involvement is extremely rare. Coleman et al. [47] also reported two autopsied cases of chronic cysticercal basal arachnoiditis causing large arterial territory infarcts and, in the second case, a hypothalamic mass. In their patient, *the diagnosis was established only at autopsy, which revealed SNCC causing basal arachnoiditis, major vessel vasculitis and infarcts. Histologically, case 1 showed degenerating racemose cysticercal cyst within the thick basal exudate. In the second case, remnants of the degenerated cysticercal cyst in the form of hooklets and calcareous corpuscles were identified within the giant cell inciting a granulomatous response to form a hypothalamic mass lesion mimicking tuberculoma.* These authors highlighted the importance of considering the non-tuberculous aetiologies of chronic basal arachnoiditis like SNCC before initiating therapy especially in countries endemic to both NCC and tuberculosis.

> Other authors [48, 49] reported stroke *as a recognised complication of NCC, occurring in 2–12% of cases, mostly in the form of small lacunar infarcts and informed about a 51-year-old Hispanic woman, which was secondary to complete occlusion of the left internal carotid and bilateral anterior cerebral arteries. Their report represents the third reported case of internal carotid artery occlusion and the first reported case of anterior cerebral artery occlusion secondary to neurocysticercosis at that time.* Another author [50] considered that ischaemic stroke *is a relatively common but under-recognised complication of NCC and it is usually caused by inflammatory occlusion of the arteries at the base of the brain secondary to cysticercotic arachnoiditis. In most cases, the involved vessels are of small diameter and the neurological picture is limited to a lacunar syndrome secondary to a small cerebral infarct. However, large infarcts related to the occlusion of the middle cerebral artery or even the internal carotid artery have also been reported* [50]. Viola et al. [57] reported a patient

who *presented with relapsed subarachnoid haemorrhage possibly linked to NCC.* In addition, they performed a *literature review of all of the reported cases of aneurysmal and non-aneurysmal haemorrhagic cerebrovascular events associated with NCC until year 2011 and identified 11 such cases. The majority of the individuals were young males (mean: 38 years; 70% males). Four cases (36%) had aneurysms. Four (36%) others had negative cerebral angiograms and therefore classified as non-aneurysmal, while the remaining three (28%) did not report sufficient information to classify them. All cases with aneurysmal haemorrhage underwent successful surgical repair of the aneurysms. Seven patients received albendazole (including three who have had surgery). Three patients died; all three presented in the pre-albendazole era.* In summary, NCC should be considered in the differential diagnosis of haemorrhagic cerebrovascular events in young patients without classical vascular risk factors who have lived or visited NCC endemic areas [57].

In 1998, using cerebral arteriography Barinagarrementeria and Cantú [27] studied 28 patients (mean age, 37 years) with subarachnoid cysticercosis admitted to their hospital from July 1993 to February 1996 and found that *15 patients had angiographic evidence of cerebral arteritis (53%); 12 of the 15 had a stroke syndrome (P = .02). Eight of the 15 patients (53%) with cerebral arteritis had evidence of cerebral infarction on MRI.* In that series, *the most commonly involved vessels were the middle cerebral artery and the posterior cerebral artery*, as we already discussed [33]. They concluded that *the frequency of cerebral arteritis in subarachnoid cysticercosis was higher than previously reported, and middle size vessel involvement is a common finding, even in those patients without clinical evidence of cerebral ischaemia.*

Some authors [58, 62] consider that NCC *is a disease with protean manifestations, which depends upon the number of parasites, their location and the degree of host inflammatory response. Most common clinical manifestations include late onset epilepsy or symptoms of intracranial hypertension and cerebrovascular complications have been reported to occur in 4–12% of patients* [58, 62]. In the majority of their cases, the diagnoses were ischaemic cerebrovascular events associated with vasculitis and/or thrombosis from surrounding cysts in both small- and large-diameter vessels. *Subarachnoid haemorrhages have been noted in SNCC and have been associated with cerebral aneurysms in some, but not all, cases* [58, 61]. Inflammatory aneurysms are usually located at distal intracranial arteries, not at bifurcations like congenital aneurysms, and are more commonly fusiform in shape. The wall of inflammatory aneurysms and parent vessels are extremely friable, and the possibility of intraoperative rupture is higher; in addition, inflammatory aneurysms are fusiform in shape so clipping of the aneurysm neck while preserving the parent artery is technically challenging [61]. As a result, *they are generally secured by wrapping* [59], *clipping of the proximal artery* [64] *or trapping* [61]. Obviously, SNCC should be considered in the differential diagnosis of aneurysmal and non-aneurysmal haemorrhagic stroke events in all patients living in regions where NCC is endemic.

4. Imagenology

Based on our experience, imagenology is the investigation of choice for confirmation of SNCC. MRI scan is better than CT scan to identify intraventricular NCC and CT is better to confirm calcified intraparenchymal NCC, and both can be used for confirmation of SNCC but

CT scan costs less; for establishing the stage of NCC, one of them are mandatory, and both are necessary before and after the treatment [65–69].

Recently Xiao et al. [70], investigated the imaging features of NCC to provide clinicians with valuable information in the diagnosis and treatment and then investigate the imagenological features of 71 consecutive cases of NCC diagnosed by CT and MRI in 5 years time; finding parenchymal cysticerci in 53 cases (92.9%), subarachnoid cysticerci in 39 cases (68.4%), ventricular cysticerci in 13 cases (22.8%) and spinal cysticerci in 1 case; 35 cases were associated with leptomeningitis, 10 cases were with hydrocephalus and they concluded that the imaging findings of the cysticerci, including their location, numbers, cystic sizes, capsular thickness, densities and signals of the scolices, as well as the peripheral oedema, have distinct value in timely making possible diagnosis of neurocysticercosis for clinicians. Similar characteristics are found in our series [1, 7, 14–18, 33, 71–89]. Combination of SNCC and INCC in the same patient as described by Hauptman [69] was also found in our series.

Apart from CT/MRI, angiographic studies sometimes are necessary to determine the imagenological features of vascular malformations, vasculitis and occlusion of blood vessels of the brain associated with NCC. In a previous study, 15 (53%) out of 28 patients with subarachnoid cysticercosis who underwent cerebral angiography had evidence of cerebral arteritis in middle size arteries (middle cerebral artery and posterior cerebral artery) [27].

> In one of the patient reported by Rocha et al. [48], MRI *demonstrated several enhancing subarachnoid cysts surrounding the occluded vessels, a right parietal racemose cyst and a left temporal large infarction area. Angiographic study showed total occlusion of left middle cerebral artery and a sub-total occlusion of right middle cerebral artery.* In the second case, CT scan *demonstrated several calcifications and a left temporal infarction area. Angiographic study showed diffuse arteritis of basilar and carotid arterial system.* In the patient reported by Levy et al. [49], the MRI demonstrated the presence of enhancing subarachnoid material surrounding these occluded cerebral arteries, providing antemortem, non-invasive documentation of the inflammatory meningeal cysticercoid reaction that was presumably responsible for the occlusive arteritis causing the cerebral infarction. In this setting, CT scan and CSF examination usually support the cause-and-effect relationship between neurocysticercosis and the cerebral infarct by showing abnormalities compatible with cysticercotic arachnoiditis. Pamplona et al. [46] *reported a case of a 43-year-old woman with an eight-month history of headaches, ataxia and loss of vision. CT and MRI showed an intraventricular cyst, causing entrapment of Monro foramina and hydrocephalus, smaller cysts at subarachnoid space in temporal lobes, Sylvian fissures, suprasellar and peri-mesencephalic cisterns, and an intra-orbital cyst. Additionally, there were acute ischaemic vascular lesions on the left thalamus and corpus callosum splenium and sub-acute ischaemic lesions of both occipital lobes.* Gilman et al. [90] reported a patient who presented with a relapsed non-aneurysmal subarachnoid haemorrhage possibly associated with subarachnoid cysticercosis and the *MRI of her brain revealed a new left subarachnoid haemorrhage involving the left suprasellar cistern, inter-peduncular cistern, left ambient cistern, and again the left Sylvian fissure. Additionally, the images showed dilatation of the lateral and third ventricles, and the aqueduct of Sylvius, with obstruction caused by cysts associated with leptomeningeal enhancement of the supracerebellar cistern.* Other authors also reported similar findings [43, 44].

Without doubt, MRI is an ideal test for investigating SNCC. However, imagenological diagnosis of SNCC is usually difficult when classical MRI sequences are used [91]. Therefore, Carrillo et al. [91] evaluated the advantages of 3D MRI sequences [fast imaging employing steady-state acquisition (FIESTA) and spoiled gradient recalled echo (SPGR)] with respect to classical sequences [fluid attenuation inversion recovery (FLAIR) and T1] in visualising *T. solium* cyst in these locations and they found that 47 *T. solium cysts located in the basal cisterns of the subarachnoid space were diagnosed in 18 Mexican patients. A pre-treatment MRI was performed on all patients, and all four sequences (FIESTA, FLAIR, T1 SPGR, and T2) were evaluated independently by two neuroradiologists.* The mentioned authors found *FIESTA sequences allowed the visualisation of cyst membrane in 87.2% of the parasites evaluated, FLAIR in 38.3%, SPGR in 23.4% and T2 in 17.0%. Therefore, the superiority of FIESTA sequences over the other three imaging methods was statistically significant (P < 0.001). Scolices were detected by FIESTA twice as much as the other sequences did, although this difference was not significant (P > 0.05). Differences in signal intensity between CSF and parasite cysts were significant in FIESTA (P < 0.0001), SPGR (P < 0.0001) and FLAIR (P = 0.005) sequences,* and they [91] concluded that, *for the first time, the usefulness of 3D MRI sequences to diagnose T. solium cysts located in the basal cisterns of the subarachnoid space was demonstrated. The routine use of these sequences could favour an earlier diagnosis and greatly improve the prognosis of patients affected by this severe form of the disease.* An accurate diagnosis of this condition is important since early treatment with steroids is advised to ameliorate the subarachnoid inflammatory reaction which may cause recurrent cerebral infarcts [50].

Acknowledgements

We thank Prof Targonska and Dr. Anwary, radiologist from Nelson Mandela Academic Hospital, and Dr. Priya Parag and her radiologist team from Inkhosi Albert Lithuli Central Hospital in Durban, South Africa, for their co-operation.

Special thanks to Ms. Christine Tronson Benner, MPH Department of Biostatistics and Epidemiology College of Public Health, University of Oklahoma Health Sciences Center for her suggestions and corrections made in this report.

Author details

Humberto Foyaca-Sibat* and Lourdes de Fátima Ibañez-Valdés

*Address all correspondence to: humbertofoyacasibat@gmail.com

Department of Neurology, Nelson Mandela Academic Hospital, Walter Sisulu University, Mthatha, South Africa

References

[1] Foyaca-Sibat H, LdeF I-V. Clinical trial of praziquantel and prednisone in rural patients with neurocysticercosis presenting recurrent epileptic attacks. The Internet Journal of Neurology. 2002;**2**:41-50. Full article available at the URL: http://www.ispub.com/journal/the_internet_journal_of_neurology/volume_1_number_2_39/article/clinical_trial_of_praziquantel_and_prednisone_in_rural_ patients_with_neurocysticercosis_presentin_with_recurrent_epileptic_attacks.html

[2] Foyaca-Sibat H, LdeF I-V. Intraventricular neurocysticercosis in HIV patients. The Internet. Journal of Neurology. 2003;**2**(1):23-31. Full article available at the URL: Full article available at the URL: The Internet Journal of Neurology http://www.ispub.com/journal/the_internet_journal_of_neurology/volume_2_number_137/article/intraventricular_neurocysticercosis_in_hiv_positive_patients. html

[3] Bandres JC, White AC Jr, Samo T, Murphy EC, Harris RL. Extraparenchymal neurocysticercosis: Report of five cases and review of management. Clinical Infectious Diseases. 1992;**15**:799-811

[4] Del Brutto OH. Albendazole therapy for subarachnoid cysticerci: Clinical and neuroimaging analysis of 17 patients. Journal of Neurology, Neurosurgery, and Psychiatry. 1997;**62**:659-661

[5] Proaño JV, Madrazo I, Avelar F, Lopez-Felix B, Diaz G, Grijalva I. Medical treatment for neurocysticercosis characterized by giant subarachnoid cysts. The New England Journal of Medicine. 2001;**345**:879-885

[6] Göngora-Rivera F, Soto-Hernández JL, González Esquivel D, Cook HJ, Márquez-Caraveo C, Hernández Dávila R, Santos-Zambrano J. Albendazole trial at 15 or 30 mg/kg/day for subarachnoid and intraventricular cysticercosis. Neurology. 2006;**66**:436-438

[7] Ibañez-Valdés LF, Foyaca-Sibat H. Refractory epilepsy in neurocysticercosis. The Internet Journal of Neurology. 2006;**5**(2):34-41. Full article available at the URL: http://www.ispub.com/journal/the_internet_journal_of_neurology/volume_5_number_2_19/article/refractory_epilepsy_in_neurocysticercosis.html

[8] Carpio A, Kelvin EA, Bagiella E, Leslie D, Leon P, Andrews H, Hauser WA. Ecuadorian Neurocysticercosis group. Effects of albendazole treatment on neurocysticercosis: A randomised controlled trial. Journal of Neurology, Neurosurgery, and Psychiatry. 2008;**79**:1050-1055

[9] Rocha MA Jr, Santos JM, Gomes EC, Rocha MA, Rocha CF, Carvalho GT, Costa BS. Treatment of cerebral cysticercosis with albendazole in elevated dosages. Arquivos de Neuro-Psiquiatria. 2008;**66**:114-116

[10] Cárdenas G, Carrillo-Mezo R, Jung H, Sciutto E, Soto HJL, Fleury A. Subarachnoid Neurocysticercosis non-responsive to cysticidal drugs: A case series. BMC Neurology. 2010;**10**:16

[11] Gubbay SS, Matz LR. Meningeal cysticercosis diagnosed in Western Australia. The Medical Journal of Australia. 1977 Apr 9;**1**(15):523-525

[12] Takayanagui OM, Odashima NS. Clinical aspects of neurocysticercosis. Parasitology International. 2006;**55**(1):111-115

[13] Bannur U, Rajshekhar V. Cisternal cysticercosis: A diagnostic problem–a short report. Neurology India. 2001;**49**(2):206-208

[14] Foyaca-Sibat H, Del Rio-Romero L, Ibañez-Valdés LF, Vega-Novoa EC, Awotedu A. Neuroepidemiological survey for epilepsy and knowledge about neurocysticercosis

at Sidwadweni location, South Africa. Electronic Journal of Biomedicine. 2004;**2**(1):40-48 http://www.biomed.edu/2004/n1/foyaca.html

[15] Foyaca-Sibat H, Del Rio-Romero A, Ibañez-Valdés LF. Prevalence of epilepsy and general knowledge about Neurocysticercosis at Ngangelizwe location, South Africa. The Internet Journal of Neurology. 2005;**4**(1): Full article available at the URL: http://www.ispub.com/journal/the_internet_journal_of_neurology/volume_4_number_1_30/article/prevalence_of_epilepsy_and_general_ knowledge_about_ neurocysticercosis at_ngangelizwe_ location_ south_africa.html

[16] Foyaca-Sibat H, Del Rio-Romero A, Ibañez-Valdés LF. Neuroepidemiological survey for epilepsy and knowledge about Neurocysticiercosis at Ngqwala location, South Africa. The Internet Journal of Neurology. 2005;**3**(2): Full article available at the URL: http://www.ispub.com/journal/the_internet_journal_of_neurology/volume_3_number_2_31/article/neuroepidemiological_survey_for_ epilepsy_and_knowledge_about_ neurocysticiercosis_at_ngqwala _ location_south_africa.html

[17] Foyaca-Sibat H, Del Rio-Romero A, Ibañez-Valdés LF. Epilepsy, Neurocysticercosis and, poverty at Mphumaze and Marhambeni locations, in South Africa. The Internet Journal of Neurology (ISSN: 1531-295X). 2007;**7**(1):8-14. Full article available at the URL: http://www.ispub.com/journal/the_internet_journal_of_neurology/volume_7_number_1_7/article/epilepsy_neurocysticercosis_and_poverty_at_mphumaze_and_marhambeni_locations_in_south_ africa.html

[18] Foyaca-Sibat H, Del Rio-Romero AI. Prevalence of epilepsy in an endemic area for Neurocysticercosis in South Africa. The Internet Journal of Neurology. (ISSN: 1531-295X). 2008;**9**(1):8-18. Full article available at the URL: http://www.ispub.com/journal/the_internet_journal_of_neurology/volume_9_number_1_6/article/prevalence_of_epilepsy_in_an_endemic_area_for_neurocysticercosis _in_ south_africa.html

[19] Cantú C, Barinagarrementeria F. Cerebrovascular complications of neurocysticercosis: Clinical and neuroimaging spectrum. Archives of Neurology. 1996;**53**:233-239

[20] Soto-Hernández JL, Gomez-Llata S, Rojas-Echeverri LA, Texeira F, Romero V. Subarachnoid hemorrhage secondary to ruptured inflammatory aneurysm: A possible manifestation of neurocysticercosis: Case report. Neurosurgery. 1996;**38**:1-3

[21] Sotelo J, Guerrero V, Rubio F. Neurocysticercosis: A new classification based on active and inactive forms. Archives of Internal Medicine. 1985;**145**:442-445

[22] Gris Iola JS, Wiederholt WC. CNS cysticercosis. Archives of Neurology. 1982;**39**:540-544

[23] Levy SA, Lillehei KO, Rubinstein D, Stears JC. Subarachnoid cysticercosis with occlusion of the major intracranial arteries: Case report. Neurosurgery. 1995;**36**:183-188

[24] Rodriguez Carbajal J, Del Brutto OH, Penagos P, Huebe J, Escobar A. Occlusion of the middle cerebral artery due to cysticercoid angiitis. Stroke. 1989;**20**:1095-1098

[25] Torrealba G, Del Villar S, Tagle P, Arriagada C, Kase CS. Cysticercosis of the central nervous system: Clinical and therapeutic considerations. Journal of Neurology, Neurosurgery, and Psychiatry. 1984;**47**:784-790

[26] terPenning B, Litchmann CD, Heier L. Bilateral middle cerebral artery occlusion in neurocysticercosis. Stroke. 1992;**23**:280-283

[27] Barinagarrementeria F, Cantú C. Frequency of cerebral arteritis in subarachnoid Cysticercosis. Stroke. 1998;**29**:123-125

[28] Camargo EC. Stroke in Latin America. Neuroimaging Clinics of North America. 2005; **15**(2):283-296

[29] Howard A, Lewandowski C. Infrequent causes of stroke. Emerg Med Clin North Amer. 2002;**20**(3):22-29

[30] Rocha MS, Brucki SM, Ferraz AC, Piccolo AC. Cerebrovascular disease and neurocysticercosis. Arquivos de Neuro-Psiquiatria. 2001;**59**(3-B):778-783

[31] Aditya GS, Mahadevan A, Santosh V, Chickabasaviah YT, Ashwathnarayanarao CB, Krishna SS. Cysticercal chronic basal arachnoiditis with infarcts, mimicking tuberculous pathology in endemic areas. Neuropathology. 2004;**24**(4):320-325

[32] Delobel P, Signate A, El Guedj M, Couppie P, Gueye M, Smadja D, Pradinaud R, Delobel P, Signate A, El Guedj M, Couppie P, Gueye M, Smadja D, Pradinaud R. Unusual form of neurocysticercosis associated with HIV infection. European Journal of Neurology. 2004 Jan;**11**(1):55-58

[33] Foyaca-Sibat H, LdeF I-V. Neurocysticercosis in HIV-positive patients. The Internet Journal of Infectious Diseases. 2003;**2**(2):15-22. Full article available at the URL: http://www.ispub.com/journal/the_internet_journal_of_infectious_diseases/volume_2_number_2 6/article/neurocysticercosis_in_hiv_positive_patients.html

[34] Serpa JA, Moran A, Goodman JC, Giordano TP, White AC Jr. Neurocysticercosis in the HIV era: A case report and review of the literature. The American Journal of Tropical Medicine and Hygiene. 2007 Jul;**77**(1):113-117

[35] Sorvillo F, DeGiorgio C, Stephen H, Waterman SH. Deaths from Cysticercosis. United Status. Emerg Infect Dis. 2007;**13**(2):230-235

[36] McCormick GF, Ciannotta S, Zee CS, Fisher M. Carotid occlusion in cysticercosis. Neurology. 1983;**33**:1078-1080

[37] Alarcón F, Hidalgo F, Moncayo J, Viñan I, Dueñas G. Cerebral cysticercosis and stroke. Stroke. 1992;**23**:224-228

[38] Lee SL, Chang GY. Recurrent braistem transient ischemic attacks due to neurocysticercosis: A treatable cause. European Neurology. 1998;**40**:174-175

[39] Wraige E, Grham J, Robb SA, Jan W. Neurocysticercosis masquerading as a cerebral infarct. Journal of Child Neurology. 2003;**18**:298-300

[40] Kohli A, Gupta R, Kishore J. Anterior cerebral artery infaction in neurocysticercosis: Evaluation by MR angiography and in vivo proton MR spectroscopy. Pediatric Neurosurgery. 1997;**26**:93-96

[41] Tellez-Zenteno JE, Or N-P, Cantú C, et al. Hemorrhagic stroke associated to neurocysticercosis. Neurología. 2003;**18**:272-275

[42] Huang PP, Choundhri HE, Jallo G, Miller DC. Inflammatory aneurysm due to neurocysticercosis. Journal of Clinical Neuroscience. 2005;**12**:585-588

[43] Lerner A, Shiroishi M, Zee C, et al. Imaging of neurocysticercosis. Neuroimag Clin N Am. 2012;**22**:659-676

[44] Kimura-Hayama E, Criales J. Neurocysticercosis: Radiologic-pathologic correlation. Radiographics. 2010;**30**:1705-1719

[45] Castillo M. Imaging of neurocysticercosis. Seminars in Roentgenology. 2004;**39**:465-473

[46] Pamplona J, Braz A, Conceição C, Rios C, Reis J. A rare case of racemose neurocysticercosis and its complications. Case report. Neuroradiol J. 2015 Aug;**28**(4):418-420

[47] Coleman N, Buitrago J, San Martin H, Hitmann B, Krishna SS. Cysticercal chronic basal arachnoiditis with infarcts, mimicking tuberculous pathology. Neuropathology. 2015 Dec;**35**(5):123-138

[48] Brucki SM, Ferraz AC, Piccolo AC. Ischemic stroke and neurocysticercosis. Arquivos de Neuro-Psiquiatria. 2002;**60**:552-557

[49] Levy AS, Lillehei KO, Rubinstein D, Stears JC. Subarachnoid neurocysticercosis with occlusion of the major intracranial arteries: Case report. Neurosurgery. 1995 Jan;**36**(1): 183-188

[50] Del Brutto OH. Cysticercosis and cerebrovascular disease: A review. Journal of Neurology, Neurosurgery, and Psychiatry. 1992 Apr;**55**(4):252-254

[51] Barinagarrementeria F, Del Brutto OH. Neurocysticercosis and pure motor hemiparesis. Stroke. 1988 Sep;**19**(9):1156-1158

[52] Barinagarrementeria F, Del Brutto OH. Lacunar syndrome due to neurocysticercosis. Archives of Neurology. 1989 Apr;**46**(4):415-417

[53] Barinagarementería F, Del Brutto OH, Otero E. Ataxic hemiparesis from cysticercosis. Archives of Neurology. 1988 Mar;**45**(3):246-246

[54] McCormick GF, Giannotta S, Zee C, Fisher M. Carotid occlusion in cysticercosis. Neurology. 1983 Aug;**33**(8):1078-1080

[55] Rodriguez-Carbajal J, Del Brutto OH, Penagos P, Huebe J, Escobar A. Occlusion of the middle cerebral artery due to cysticercotic angiitis. Stroke. 1989 Aug;**20**(8):1095-1099

[56] Barinagarrementeria F, Cantú C. Frequency of cerebral arteritis in subarachnoid cysticercosis: An angiographic study. Stroke. 1998 Jan;**29**(1):123-125

[57] Viola GM, White AC, Serpa JA. Hemorrhagic cerebrovascular events and Neurocysticercosis: A case report and review of the literature. The American Journal of Tropical Medicine and Hygiene. 2011 Mar 4;**84**(3):402-405. DOI: 10.4269/ajtmh.2011.10-0429

[58] Alarcon F, Hidalgo F, Moncayo J, Vinan I, Duenas G. Cerebral cysticercosis and stroke. Stroke. 1992;**23**:224-228

[59] Soto-Hernandez JL, Gomez-Llata Andrade S, Rojas-Echeverri LA, Texeira F. Romero subarachnoid hemorrhage secondary to a ruptured inflammatory aneurysm: A possible manifestation of neurocysticercosis: Case report. Neurosurgery. 1996;**38**:197-199 discussion 9-200

[60] Huang PP, Choudhri HF, Jallo G, Miller DC. Inflammatory aneurysm and neurocysticercosis: Further evidence for a causal relationship? Case report. Neurosurgery. 2000;**47**:466-467 discussion 7-8

[61] Kim IY, Kim TS, Lee JH, Lee MC, Lee JK, Jung S. Inflammatory aneurysm due to neurocysticercosis. Journal of Clinical Neuroscience. 2005;**12**:585-588 [PubMed] 10. Zee CS, Segall HD, Miller C, Tsai FY, Teal JS, Hieshima G, Ahmadi J, Halls J. Unusual neuroradiological features of intracranial cysticercosis. Radiology. 1980;**137**:397-407

[62] Garcia HH, Del Brutto OH. Neurocysticercosis: Updated concepts about an old disease. Lancet Neurology. 2005;**4**:653-661

[63] Nash TE, Singh G, White AC, Rajshekhar V, Loeb JA, Proano JV, Takayanagui OM, Gonzalez AE, Butman JA, DeGiorgio C, Del Brutto OH, Delgado-Escueta A, Evans CA, Gilman RH, Martinez SM, Medina MT, Pretell EJ, Teale J, Garcia HH. Treatment of neurocysticercosis: Current status and future research needs. Neurology. 2006;**67**:1120-1127

[64] Zee CS, Segall HD, Miller C, Tsai FY, Teal JS, Hieshima G, Ahmadi J, Halls J. Unusual neuroradiological features of intracranial cysticercosis. Radiology. 1980;**137**:397-407

[65] Iwanowski L, Wislawski J. Neuropathologic analysis of 8 undiagnosed cases of cerebral cysticercosis. Neurologia i Neurochirurgia Polska. 1987;**21**:390-395

[66] Carpio A, Escobar A, Hauser WA. Cysticercosis and epilepsy: A critical review. Epilepsia. 1998;**39**:1025-1040

[67] Garcia HH, Gonzalez AE, Evans CA, et al. *Taenia solium* cysticercosis. Lancet. 2003;**362**: 547-556

[68] Rodriguez S, Dorny P, Tsang VC, Pretell EJ, Brandt J, Lescano AG, Gonzalez AE, Gilman RH, Garcia HH. Detection of *Taenia solium* antigens and anti-*T. solium* antibodies in paired serum and cerebrospinal fluid samples from patients with intraparenchymal or extraparenchymal neurocysticercosis. The Journal of Infectious Diseases. 2009;**199**:1345-1352. DOI: 10.1586/14737175.2014.890892

[69] Hauptman JS, Hinrichs C, Mele C, Lee HJ. Radiologic manifestations of intraventricular and subarachnoid racemose neurocysticercosis. Emergency Radiology. 2005 Apr;**11**(3):153-157

[70] Xiao A, Zeng H, Xiao J, Zhang X, You C. Imaging features of neurocysticercosis: Analysis of consecutive 57 patients in 5 years. Turkish Neurosurgery. 2015 Dec 7. DOI: 10.5137/1019-5149.JTN.16209-15.0

[71] Humberto Foyaca Sibat and Lourdes de Fátima Ibañez Valdés (2013). Uncommon Clinical Manifestations of Cysticercosis, Novel Aspects on Cysticercosis and Neurocysticercosis, Prof. Humberto Foyaca Sibat (Ed.), InTech, DOI:10.5772/53078. http://www.intechopen.com/books/novel-aspects-on-cysticercosis-and-neurocysticercosis/uncommon-clinical-manifestations-of-cysticercosis

[72] Foyaca-Sibat H, Ibañez-Valdés L. Pseudoseizures and epilepsy in Neurocysiticercosis: Some advice for family doctors. The Internet Journal of Neurology. 2003;**2**(2). Available on line at the URL: https://ispub.com/IJN/2/2/3786): Accessed: 2017-March-11

[73] Humberto Foyaca-Sibat and Lourdes de Fátima Ibañez Valdés (2011). Treatment of epilepsy secondary to Neurocysticercosis, Novel Treatment of Epilepsy, Prof. Humberto Foyaca-Sibat (Ed.), InTech, DOI: 10.5772/31465. Available from: http://www.intechopen.com/books/novel-treatment-of-epilepsy/treatment-of-epilepsy-secondary-to-neurocysticercosis

[74] Foyaca SH, VLdeF I. Clinical trial of praziquantel and prednisone in rural patients with neurocysticercosis presenting recurrent epileptic attacks. The Internet Journal of Neurology. 2002;**1**(2). Available from: http://www.ispub.com/ostia/index.php?xmlFilePath=Journals/ijn/vol1n2/ncc.xml): Accessed: 2017-March-03

[75] Humberto Foyaca-Sibat and Lourdes de Fátima Ibañez Valdés (2011). Clinical features of epilepsy secondary to Neurocysticercosis at the insular lobe, Novel Aspects on Epilepsy, Prof. Humberto Foyaca-Sibat (Ed.), InTech, DOI: 10.5772/19476. Available from: http://www.intechopen.com/books/novel-aspects-on-epilepsy/clinical-features-of-epilepsy-secondary-to-neurocysticercosis-at-the-insular-lobe

[76] Humberto Foyaca Sibat and Lourdes de Fátima Ibañez Valdés (2013). Introduction to Cysticercosis and its historical background, Novel Aspects on Cysticercosis and Neurocysticercosis, Prof. Humberto Foyaca Sibat (Ed.), InTech, DOI: 10.5772/50318. Available from: http://www.intechopen.com/books/novel-aspects-on-cysticercosis-and-neurocysticercosis/introduction-to-cysticercosis-and-its-historical-background

[77] Foyaca SH, Ibanez-Valdes LF. Intraventricular neurocysticercosis in HIV positive patients. The Internet Journal of Neurology. 2003;**2**(1). Available from: http://www.ispub.com/ostia/index.php?xmlFilePath=journals/ijn/vol2n1/ncc.xml): [Accessed: 2017-March-07]

[78] Foyaca SH, Ibanez-V. LF. Vascular dementia type Binswanger's disease in patients with active neurocysticercosis. Electronic Journal of Biomedicine. 2002;**1**(1):1-12 Available from: http://www.uninet.edu/biomed/rebio/reb/2002/n1/foyaca.html Accessed: 2017-March-13

[79] Humberto Foyaca Sibat and Lourdes de Fátima Ibañez Valdés (2013). What is a low frequency of the disseminated Cysticercosis suggests that Neurocysticercosis is going to disappear? Novel Aspects on Cysticercosis and Neurocysticercosis, Prof. Humberto Foyaca Sibat (Ed.), InTech, DOI: 10.5772/51395. Available from: http://www.intechopen.com/books/novel-aspects-on-cysticercosis-and-neurocysticercosis/what-is-a-low-frequency-of-the-disseminated-cysticercosis-suggests-that-neurocysticercosis-is-going-to-dissapear?

[80] Humberto Foyaca-Sibat (2011). Epilepsy secondary to parasitic Zoonoses of the brain, Novel Aspects on Epilepsy, Prof. Humberto Foyaca Sibat (Ed.), DOI: 10.5772/31463. Available from: http://www.intechopen.com/books/novel-aspects-on-epilepsy/epilepsy-secondary-to-parasitic-zoonoses-of-the-brain

[81] Humberto Foyaca Sibat, María Carolina Salazar Campos and Lourdes de Fátima Ibañez Valdés (2013). Orbital Cisticercosis. A challenger for neurologists, ophthalmologists, Neuro-Opthalmologists, and general practitioners, Novel Aspects on Cysticercosis and Neurocysticercosis, Prof. Humberto Foyaca Sibat (Ed.), InTech, DOI:10.5772/52515. Available from: http://www.intechopen.com/books/novel-aspects-on-cysticercosis-and-neurocysticercosis/orbital-cisticercosis-a-challenger-for-neurologists-ophthalmologists-neuro-opthalmologists-and-general- practtioner

[82] Del Rio A, Foyaca-Sibat H, LdeF I-V. Epidemiological survey about socio-economic characteristic of Mpindweni location, South Africa. The Internet Journal of Neurology. 2005;**4**(2) [Accessed: 2017-March-16] http://www.ispub.com/journal/the_internet_journal_of_neurology/volume_4_number_2_27/article/epidemiological_survey_about_socio_economic_characteristic_of_mpindweni_location_south_africa.html): [Accessed: 2017-March-17]

[83] Foyaca-Sibat H, LdeF I-V. Insular Neurocysticercosis: Our finding and review of the medical literature. The Internet Journal of Neurology. 2006;**5**(2): http://www.ispub.com/journal/the_internet_journal_of_neurology/volume_5_number_2_19/article/insular_neurocysticercosis_our_findings_and_review_of_the_medical_literature.html [Accessed: 2017-March-21]

[84] Foyaca-Sibat H, LdeF I-V, Del Rio IA. Prevalence of epilepsy and general knowledge about Neurocysticercosis at Ngangelizwe location, South Africa. The Internet Journal of Neurology.(ISSN: 1531-295X). 2005;**4**(1):23-37 http://www.ispub.com/journal/the_internet_journal_of_neurology/volume_4_number_1_30/article/prevalence_of_epilepsy_and_general_knowledge_about_neurocysticercosis_at_ngangelizwe_location_south_africa.html [Accessed: 2017-March-10]

[85] Del Rio AR, Foyaca-Sibat H, Ibañez Valdés LF. Neuroepidemiological survey for epilepsy, knowledgeaboutepilepsy,NeurocysticercosisandHIV/AidsattheMakaulaVillageinSouth Africa. The Internet Journal of Neurology. (ISSN: 1531-295X). 2007;**7**(3):41-49. http://www.ispub.com/journal/the_internet_journal_of_neurology/volume_7_number_2_5/article/neuroepidemiological_survey_for_epilepsy_knowledge_about_epilepsy_neurocysticercosis_and_hiv_aids_at_the_makaula_village_in_south_africa.html [Accessed: 2017-March-18]

[86] Del Rio-Romero AI, Foyaca-Sibat H, Ibañez Valdés LF. Neuroepidemiology findings as contributors for epilepsy due to Neurocysticercosis at Mngceleni location, South Africa. The Internet Journal of Neurology. (ISSN: 1531-295X). 2008;**9**(1):33-40. http://www.ispub.com/journal/the_internet_journal_of_neurology/volume_9_number_1_6/article/neuroepidemiology_findings_as_contributors_for_epilepsy_due_to_neurocysticercosis_at_mngceleni_location_south_africa.html [Accessed: 2017-March-12]

[87] Foyaca-Sibat H, Ibañez Valdés LF, Moré-Rodríguez J. Parasitic Zoonoses of the brain: Another challenger? The Internet Journal of Neurology. 2010;**12**(2): http://www.ispub.com/journal/the_internet_journal_of_neurology/volume_12_number_2_4/article/parasitic-zoonoses-of-the-brain-another-challenger.html [Accessed: 2017-March-19]

[88] Foyaca Sibat H, Ibañez Valdés Lde F. Treatment of epilepsy secondary to neurocysticercosis. 2011 Chapter V. Treatment Approach to Epilepsy. Text Book I ISBN 979-953-307-011-6 (Ed: Prof. H Foyaca Sibat) pages:25-47 INTECH OPEN ACCESS. Rijeka 2011 More information available at the URL: http://www.intechweb.org/

[89] Foyaca Sibat H, Ibañez Valdés Lde F. Insular lobe seizures secondary to insular lobe neurocysticercosis 2011 chapter III. Clinical Manifestation of Epilepsy. Text Book II [ISBN 978-953-307-678-2] (Ed: Prof. H Foyaca Sibat) pages: 20-40, Jun INTECH OPEN ACCESS Rijeka, More information available at the URL: http://www.intechweb.org/

[90] Gilman RH, Martinez SM, Medina MT, Pretell EJ, Teale J, Garcia HH. Treatment of neurocysticercosis: Current status and future research needs. Neurology. 2006;**67**:1120-1127

[91] Carrillo Mezo R, Lara García J, Arroyo M, Fleury A. Relevance of 3D magnetic resonance imaging sequences in diagnosing basal subarachnoid neurocysticercosis. Acta Tropica. 2015 Dec;**152**:60-65. DOI: 10.1016/j.actatropica.2015.08.017 Epub 2015 Aug 29]

Permissions

All chapters in this book were first published in SEIZURES, by InTech Open; hereby published with permission under the Creative Commons Attribution License or equivalent. Every chapter published in this book has been scrutinized by our experts. Their significance has been extensively debated. The topics covered herein carry significant findings which will fuel the growth of the discipline. They may even be implemented as practical applications or may be referred to as a beginning point for another development.

The contributors of this book come from diverse backgrounds, making this book a truly international effort. This book will bring forth new frontiers with its revolutionizing research information and detailed analysis of the nascent developments around the world.

We would like to thank all the contributing authors for lending their expertise to make the book truly unique. They have played a crucial role in the development of this book. Without their invaluable contributions this book wouldn't have been possible. They have made vital efforts to compile up to date information on the varied aspects of this subject to make this book a valuable addition to the collection of many professionals and students.

This book was conceptualized with the vision of imparting up-to-date information and advanced data in this field. To ensure the same, a matchless editorial board was set up. Every individual on the board went through rigorous rounds of assessment to prove their worth. After which they invested a large part of their time researching and compiling the most relevant data for our readers.

The editorial board has been involved in producing this book since its inception. They have spent rigorous hours researching and exploring the diverse topics which have resulted in the successful publishing of this book. They have passed on their knowledge of decades through this book. To expedite this challenging task, the publisher supported the team at every step. A small team of assistant editors was also appointed to further simplify the editing procedure and attain best results for the readers.

Apart from the editorial board, the designing team has also invested a significant amount of their time in understanding the subject and creating the most relevant covers. They scrutinized every image to scout for the most suitable representation of the subject and create an appropriate cover for the book.

The publishing team has been an ardent support to the editorial, designing and production team. Their endless efforts to recruit the best for this project, has resulted in the accomplishment of this book. They are a veteran in the field of academics and their pool of knowledge is as vast as their experience in printing. Their expertise and guidance has proved useful at every step. Their uncompromising quality standards have made this book an exceptional effort. Their encouragement from time to time has been an inspiration for everyone.

The publisher and the editorial board hope that this book will prove to be a valuable piece of knowledge for researchers, students, practitioners and scholars across the globe.

List of Contributors

Lourdes de Fátima Ibañez-Valdés and Humberto Foyaca-Sibat
Department of Neurology, Nelson Mandela Academic Central Hospital, Walter Sisulu University, Mthatha, South Africa

Adrianna Ranger
Department of Clinical Neurological Sciences, Division of Neurosurgery, Children's Hospital-London Health Sciences Center, Western University, London, Ontario, Canada

David Diosy
Department of Clinical Neurological Sciences, Division of Neurology, London Health Sciences Center, Western University, London, Ontario, Canada

Birute Tumiene and Algirdas Utkus
Department of Human and Medical Genetics, Centre for Medical Genetics, Vilnius University, Vilnius, Lithuania

Vaidutis Kučinskas
Department of Human and Medical Genetics, Centre for Human Genomics, Vilnius University, Vilnius, Lithuania

Aleš Maver and Borut Peterlin
Clinical Institute for Medical Genetics, Division of Gynecology, University of Ljubljana Medical Centre, Ljubljana, Slovenia

Ayşe Kutlu and Serap Mülayim
Department of Neurology, Faculty of Medicine, Kocaeli University, Kocaeli, Turkey

Sandra Orozco-Suarez, Iris Feria-Romero and Israel Grijalva
Unidad de Investigación Médica en Enfermedades Neurológicas, Hospital de Especialidades "Dr. Bernardo Sepúlveda", Centro Médico Nacional Siglo XXI, Instituto Mexicano del Seguro Social, Mexico City, Mexico

Angélica Vega-Garcia
Unidad de Investigación Médica en Enfermedades Neurológicas, Hospital de Especialidades "Dr. Bernardo Sepúlveda", Centro Médico Nacional Siglo XXI, Instituto Mexicano del Seguro Social, Mexico City, Mexico
Universidad Autónoma Metropolitana (UAM), Mexico City, Mexico

Lourdes Arriaga-Pizano
Unidad de Investigación Médica en Inmunología, Hospital de Especialidades "Dr. Bernardo Sepúlveda", Centro Médico Nacional Siglo XXI, Instituto Mexicano del Seguro Social, Mexico City, Mexico

Emmanuel Rodriguez-Chavez
Servicio de Neurología, Hospital de Especialidades "Dr. Antonio Fraga Mouret", Centro Médico Nacional, La Raza, Instituto Mexicano del Seguro Social, Mexico City, Mexico

Svetlana A. Dolina
Advanced Neuroprotective Systems LTD., Ness-Ziona, Israel

Jonathan Bidwell and Elizabeth D. Mynatt
Georgia Institute of Technology, School of Interactive Computing, Atlanta, GA, USA

Eliana Kovich and Cherise Frazier
Children's Healthcare of Atlanta, GA, USA

Cam Escoffery
Emory University, Rollins School of Public Health, Atlanta, GA, USA

Humberto Foyaca-Sibat and Lourdes de Fátima Ibañez-Valdés
Department of Neurology, Nelson Mandela Academic Hospital, Walter Sisulu University, Mthatha, South Africa

Index

www.ingramcontent.com/pod-product-compliance
Lightning Source LLC
LaVergne TN
LVHW060601210926
848485LV00005B/1351